Digestive Health with REAL Food

a practical guide to an anti-inflammatory, low-irritant, nutrient-dense diet for IBS & other digestive issues

By Aglaée Jacob, M.S., R.D.

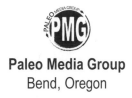

Paleo Media Group
Bend, Oregon

www.paleomediagroup.com

First Published in 2013 by Paleo Media Group LLC
www.paleomediagroup.com

ISBN 13: 978-0-9887172-0-6

Book design by Kate Miller, Kate Miller Design
Food photography by Savannah Wishart
Illustrations by Aglaée Jacob

Printed in USA

Dedication

To everyone suffering from digestive issues and feeling abandoned by conventional medicine.

Gratitude

First, I am truly grateful for my health struggles. As strange as it may seem, I now see the positive side of what this challenging period of my life has brought me. Although I have been through some rough times, my personal health issues have opened the door to a new field of holistic health and nutrition for me, now allowing me to help other people dealing with similar struggles. My own health issues made me a more understanding and knowledgeable health care provider.

I want to thank all the health and nutrition experts in the REAL food community. There are too many to name here, but leaders of the Paleo community, Weston A. Price Foundation and the experts behind the GAPS, SCD, and low-FODMAP diets have each taught me so much. You have allowed me to further my education, heal myself, and develop a nutritional approach to help others.

A special acknowledgement to Cain Credicott, editor of Paleo Magazine, for believing in me and enthusiastically working for the publication of this book. I also thank Ray Sylvester, editor of this book, Kate Miller, graphic designer and Savannah Wishart, food photographer, for your hard work. You all played essential roles in the arduous but so rewarding process of making this book come to life.

I am grateful for the thousands of people who have supported me in the last years, visiting my website, sharing their stories, and helping me continue to learn more every day.

Merci à ma famille, mes parents Hélène et Gilles et mon frère Ludovic, pour toujours me supporter dans toutes mes folles aventures. Vous avoir derrière moi me donne la force de continuer de foncer chaque jour.

Finally, an enormous heartfelt MERCI to my always loving and supportive husband, Jonathan. I would not be here without you. Je t'aime tellement!

Table of Contents

Introduction

Health Starts In The Gut!

The roots of optimal health lie in your intestines. You simply can't be healthy if your digestion isn't working properly. It's in the gut that your body extracts the nutrients it requires while keeping out harmful compounds. It's also where most of your immune system resides. Bloating, constipation, diarrhea, abdominal pain, and excessive flatulence are all warning signs that something has gone wrong in your gut. Inflammatory bowel disease (IBS) symptoms shouldn't be a diagnosis, but a clue that you need to look for more answers.

"All diseases start in the gut." – Hippocrates

It can be discouraging when doctors tell you what you eat has nothing to do with your digestive problems or to follow an "everything in moderation" path. There are many books about irritable bowel syndrome (IBS) claiming that a gluten-free or low-FODMAP diet is the solution. Others promote high-fiber foods, a vegetarian approach, or a low-fat diet. Unfortunately, all of these diets are reductionist, isolating specific, potentially problematic compounds without looking at the whole picture. Many of these diets also fail to emphasize the importance of healing your gut to not only manage your symptoms but to allow you to improve your food tolerance and recover your optimal digestive health.

Nobody knows what you should eat, but your body will tell you if you learn how to listen. This book provides a practical, step-by-step guide to a REAL-food-based approach help you recover your digestive health naturally. The protocol described in this book is the most comprehensive approach to building your personal optimal diet.

The approach I propose is effective because it shows you how to eliminate all processed and fake foods, which often contain irritants, allergens, and inflammatory and hard-to-digest ingredients that can contribute to digestive problems. You might be surprised at how many of these processed foods are already in your meals, even if you think you're already eating healthfully.

The first step of the nutritional protocol in this book will help you "reset" your digestive system—like putting it in a cast for a few weeks to allow it to heal so it can better "signal" you when eating specific foods. Afterward, you'll be able to figure out whether grains (with or without gluten), dairy, cruciferous vegetables, and other foods are right for you. And by creating your own optimal diet in the final phase, you'll regain control of your symptoms, your gut will be able to heal, and your quality of life and health should reach a new level.

It's critical to tackle your digestive issues from as many angles as possible. A holistic approach isn't necessarily easy, but it will help you get the best results. You may have tried other dietary modifications in the past without success. Unlike narrow diets that tell you what to eat and what not to eat, this book explains why certain foods are problematic for some people and how to determine if they are problematic for you. Unlike other diets you may have followed, this plan will help you discover and build your own optimal diet.

This book presents everything I wish I had known when I started experiencing my own digestive issues, and represents everything I have learned in the last several years of intensively researching the topic of digestive health and assisting many fellow sufferers to get their symptoms under control.

Chapter 1 will review the basic functioning of a healthy digestive system, including the importance of stomach acid, gut flora, and the leaky gut concept. In Chapter 2, we'll discuss the many ways your digestion can go wrong. You'll learn more about non-celiac gluten sensitivity, SIBO, and FODMAP intolerance, along with many other digestive disorders.

Food can either compromise your gut health or help it function more optimally, and Chapters 3 and 4 will cover different foods and food groups to help you understand what you should and shouldn't eat. Everyone is different and individual tolerance varies, but understanding the foods that are more likely to be problematic can help you better understand how your digestive system reacts to what you eat.

"Every time you eat or drink, you are either
feeding disease or fighting it."

– Heather Morgan, M.S., N.L.C.

In Chapter 5, it's time for action! You will learn how to proceed with the elimination diet protocol to start building your personal optimal diet.

Food is the central factor in digestive health, but supplements and the mind-body connection also play a big role. Chapter 6 addresses supplements, including homemade bone broth, fermented foods, glutamine, omega-3 fats, and vitamin D that can help support your digestive and overall health.

Chapter 7 covers the importance of taking care of your mind with tips on stress management, sleep, and exercise, which should constitute an integral part of your gut-healing program.

Your new way of eating shouldn't prevent you from eating out and traveling. All you need is a little planning. Chapter 8 will help you develop strategies to live your life to the fullest without having to worry about digestive problems or limited food tolerance.

Don't skip Chapter 9! It includes helpful and practical troubleshooting tips to help you address cravings and fatigue, in addition to helping you understand why symptoms can return and how to deal with them.

In Chapter 10 you'll find several meal, snack, and treat recipes and ideas to help you stay excited about eating REAL food. You'll never again have the excuse of saying you don't know what to eat!

Chapter 11 gives you an idea what a week of eating on the elimination and reintroduction phase looks like. It also details how much you need to eat to ensure you get enough calories. Too many people fail at following an elimination diet because they forget that it's about eliminating problematic foods—not calories! The nutritional protocol suggested in this book is far from a starvation diet, and this chapter will help you make sure you're eating enough.

"A well-functioning gut with healthy gut flora holds
the roots of our health. And, just as a tree with sick roots
is not going to thrive, the rest of the body cannot thrive
without a well-functioning digestive system."

– Dr. Natasha Campbell-McBride

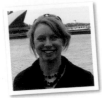

My Story

For most of my life, I didn't know much about digestive issues, apart from what I learned about IBS and other gastrointestinal conditions during my dietitian training. This changed when I became my very first client. I got very sick after a trip to the Peruvian jungle, and my digestive system never fully recovered.

Bloating, abdominal pain and cramping, diarrhea, gas, brain fog, lack of concentration, depression, headaches, skin rash, and insomnia became part of my life. The symptoms were on and off at first, but kept worsening to a point where I experienced them nonstop. After a couple of months, I consulted a medical doctor who told me that I was eating too much animal-based food. This advice wasn't very helpful and I later found out that this doctor was vegan and had a strong bias against meat.

Fortunately, though, he referred me to a gastroenterologist (also known as a gastrointestinal or GI doctor) who was finally able to diagnose me with a parasite infection (Blastocystis hominis). Many doctors believe that this type of parasite is nonpathogenic (does not cause disease), but fortunately, my GI doctor felt that my symptoms warranted treatment. I received a first course of antibiotics, then a second one, but my symptoms returned despite eradicating the bug. I had already started eating a gluten-free, grain-free, legume-free, and dairy-free diet, but it didn't make a big difference. After ruling out celiac disease (although it can't be truly ruled out since these tests aren't reliable if you're not eating gluten, as you'll learn later), post-infectious IBS became my new problem. Many IBS cases can be traced back to a gastrointestinal infection, as you'll learn in Chapter 2. The GI doctor couldn't offer much to alleviate my symptoms, but she suggested I look into fructose malabsorption. I was fortunate to be in Australia at the time, where awareness about food sensitivities was greater than in North America.

As soon as I returned home, I started doing some research. I knew I didn't want to spend the rest of my life living like I had been. Even though IBS is not life threatening, I knew it couldn't be good for my body to be in so much distress day after day. I knew I didn't want to live like that for the rest of my life. And I knew there had to be something I could do about it. The food we eat every day is in direct contact with our intestines, for better or worse. I really hoped it would be possible to soothe the inflammation and provide nourishment to heal my gut. I started researching fructose malabsorption, as well as FODMAPs (more on these later) and food-chemical intolerances. I experimented with low-fructose, low-FODMAP, and low-food-chemical diets, combined with my already gluten-free, dairy-free diet. I got to the point where I ate just five foods: chicken, meat, eggs, ghee, and very small amounts of green beans, seasoned only with unrefined salt. It was restrictive, but it helped me start to feel significantly better. It showed me that there was a link between my diet and my symptoms.

I then stumbled upon the concept of small intestinal bacterial overgrowth (SIBO) and decided to get tested. SIBO made a lot of sense considering that I reacted to almost all carbohydrate-containing foods (SIBO symptoms are due to excessive intestinal fermentation of all types of sugars and starches). The results of the breath test were positive and I was relieved to finally know what was wrong with me.

I started on a course of natural antibiotics and embarked on a modified version of the GAPS diet (see Chapter 3). I sometimes wonder if I had had SIBO all along and that perhaps the parasite was not really responsible for my symptoms, but simply hid a more profound gut-dysbiosis problem (gut flora imbalance). In any case, I had finally started feeling better and was able to slowly improve my food tolerance and variety.

I now manage to stay 100-percent symptom free. I also believe that my new way of eating gave me the added bonus of making me healthier overall. Even though I now know that I can't eat foods I thought I once couldn't live without, like oatmeal, peanut butter, cheese, bread, and sugar, I don't even want to eat these foods anymore. I have found a tasty new way of eating that has helped me recover my digestive health and get my life back.

I wrote this book to help some of the millions of people, like you and me, who suffer and are given bad dietary advice, or told that diet has nothing to do with their digestive health. You've been waiting long enough: It's your turn now! There is nothing like finally understanding the cause of your digestive problems and being able to fix them by eating REAL, nourishing foods that help your digestive system heal itself and your body to function at its full potential.

From my own experience and my work with other fellow sufferers, I have developed a comprehensive and effective approach that should help you see results within a few weeks—without having to eat just five foods or make the same mistakes I did! Whether you have IBS, celiac disease, Crohn's disease, ulcerative colitis, reflux, or any other gastrointestinal problem(s)—and despite your doctor's advice that there's nothing you can do—REAL food may be just what you need to get your symptoms under control and start living the life you deserve.

Chapter 1: The Basics of Digestion

Digestion 101

Your digestive system is more than a simple tube through which food travels. Digestion starts in your mouth and continues through your esophagus, stomach, small intestines, and colon. Your liver and pancreas also participate by delivering enzymes and bile to facilitate the breakdown of food. The main goal of digestion is to sort the good from the bad so your body can extract the nutrients you need and excrete what may be harmful. A lot happens between the time you put food in your mouth and when the remaining wastes are eliminated in the toilet.

To understand what's going wrong with your digestion, it's important to know how healthy digestion works. The digestion process is complex, so to better understand it, let's see what happens after you eat a "balanced" meal of fat, protein, and carbohydrates, the three main macronutrients from which your body extracts energy: a stir-fry of vegetables and chicken served with rice and cooked in vegetable oil. The vegetables provide a little bit of carbohydrate, particularly in the form of fiber; the chicken is mostly protein; rice is mostly carbohydrate in the form of starch; and the vegetable oil is 100-percent fat.

Table 1 provides an overview of what distinguishes fat, protein, and carbohydrates:

Table 1: Macronutrients

	Roles	Sub-Categories		Examples
Carbohydrates	• Carbohydrates (both sugar and starches) are converted to sugar • Provide a source of quick energy • Unneeded carbohydrates are stored as glycogen in your liver and muscles or converted to fat in your body fat stores for later use • Insoluble fiber gives bulk to your stools • Soluble fiber keeps your stools moist	Sugars		Table sugar, high-fructose corn syrup, honey
		Starches		Bread, rice, potato, anything made from flours
		Dietary fiber	Insoluble	Vegetables and fruits (especially in the skin), whole grains
			Soluble	Eggplant, okra, apples, citrus fruits, flaxseed, psyllium, legumes, oatmeal, barley
Protein	• Long molecules made of small building blocks called amino acids • Repair and maintenance of all your organs, skin and muscles • Most satiating of all nutrients	Complete		Meat, poultry, fish, eggs
		Incomplete		Soy, legumes, grains
Fats	• Facilitate the absorption of fat-soluble nutrients (vitamins A, D, E, and K, CoQ10) • Some fats contribute to the good functioning of the brain and nervous system • Provide a sustainable source of energy • Promote satiety • Processed fats (trans fats and oxidized fats) promote oxidative damage and are associated with aging and chronic diseases (heart disease, diabetes, cancer, etc.)	Saturated (SFA)		Butter, coconut oil, animal fat
		Monounsaturated (MUFA)		Avocado, olive oil, almonds
		Polyunsaturated (PUFA)		Sunflower oil, corn oil, flaxseeds, fish oils (omega-3 fats)
		Trans fats		Margarine, shortening, hydrogenated oils

The digestion process begins before you even start eating; thinking about eating and smelling appetizing foods "primes" your body to digest. But it's in your mouth, when you chew your food and mix it with saliva, that the concrete digestion process is really initiated. The act of chewing breaks down food to make it easier for your stomach and intestines to digest it. Saliva coats your food to make it easier to swallow. It also contains an enzyme (amylase) that starts to break down the starches in the rice.

After swallowing, the food travels down the esophagus into your stomach. The stomach churns the food for a little while and mixes it with hydrochloric acid and enzymes that digest the protein (pepsin) of your chicken. The churning action and acidity of your stomach help to turn your meal into a paste that will be even easier to digest. After a few hours, small amounts of your now-puréed meal are released gradually into the first part of your small intestines.

When the stir-fry arrives in your small intestines, its acidity triggers the release of bile from your liver and digestive enzymes from your pancreas. Since the fat in the oil of your stir-fry doesn't mix with water, bile mixes with the fat to make it easier to digest in the water-based environment of your digestive tract.

Your pancreas produces enzymes that digest the protein of the chicken (protease), the starches of the rice (amylase), and the fat of the vegetable oil (lipase). The cells lining your small intestines also contribute by producing enzymes that break the small chunks of chicken protein into amino acids (peptidases) and that break down sugars and incompletely digested starches (disaccharidases like lactase, sucrose, and maltase).

Humans don't have the enzymes necessary to digest fiber, so it makes its way intact to the colon. In your small intestines, the amino acids of the protein of the chicken, the sugars derived from the carbohydrates in the rice and vegetables, and the fatty acids from the fats in the vegetable oils, as well as various vitamins and minerals, are absorbed into your body and circulated into your bloodstream.

After your body has taken all the nutrients it needs from your meal, the leftovers, which resemble nothing like your stir-fry, enter your colon (large intestines). Whatever you were not able to digest from your vegetables (primarily fiber) is fermented by the bacteria that make up your gut flora, and most of the remaining liquid is reabsorbed to compact your stools and make them solid. Your colon then acts as a storing place for your stools for a few hours or even a few days in some cases. And you know how the story ends!

Figure 1

the digestive system

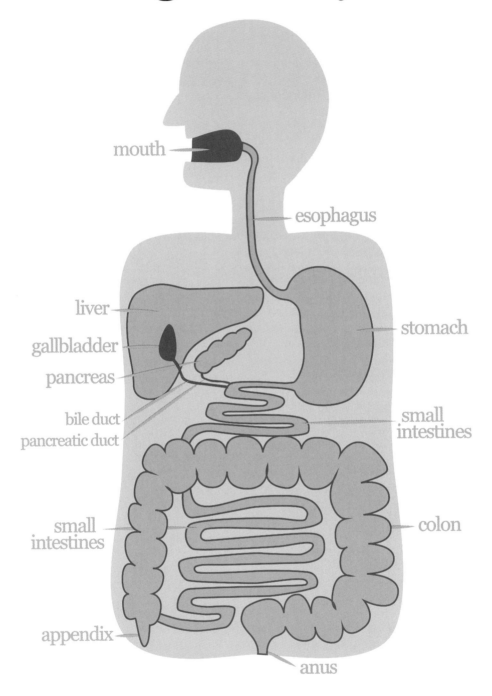

The next table provides a condensed version of the most important steps of the digestive process:

Table 2: Digestion 101

Organs	Digestion 101
Mouth	• Chewing reduces your bites of food into smaller, easier-to-digest particles. • Some enzymes (amylase) found in your saliva start breaking down starches (carbohydrates). • Your taste buds help you enjoy the taste of your food. • Signals are sent to your brain to notify your body that energy and nutrients are on their way.
Esophagus	• Permits food to travel from your mouth to your stomach.
Stomach	• Acts as a reservoir for all the foods you ate at your last meal or snack. • Produces hydrochloric acid (stomach acid) to facilitate digestion and kill potentially harmful bacteria and microorganisms. • Produces pepsin, a digestive enzyme that starts to break down protein. • Churns your food and mixes it with stomach acid and digestive juices from your stomach. • Releases its contents gradually into the small intestines (fat stays the longest in your stomach and carbohydrates the shortest).
Small Intestines	• Divided into three parts called the duodenum, jejunum, and ileum (in order from the stomach to the colon). • Covered with villi that increase the surface area of your intestines to maximize absorption—think of them as a carpet covering the inside of your intestines, increasing their surface area to 200 square meters, the size of the singles area of a tennis court or 100 times the area of your skin. • Receive the acidic content of the stomach, called chyme, which triggers the release of bicarbonate ions from the pancreas to bring the stomach contents' pH closer to neutral. • The acidic chyme entering the small intestines stimulates a cascade that triggers the release of digestive enzymes from the pancreas and bile from the gallbladder (which is connected to your liver). • Produce digestive enzymes to break down various sugars (including lactose), peptides (small chunks of protein), and small pieces of starches into smaller, easier-to-absorb particles.
Pancreas	• Produces a variety of digestive enzymes that break down starches (carbohydrates), protein, and fat. • Releases these enzymes in the upper part of the small intestines through the pancreatic duct. • Produces insulin, especially if you eat carbohydrates, to help your body utilize this quick form of energy by either 1) using carbohydrates for fuel, 2) storing them as glycogen in your liver and muscles, or 3) converting them to fat and placing them in your fat stores for later use.
Gallbladder	• Stores the bile produced by the liver. • Squeezes its bile out into the small intestines through the bile duct whenever you eat fat • Its bile acids emulsify fat (remember that fat and water don't mix; bile salts help transform big fat droplets into smaller droplets to make fat digestion easier).
Colon	• Contains the most bacteria in the digestive system, which ferment whatever is left undigested. • Reabsorbs water to make your stools solid. • Acts as a reservoir for the undigested material, fiber, and wastes that will be evacuated in your stools.

The Importance of Stomach Acid

You read that right: Stomach acid is very important. Many people believe stomach acid is bad and that too much of it causes heartburn and acid reflux, but this is generally not the case. In fact, most people don't produce enough stomach acid, which is crucial for proper digestion. Ever heard someone say they can't stomach meat or that it sits like a rock in their stomach for hours? A lack of adequate stomach acid is likely the problem. As we get older, our stomach can lose its ability to produce enough hydrochloric acid. Low stomach acid, or hypochlorhydria, is not something you hear about often, but it's very common and can contribute to many digestive problems. A lack of stomach acid can have serious consequences and can contribute to malnutrition, nutrient deficiencies, and gastrointestinal infections. Since stomach acid is one of your first lines of defense against invaders, not having enough can put you at risk of food poisoning or other infections from harmful parasites, bacteria, or viruses. Low stomach acid can also promote the overgrowth of bacteria or yeast in your small intestines. Three quarters of adults over 60 have low stomach acid—and just a single dose of proton-pump inhibitors, the most commonly prescribed type of antacid medication, is enough to reduce stomach acid production by more than 90 percent.

Table 3: The pH Scale and Stomach Acid

pH basics

pH is the tool used to classify the degree of acidity or alkalinity of different substances on a scale of 0 to 14. The closer the pH is to zero, the more acidic it is. In other words, a lower pH in your stomach indicates greater stomach acid levels while a higher pH indicates a lower level.

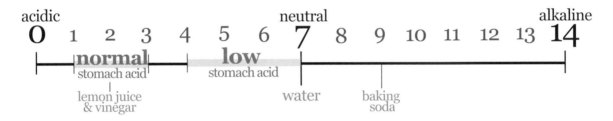

- Water has a neutral pH of 7.

- The hydrochloric acid produced by your stomach has a pH of ~0.8.

- Normal stomach acid corresponds to a pH ranging between 1 and 3 between meals.

- Low stomach acid (hypochlorhydria) corresponds to a pH between 4 and 7.

NUTRIENT ABSORPTION

The first role of stomach acid is to activate the enzyme pepsin, which is responsible for starting to break down protein in your stomach. One study showed that a normal acidity level in your stomach (pH of 2.5) allows you to break down 75 percent of beef protein. Without enough stomach acid, you can't properly digest the protein you eat. If the pH of your stomach reaches 5 (remember that the higher the pH, the less acidic), as is often the case in people taking antacids, only 25 percent of beef protein can be broken down, according to the same study. Inadequate protein digestion can result in the development of deficiencies in amino acids, the building blocks of protein. These deficiencies can in turn impair your body's production of neurotransmitters, the chemical messengers that help your brain cells communicate, and can even lead to depression, forgetfulness, and other mental problems over time.

The acidity of the stomach contents entering your small intestines then triggers the release of the bile from the gallbladder, which is crucial for the digestion of fat and the assimilation of fat-soluble nutrients. Insufficient acidity in your stomach can also therefore result in malnutrition and deficiencies in omega-3 fatty acids and vitamins A, D, E, and K, as well as inadequate absorption of the antioxidants CoenzymeQ10 (CoQ10), lycopene, tocopherols, and alpha- and beta-carotene.

Stomach acid starts the cascade required for healthy digestion by enhancing all the other steps of the digestive process. In addition to its roles in protein and fat digestion, hydrochloric acid is also important in absorbing many important vitamins and minerals. Studies have shown the importance of stomach acid for proper absorption of the minerals iron, calcium, and zinc, as well as vitamins B_6, B_9 (folate), and B_{12}. It's probable that stomach acid also plays a role in the absorption of any nutrients that are bound to protein, such as vitamins A, E, B_1 (thiamine), B_2 (riboflavin), and B_3 (niacin), although studies haven't yet been conducted on the impact of stomach acid on the absorption of these nutrients.

INFECTION PREVENTION

One of the main roles of a low pH in the stomach is to prevent infections. This is sometimes referred to as the "stomach acid barrier" because it truly acts as a barrier against infections. Most bacteria, parasites, and other microbes can't survive in the acidic milieu of the stomach. If you don't have enough stomach acid, you are more likely to get infected with *Salmonella, Campylobacter, Cholera, Listeria, C. Difficile, Giardia*, and other nasty bugs. Not having enough stomach acid can also result in an overgrowth of so-called "good" bacteria in your small intestines, a condition called small intestinal bacterial overgrowth (SIBO). Gut-friendly bacteria are important but too many of them in the wrong place can cause big digestive problems, as you'll see in Chapter 2.

FOOD SENSITIVITIES

Many digestive symptoms are actually associated with food sensitivities, which can be due in part to inadequate levels of stomach acid. Do you know how researchers make mice allergic to certain foods for the purposes of their studies? One of the most popular methods involves giving the mice encapsulated proteins from dairy, nuts, or eggs. The capsule acts as a barrier and prevents the proteins from being broken down properly and digested by the acid in the mouse's stomach. Result? The proteins move virtually intact into the intestines, potentially triggering an allergic reaction or the development of food sensitivities. Proteins are not meant to appear undigested in your intestines. If they do, they can confuse your immune system and trigger unpleasant reactions.

And this doesn't happen only in mice. If the pH in your stomach isn't acidic enough, the pepsin in your stomach won't be able to do its job effectively. If you have low stomach acid, you won't be able to properly digest most of the protein you eat. Large molecules of incompletely digested protein will make their way into your intestines, carrying with them the potential to induce the development of food allergies, sensitivities, and intolerances. Because of this, antacid medications, which make your stomach less acidic, are actually associated with a higher risk of developing food intolerances. You need adequate stomach acid to digest your food; incomplete digestion can cause big problems for your digestive health.

CAUSES OF LOW STOMACH ACID

Antacids, years on a vegetarian diet, stress, and certain gastrointestinal infections (such as *H. pylori*) can all reduce normal stomach-acid secretion and alter the normal pH of your stomach, compromising your digestion and health. The most common symptoms of low stomach acid (hypochlorhydria) include:

- Acid reflux, heartburn, and gastroesophageal reflux disease (GERD)
- Frequent belching after eating
- Indigestion or upset stomach after a meal
- Excessive feeling of fullness after eating
- Flatulence and gas
- Constipation or diarrhea
- Intestinal infections (parasites, yeasts, candida, bacteria)
- Small intestinal bacterial overgrowth (SIBO)
- Undigested food in stools
- Food sensitivities and intolerances
- Nutrient deficiencies
- Anemia

Don't these symptoms sound strangely similar to IBS and other common digestive problems?

Tests to check stomach-acid levels are not done routinely, but you can ask your doctor to get tested. The best test is the Heidelberg Stomach Acid Test. It's not cheap, averaging around US$350, and is unfortunately rarely covered by health insurance. Even if your doctor has diagnosed you with acid reflux or GERD, it's unlikely he or she will refer you for this test automatically. Request it if you want to know whether your problems are really due to too much stomach acid. The results may surprise you.

Some people also resort to a home test to evaluate their stomach acid level: the baking soda test. The validity of this test is not supported by any studies or evidence, but it can be worth a try. All you have to do is mix one-quarter teaspoon (one milliliter) of baking soda in a small glass of cold water and drink it first thing in the morning before breakfast. Watch the clock and time how long it takes before you belch. If you belch within the first two or three minutes, you probably have enough stomach acid. If it takes between three and five minutes, your stomach-acid levels are probably low, and if it takes more than five minutes, you are likely to have very low stomach-acid levels. It's best to repeat this test on at least three different mornings to average the results and get a better sense of your stomach-acid levels.

If you have low stomach acid, you can supplement with betaine HCl to replace the acid your stomach doesn't produce, or take digestive bitters to increase your stomach-acid production (see Chapter 6 for more details). Achieving the right level of acidity in your stomach can make a difference in alleviating your digestive problems, improving nutrient absorption, preventing gastrointestinal infections, and reducing some of your food sensitivities.

The Gallbladder

Your gallbladder has the important role of storing the bile produced by your liver. This organ can reach the size of a small pear when full, but it flattens out completely after squeezing out its bile following the ingestion of fat. Bile is crucial for properly digesting and absorbing fat and fat-soluble nutrients. If your gallbladder has been removed, the bile will simply drip continuously from your liver into your small intestines instead of being stored and dumped all at once when you eat fat.

Even though it's possible to live without a gallbladder, it's certainly not ideal. Missing this important organ can worsen digestive issues by forcing you to eat a low-fat diet. Low-fat diets are by definition high in carbs, and many carb-containing foods such as grains, dairy, and fruit can cause bloating, abdominal pain, gas, diarrhea, or constipation (as you'll discover in the following chapters).

A few studies even indicate that some types of gallbladder issues have an autoimmune component. Considering that many autoimmune diseases seem to be aggravated by gluten, your diet has a huge role to play in your digestive health, whether you still have your gallbladder or had it removed. If you have gallbladder issues, sticking to REAL food that is naturally free of gluten and other ingredients that can be inflammatory, irritating, or allergenic can help you get your problem under control.

If your gallbladder has already been removed, the approach proposed in this book may still be beneficial for you, although a few tweaks may be needed to facilitate fat digestion (as explained in more detail later on). Supplementing with ox bile or using fats that don't require bile to be digested, such as the medium-chain triglycerides found in coconut oil, are examples of things you can do to better tolerate fat without a gallbladder. Properly digesting fat is crucial for both your overall and digestive health.

Your Gut Flora

If you think you're alone in your fight against digestive problems, think again. A very large number of microorganisms forming your gut flora (gut microbiota) live in your intestines. Although your gut flora can change over time, you're pretty much stuck with it, for better or for worse. A healthy gut flora can help your digestion run smoothly, while an unbalanced gut flora (gut dysbiosis) can lead to many digestive issues and even negatively affect your overall health.

The number of bacteria living on your body and inside your gut is huge: 100 trillion bacteria. This is the same as 100,000 billion: a 1 followed by 14 zeros! It would take you thousands of years to count up to that number (counting one digit per second, 24/7)! Your body actually holds 10 times more bacteria than it has human cells. You're outnumbered in your own body!

The composition of your gut flora can vary depending on your diet, lifestyle, and age, but at any given time you're carrying the equivalent of three to four pounds of bacteria. Even 60 percent of the weight of your stools is bacteria! The bacteria that live in your gut can have a tremendous influence on your health. It's estimated that at least 800 species and 7,000 different strains of bacteria live in your intestines, but the majority of them have yet to be identified.

Most of the microorganisms residing in the gastrointestinal tract of healthy people are commensal (gut friendly), which means that they don't normally harm you and can even contribute to optimal health. In exchange for providing them a safe environment to live in, gut-friendly bacteria protect you against infections from pathogenic (harmful) microorganisms, in addition to stimulating your immune system, metabolizing dietary carcinogens, synthesizing some vitamins, and helping you better digest your foods. In addition, the good bacteria in your GI tract can also produce short-chain fatty acids (SCFAs), especially if your diet is rich in vegetables and fruits, which contribute to the health of the cells of your gut lining and provide you with an extra source of energy.

Figure 2

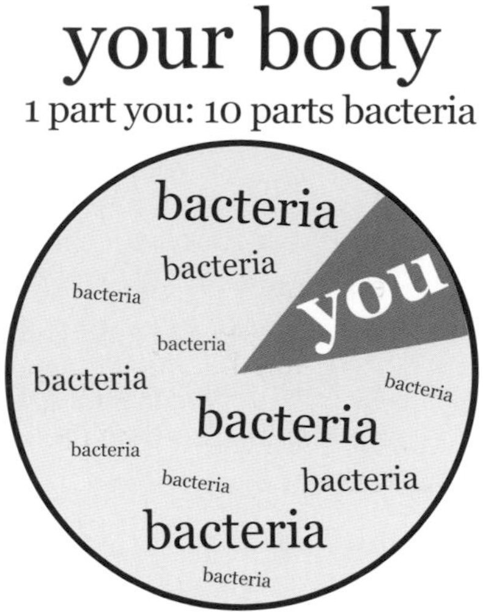

your body
1 part you: 10 parts bacteria

WHY IS A HEALTHY GUT FLORA SO IMPORTANT?

- Promotes immunity
- Prevents gastrointestinal infections
- Reduces inflammation
- Metabolizes dietary carcinogens and heavy metals
- Synthesizes some nutrients (vitamins K and B12, biotin, short-chain fatty acids)
- Contributes to digestion
- Regulates body weight
- Protects the integrity of your gut lining

Between 70 and 80 percent of your immune system is located in your gut. A healthy gut flora communicates with your immune system to help it distinguish good microorganisms from bad. This helps your body know which bacteria to destroy and which to protect to maintain a healthy balance in your intestines. If your digestion isn't working properly, chances are your immune system isn't, either. An incompetent immune system not only puts you at greater risk of getting sick, but it also increases your likelihood of developing food sensitivities and autoimmune disorders. Your gut flora also protects the integrity of the intestinal lining to prevent abnormal intestinal permeability (known as leaky gut), which can lead to further food intolerances and contribute to the development or worsening of autoimmune disorders.

GUT DYSBIOSIS IS ASSOCIATED WITH:

- IBS
- Celiac disease
- Inflammatory bowel disorders (Crohn's disease and ulcerative colitis)
- GERD
- Some cancers
- Obesity
- Allergies and food sensitivities
- Heart diseases
- Mental disorders (autism, schizophrenia, anxiety, depression)
- And many more

Many factors can influence your gut flora over the course of your life. Your digestive tract was completely sterile until birth, when it was colonized either by the bacteria from your mother's flora if you were born naturally or from any bacteria in your environment if you were born via C-section. The foods you eat throughout your life, infections, and the use of medications, especially antibiotics, can all drastically alter your gut flora balance. Studies show that a single course of antibiotics can result in a loss of the biodiversity of your gut flora within three to four days. Although your gut flora can slowly start to restore itself once you discontinue your antibiotics, researchers have shown that it usually never returns fully to its initial composition. Table 4 lists many factors that can affect your gut flora positively or negatively. In the next chapters, you will learn how you can try to improve your gut flora to optimize your digestion, reduce food sensitivities, and improve your overall health by choosing the right foods (including fermented foods) and using probiotic supplements.

Table 4: Factors that Influence Gut Flora

Things that Disrupt Your Gut Flora	Things that Improve Your Gut Flora
• C-section birth	• Natural vaginal birth
• Bottle feeding (infant formula)	• Breast feeding (human breast milk)
• Antibiotics and other medications	• Probiotic supplements (live bacteria)
• GI infections (food poisoning, traveler's diarrhea, gastroenteritis)	• Fermented foods (probiotics + prebiotics)
• Poor diet (rich in refined carbohydrates and inflammatory fats, low in vegetables)	• Prebiotics (food for bacteria)
• Chronic stress	
• Environmental toxins	
• Digestive problems (low stomach acid)	
• Excessive hygiene (antibacterial products)	

The Gut-Brain Axis

Your gastrointestinal system is the oldest and most evolved organ in your body. In fact, there are more nerve tissues in your digestive system than in your brain. The nerve system in your gastrointestinal tract is so complex that it's the only organ that can work completely independently of the brain. This complex system, and its impact on your brain and body, is often referred to as the brain-gut axis. From regulating your food intake to the metabolism of glucose and fat, bone metabolism, and mental health, the gut-brain axis appears to play many important roles, many of which have yet to be elucidated.

Even though the gut-brain axis is extremely complex, you've probably already experienced the strong connection between your gut and your brain in your personal life. Have you ever noticed that stress can affect your bowel movements? Or had butterflies in your stomach before speaking in public? Perhaps you've sometimes just had a gut feeling about something. It's no coincidence that emotions and feelings often seem to be connected with our digestive system.

There is a strong connection between our brain and intestines, and it works both ways. Stress can harm your gut flora and even damage your intestines, while bloating and problems with bowel movements can result in depression, anxiety, and other mental disorders. In fact, 50 to 90 percent of people with IBS report experiencing one of these mental conditions.

This might be due, in part, to the altered serotonin levels found in the guts of people with digestive issues. Serotonin is an important neurotransmitter found in your brain that helps you feel happy, calm, and relaxed. What many people don't know, however, is that 95 percent of the serotonin in your body is actually found in your GI tract. The serotonin in your gut influences the communication between your gut and your brain, and affects intestinal motility, fluid secretion in your digestive system, and the sensation of pain in your abdomen. People with IBS have abnormal serotonin levels in their gut, which further reinforces the importance of the gut-brain axis. Chapter 7 addresses the mind-body connection, because you can't expect to improve your digestive health without also taking care of your mind.

Intestinal Permeability: When Your Gut Goes Leaky

Your intestines constitute an important barrier—and the largest one—between your body and the environment. The surface of your small intestines is so big that it corresponds to 100 times the surface area of your skin. Like your skin, your intestines have the role of protecting you against invaders like harmful microorganisms and toxins.

Did you know that what's inside your digestive system is actually outside your body? It's only when nutrients are absorbed and circulated in your bloodstream that they truly enter your body. One of the roles of your digestive system is to meticulously sort the good from the bad in the food you eat, making sure that only the beneficial stuff, such as nutrients, enters the body, and keeping out bacteria, toxins, and waste products until they can be flushed away.

Your gut lining is made of a single layer of epithelial cells that are, amazingly, all that keeps what's in your intestines from reaching your bloodstream. This microscopic cellular barrier is all that separates you from the outside world, and it sticks together with the help of what are called tight junctions. Tight junctions form connections like "holding hands" to form your gut lining, opening when necessary to let in nutrients. If your intestinal lining is compromised, some of the cells lining your gut can become too weak to hold hands. Some of the tight junctions can break, allowing incompletely digested nutrients, toxins, and bacteria to enter your bloodstream (see Figure 3). This is called increased intestinal permeability, or leaky gut.

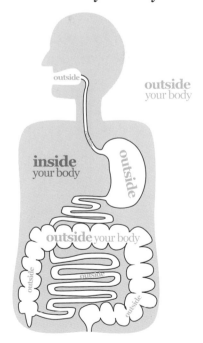

what is INSIDE your digestive system is OUTSIDE your body

Figure 3

normal and abnormal intestinal permeability

a. normal intestinal permeability

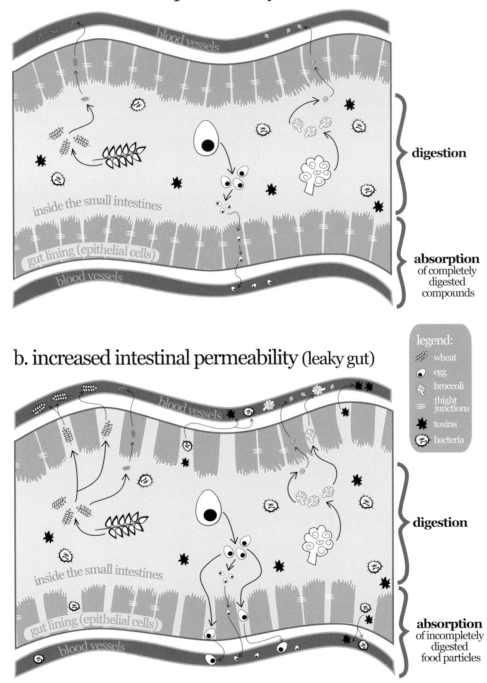

b. increased intestinal permeability (leaky gut)

a. In a healthy digestive system, the nutrients in food are digested completely into their smallest elements (glucose, fructose, and galactose for carbohydrates, and amino acids for protein, for example) before being absorbed into the bloodstream. The tight junctions of the intestinal lining act like closed doors that prevent toxins, bacteria, and incompletely digested food particles from passing into the bloodstream.

b. With impaired intestinal permeability (leaky gut), the tight junctions don't function as they should, as though the doors have been left open. If your gut is leaky, incompletely digested food particles, toxins, and bacteria in your intestines can pass directly into your bloostream. These compounds can overwhelm your immune system, trigger food sensitivities, and affect the functioning of your body (causing or worsening headaches, joint pain, skin problems, brain fog, autoimmune conditions, etc.).

If you have a leaky gut, part of what should be eliminated in your stool finds its way into your body, where it can cause all kinds of problems. Poop isn't meant to be in your blood! People with digestive problems such as IBS, SIBO, Crohn's disease, and celiac disease, as well as conditions such as asthma, urticaria, schizophrenia, cancer, lupus, and other autoimmune conditions often suffer from a leaky gut. Studies even show that the development of a leaky gut is the first step preceding the appearance (or relapse) of an autoimmune condition such as Hashimoto's thyroiditis, type 1 diabetes, rheumatoid arthritis, celiac disease, and multiple sclerosis.

One of the best hypotheses to explain the connection between a leaky gut and autoimmune diseases is called molecular mimicry. If your intestines are too permeable, they can act like a broken colander, allowing substances that should remain in the stool to sneak into your body. Your immune system responds by attacking these unwanted substances, but over time, the immune system can be overwhelmed and start confusing your own cells with some of the harmful substances leaking from your gut (if you're genetically predisposed to autoimmune disease). The body may thus start fighting its own tissues and organs: the intestines if you have celiac disease, your pancreas if you have type 1 diabetes, and your joints if you have rheumatoid arthritis. Taking care of your digestive health is a critical measure to keep autoimmune disorders at bay. If you're already affected by an autoimmune condition, addressing a leaky gut can make a tremendous difference in managing your symptoms and preventing a worsening of your condition.

As Hippocrates said, "All disease begins in the gut." And many "alternative" health practitioners associate a leaky gut with a wide variety of conditions, including eczema, acne, asthma, joint pain, anxiety, and autism. More studies are needed to determine whether a connection truly exists between the leaky gut and each of these different health conditions, but taking steps to improve your gut health certainly can't hurt your digestive health and may even offer you health benefits beyond your gastrointestinal system. Table 5 details the most common symptoms that indicate leaky gut.

Table 5: Symptoms of Leaky Gut

Symptoms of Increased Intestinal Permeability (Leaky Gut)
• Fatigue
• Food sensitivities
• Gastrointestinal problems (bloating, abdominal pain, diarrhea, constipation)
• Autoimmune conditions (celiac disease, multiple sclerosis, rheumatoid arthritis, Hashimoto's thyroiditis, type 1 diabetes, ulcerative colitis, Crohn's disease, endometriosis)
• Joint pain
• Headaches and migraines
• Skin problems (hives, eczema, rashes, mouth ulcers)
• Concentration issues (brain fog, fatigue, confusion, memory loss)
• Respiratory problems (asthma)
• Depression
• Anxiety
• Behavioral problems (autism, ADHD, dyslexia)
• Fertility problems
• Weight abnormalities (underweight or overweight)
• Adrenal fatigue
• Liver problems
• Nutritional deficiencies

WHAT MAKES YOUR GUT LEAKY?

Stress, gastrointestinal infections, alcohol, smoking, inflammation, and a poor diet can all disrupt the integrity of your gut lining. A porous gut lining can allow potentially harmful substances that should be evacuated in your stool to be absorbed into your body. Studies also indicate that gluten, by stimulating the secretion of zonulin, can impair tight junctions and negatively affect intestinal permeability in gluten-sensitive people.

The first step to repair a leaky gut and reach optimal digestive health with REAL food is to eliminate the foods that are contributing to your symptoms. The second step is to nourish your intestines and body to allow your health to reach its full potential. Besides eliminating the factors that can cause your small intestines to become too permeable, there are also several strategies you can implement to improve your intestinal permeability and heal a leaky gut. Probiotics, relaxation, and specific nutrients (glutamine, zinc, and vitamin A) can all help your intestines regain their natural integrity.

Table 6 lists the factors that can positively and negatively affect intestinal permeability.

Table 7: Factors that Affect Intestinal Permeability

Increase Intestinal Permeability (Contribute to Leaky Gut)	Improve Intestinal Permeability (Heal Leaky Gut)
• Chronic stress • Inflammation • Alcohol • High-intensity exercise • GI infections (*H. pylori*, parasites, food poisoning, etc.) • Bacterial overgrowth (SIBO) • Gluten (through zonulin release) • Toxins, lectins, and saponins (in the environment and in some foods like grains) • Bisphenol A (BPA) in plastics • Some medications (NSAIDs, etc.) • Poor diet (rich in sugar, refined carbohydrates, inflammatory ingredients and foods you are sensitive to) • Malnutrition (nutritional deficiencies) • Smoking	• Reducing or addressing factors that increase intestinal permeability (see left column) • Treatment of GI infections and bacterial overgrowth (SIBO) • Relaxation • Homemade bone broth (gelatin) • L-glutamine (amino acid) • Some nutrients (vitamin A, zinc) • Probiotics (supplements and fermented foods) • Elimination of inflammatory, irritant, allergenic, and fermentable foods • Colostrum ("first milk")

HOW DO I KNOW IF I HAVE LEAKY GUT?

If you have an autoimmune condition or food sensitivities, you can suspect that your intestinal permeability isn't normal. Leaky gut is also seen frequently in people with IBS, IBD, celiac disease, and other digestive disorders. The good news is that the protocol in this book will help you both manage your symptoms and improve the permeability of your intestines. Even though many people are still suspicious of the leaky gut concept, you can't go wrong by eliminating factors that can compromise your gut lining and adopting strategies to improve your gut health. And you definitely have more to gain than to lose since these dietary and lifestyle changes come with no side effects.

If you really want to know if your gut is leaky, a test called the lactulose-mannitol test can determine your degree of intestinal permeability. At the beginning of the test, you'll be given a small amount (about five grams each) of lactulose and mannitol and your urine will be collected for the next five to six hours. Both lactulose and mannitol are sugars, but only mannitol is small enough to be absorbed and show up in the bloodstream of healthy people. Lactulose is a larger molecule that your body cannot absorb (it's sometimes used to treat constipation because of its ability to draw water into your colon and make your stools moister). If you have a leaky gut, some of the large lactulose molecules will be able to pass through your intestinal cells into your bloodstream. Since your body can't use lactulose, your kidneys will eliminate it into your urine within a few hours.

Measuring lactulose levels in your urine can therefore indicate if you have a leaky gut and the degree of the problem (the more lactose, the leakier your gut). It's important to heed the test conditions: sugars must be taken correctly, and urine collected appropriately and sent to the lab without delay. This is a good test to do now and a few months after starting the plan in this book to evaluate changes in your intestinal permeability. You can ask your doctor for a referral or order the test online for around US$150.

Poop 101

Poop may not be a popular topic of discussion, but it can't be ignored when examining your digestive health. In fact, your stool is one of the best gut-health indicators, but how often do doctors show interest in the regularity and consistency of their patients' bowel movements? Defecation is something of a taboo topic, but it's no secret that everyone has to poop!

The Bristol stool chart (or Meyers Scale), developed in the UK, is used to classify stools by appearance using numbers instead of unappetizing descriptions. This chart is a great way to track your progress toward your own optimal diet. The "poop chart" below has been adapted from the original Bristol Stool chart and lists seven main types of stool (see Figure 4,) as well as two subtypes. The ideal stool should look like a type 3 or 4, while the examples at either end of the chart are less ideal. If you usually have stools that look like either one of the extremes, anything closer to the middle of the chart is a sign that your digestive health is moving in the right direction. Your daily number of bowel movements is another important factor in determining if your digestion is working properly. Going too often or not going regularly are signs that your digestion is suffering.

HOW OFTEN SHOULD YOU POOP?

There are no clear guidelines about how often you should have a bowel movement, but most doctors would agree that at least once a day, and up to two or three times, is preferable. Skipping a day, or even a few days, is usually associated with types 1 and 2 on the Poop chart. These types of stools are usually harder to pass and can cause straining. Stools consist of a lot of toxins and waste products that your body needs to eliminate on a daily basis to reduce its time of exposure to these potentially harmful substances.

On the other hand, more than two or three bowel movements per day is usually associated with stool types 5, 6, or even 7, and can indicate that things are moving too quickly through your intestines. An accelerated transit may not give your digestive system enough time to absorb the important nutrients your body needs.

THE PERFECT POOP:

- Frequency: One to three daily bowel movements
- Consistency: Type 3 or 4 on the Poop chart (see next page)

Tracking not only the frequency but also the appearance of your stools is a good way to determine if your dietary changes are helping you move in the right direction.

Figure 4

the poop chart

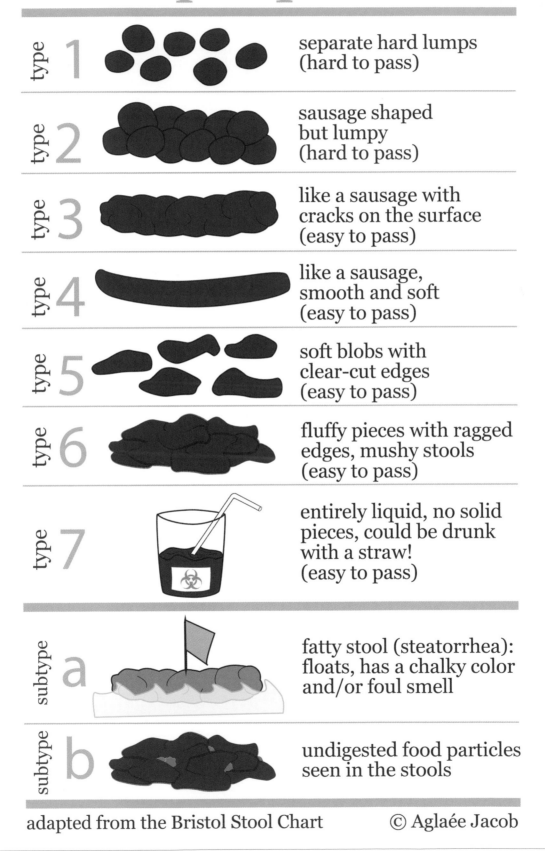

type	1	separate hard lumps (hard to pass)
type	2	sausage shaped but lumpy (hard to pass)
type	3	like a sausage with cracks on the surface (easy to pass)
type	4	like a sausage, smooth and soft (easy to pass)
type	5	soft blobs with clear-cut edges (easy to pass)
type	6	fluffy pieces with ragged edges, mushy stools (easy to pass)
type	7	entirely liquid, no solid pieces, could be drunk with a straw! (easy to pass)
subtype	a	fatty stool (steatorrhea): floats, has a chalky color and/or foul smell
subtype	b	undigested food particles seen in the stools

adapted from the Bristol Stool Chart   © Aglaée Jacob

In addition to paying attention to the frequency and consistency of your bowel movements, it's important to look for other details that can provide information about your digestive health.

EFFORT

When you feel a bowel movement coming, you shouldn't feel the need to run to the nearest bathroom. On the other hand, having to sit on the toilet for 15 minutes while reading the journal before anything starts moving isn't normal, either. Once you are seated on the toilet, you shouldn't have to think or concentrate too much on the task at hand; it should start naturally, almost as soon as you sit down, and the stools should pass effortlessly and without discomfort. If you feel like you're giving birth every time you have a bowel movement, something isn't right! Once you're finished, you should feel relieved. A sense of incomplete evacuation is a sign of sub-optimal bowel movements.

FATTY STOOLS

Stools that float, have a chalky or pale color, look oily, or have a particularly foul smell are not normal. These signs indicate steatorrhea (fatty stools or subtype a on the poop chart), which means you're unable to digest and absorb fat properly. This can be due to a lack of stomach acid or to gallbladder problems. Supplementing with betaine HCl (stomach acid) and ox bile, respectively, can help address this problem. Absorbing the fat you eat is critical. Fat is one of the best sources of energy, and allows your body to absorb important fat-soluble nutrients such as vitamins A, D, E, and K, as well as several other fat-soluble antioxidants.

GOING GREEN

Green poop can indicate a malabsorption problem or issues with your gallbladder and bile production. Bile is naturally green, but it becomes brown as it moves through your intestines because of the action of bacteria on bile salts in your intestines. If your stools are green, it probably means that things are moving through your system too quickly and that you're not properly absorbing the nutrients in your food.

LEFTOVERS

You shouldn't see undigested food in your stools (subtype b on the poop chart). If you can recognize part of your dinner in your stools, it's a sign you aren't chewing your food well enough, that you don't have enough stomach acid, or that you simply can't tolerate that food. This is especially common with raw vegetables. If type b stools are showing up for you, it might be a good idea to avoid hard-to-digest salads and crudités and try eating your vegetables thoroughly cooked and even puréed for a while to facilitate digestion. Preparing your vegetables this way can help your intestinal health improve more quickly, as well as allow you to better absorb the nutrients in these vegetables. You'll learn more about strategies to improve your digestion in the next chapters.

BLACK, RED, AND OTHER POOP PALETTES

You shouldn't see mucus in your stools or in the toilet, nor should you see anything clear, white, or yellow that looks gooey. This is a sign of inflammation in your intestines, and possibly even a gastrointestinal infection. Sandy poop (grainy texture) can also indicate a parasite infection, food sensitivities, or something more serious like colon cancer. Don't ignore these signals, and consult your doctor if they don't resolve despite your dietary changes.

Blood in your stools is also a bad sign. Fresh, bright-red blood on the toilet paper is probably caused by hemorrhoids. If it persists or increases, talk to your doctor. Black stools can reveal the presence of a deeper bleeding inside your gastrointestinal tract, warranting further investigation by a medical professional. Be aware, however, that beets, tomatoes, blueberries, black licorice, and iron pills can also affect the color of your stools.

> Daily bowel movements that look like a type 3 or 4 on the poop chart are one of the many benefits you can get from optimizing your diet. Striving for perfect stools is striving for healthy digestion.

The time it takes for food to travel from your mouth to the toilet is known as transit time. Your transit time should be around 12 to 24 hours. A longer transit time indicates constipation and a longer exposure time for your body to the toxins and waste products in your stools. A rapid transit time (less than 12 hours) points toward diarrhea and malabsorption. Even if bowel movements occur right after eating, those stools are not the remnants of your last meal but of what you ate in the preceding 12 to 24 hours (assuming a normal transit time).

Figure 5

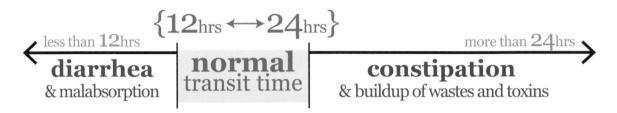

If food travels too quickly through your digestive tract, whether you have diarrhea or not (subtypes 5, 6, or 7 on the chart), you could be at risk for malabsorption and nutrient deficiencies. A transit time of less than 12 hours indicates that your body doesn't have enough time to absorb the nutrients in the food you eat. On the opposite end of the spectrum, if it takes 36 to 48 hours or longer for food to traverse your digestive tract, your body can be exposed to toxins and other undesirable substances in your intestines for too long. A long transit time also often results in dry, hard-to-pass stools, along with straining and hemorrhoids that can worsen constipation.

TEST YOUR TRANSIT TIME

How do you know how long your transit time is? If you have daily bowel movements and don't see undigested foods in your stools, your transit time is likely to be normal. But if you suspect your transit time is abnormal, you can do a simple test to measure it at home without any fancy equipment. This test is not super accurate, but it can give you a rough idea of your transit time. All you need are white sesame seeds. Mix roughly two tablespoons of whole seeds in a small glass of water and drink it. Write down the day and time on your calendar. Whole sesame seeds are not digested at all in humans and will therefore be evacuated intact in your stools (and white seeds are more visible). Check your stools in the following hours and days until you see them, then calculate how long it took for the sesame seeds to travel through your system. That's your transit time. You can also substitute with sunflower seeds, corn kernels, or beets. If you have a food sensitivity or allergy to any of these foods, however, skip this test.

Optimal Digestion

If you're reading this book, your digestion is probably not what you'd like it to be. Some people experience so many digestive problems that they forget what optimal digestion should feel like. The criteria used to define optimal digestion may vary slightly depending on whom you ask, but most gastrointestinal health experts would likely agree that optimal gut health involves most of the following criteria:

Table 6: Optimal Digestion

Aspects of Optimal Digestion	Specific Criteria
Effective Digestion and Absorption of Food	• Normal stomach acid levels, bile production, and digestive-enzyme secretion • Absence of malnutrition, nutrient deficiencies, and dehydration • Regular bowel movements (at least once per day) • Normal stool consistency (type 3 or 4 on the poop chart) • Normal transit time (12 to 24 hours)
Absence of Gastrointestinal Problems	• No abdominal pain, bloating, diarrhea, constipation, acid reflux, nausea, or vomiting • No carbohydrate intolerance (fructose, lactose, sugar, starch) • Normal intestinal permeability (no leaky gut) • Absence of gastrointestinal disorders (celiac disease, Crohn's disease, and other inflammatory bowel disorders) or good management of the condition(s) • Absence of inflammation
Healthy Gut Flora	• No bacterial or yeast overgrowth • No infections from parasites, fungi, viruses, or pathogenic bacteria • Normal composition and diversity of gut flora
Strong Immune Status	• Intact intestinal barrier (no leaky gut) • Normal levels of antibodies • Normal activity of the immune system • Normal food tolerance (absence of abnormal food sensitivities) • Absence of autoimmune conditions or good management of the condition(s)
Well-Being	• Good quality of life • Absence of depression or other mood disorders

*Adapted from Bischoff SC. 'Gut health': a new objective in medicine? BMC Med. 2011;9:24.

Even if your digestive health is far from optimal at the moment, this isn't set in stone. The food you eat or don't eat can have a huge impact on the factors in the table above. After learning about different digestive disorders in Chapter 2, Chapters 3, 4, and 5 will tell you all about the foods to seek and avoid, and the approach to use to figure out what your body wants and needs. Not everyone may be able to reach perfect digestive health, but a diet based on REAL food can help you get closer to that ideal.

Chapter 2: When Digestion Goes Wrong

The digestion process is complex and involves many steps. If something goes wrong along the way, it can manifest as one of several problems. Since you're reading this book, chances are you have a good idea of some of the following problems and how they can affect your quality of life: Passing enough gas to be accused of contributing to global warming. Spending more time cuddling your hot water bottle than your significant other. Getting your exercise in by running to the bathroom multiple times a day. Wearing stretchy or loose clothing to accommodate your bloated belly. Or saving on toilet paper by having a #2 just once a week. Does any of this sound familiar?

Living with digestive problems like bloating, gas, abdominal pain, diarrhea, and constipation day after day is no fun. Many people suffering with these issues come to a point where they fear socializing and even avoid eating out or traveling. Some people force themselves to fast the day before appointments or public events to try to avoid embarrassing situations. Have your bowels taken control of your life?

In addition to these obvious and unpleasant symptoms, digestive problems can also have repercussions on your overall health. If your intestines now seem to be ruling your life, you may also be depressed, lack energy, and feel unable to live life to the fullest. You may develop nutrient deficiencies, have troubles with your weight, and experience aches and pains you didn't use to have. To make matters worse, your friends and family may argue that you're just imagining it, that you "just have a sensitive stomach," or that you complain too much. Many people simply don't understand how miserable digestive problems can make you feel. I've been on both sides of the fence (see my story in the introductory chapter). I once thought IBS couldn't be more than just "unpleasant" until I experienced it myself. Now I know it can be pure torture.

Digestive problems are one of the top reasons for consulting a doctor, but most health practitioners don't really know what to do about these issues. This is a shame, since an estimated 25 to 35 million people in the United States alone (10 to 15 percent of the population) suffer from IBS, the most commonly diagnosed gastrointestinal disorder. Digestive disorders affect both men and women of all ages, including children. Worldwide, this figure ranges between nine and 23 percent of the population, which means that it affects at least one in 10 (and even up to one in four) of the people around you. Many of them have probably decided to keep these problems to themselves considering the unfortunate lack of understanding from the both the general public and the medical community.

Although symptoms like bloating, abdominal pain, or abnormal bowel movements are real problems, they're not very specific. Extensive testing is therefore required in order to find the underlying cause of these digestive issues. Is it a GI infection? Celiac disease? Crohn's disease? And if your doctor doesn't find anything, the resulting diagnosis is usually irritable bowel syndrome (IBS).

Irritable Bowel Syndrome (IBS)

IBS is by far the most commonly diagnosed digestive disorder, but it's highly misunderstood. IBS symptoms can include bloating, gas, abdominal pain, diarrhea, constipation, and alternating constipation and diarrhea. Although IBS is a common diagnosis, it is not normal. If you've been dealing with IBS symptoms for more than a few weeks or months, it's important to consult your doctor for more testing. IBS may not be life threatening, but it can affect your health and quality of life.

Before you can be diagnosed with IBS, your doctor first needs to ensure you don't suffer from another serious condition such as celiac disease, an inflammatory bowel disease such as Crohn's disease or ulcerative colitis, or colon cancer. If your intestines appear healthy but aren't functioning as well as they should, your doctor will compare your symptoms with a set of criteria called the Rome III criteria. The Rome III criteria were developed by a group of gastroenterologists to diagnose digestive disorders, such as IBS, that do not present with physical abnormalities. You may be diagnosed with IBS if:

You've been dealing with abdominal pain/discomfort for at least three days during *at least three of the past six months and*

Your symptoms meet at least two of these three criteria:

- Relieved by bowel movements
- Accompanied by a change in the frequency of your bowel movements
- Accompanied by a change in the consistency/appearance of your bowel movements.

In other words, IBS isn't really a condition, but a collection of symptoms. It's also a diagnosis of exclusion since it is diagnosed only once your doctor has confirmed that you don't have any other conditions that could cause similar symptoms. Researchers are trying to identify a marker that could be measured to diagnose and treat IBS more easily, but it hasn't been found yet (if it exists at all).

It's also important to know that even if your intestines may appear perfectly healthy with IBS, a large number of people diagnosed with IBS still have high levels of inflammation, which explains why an anti-inflammatory diet can be very helpful for people with digestive problems. Many people with IBS also seem to have increased intestinal permeability (leaky gut) and altered gut flora (gut dysbiosis), which explains the various food sensitivities associated with IBS and the systemic symptoms that often accompany the digestive ones.

The current treatment options for IBS are inadequate, to say the least. There is no cure for IBS and the best available treatments simply aim at covering up symptoms of diarrhea and constipation without correcting their underlying causes, like putting a bandage on a wound from which the splinter hasn't been removed. On top of not correcting the problem at the source, many of the medications prescribed to reduce abdominal pain can worsen constipation or cause other unpleasant side effects, which are then treated with more medications. Whether you choose to give medications a try or not, the standard IBS prescription almost always includes:

- Managing your stress
- Eating more fiber

Managing stress may help because of the important connection between your brain and your intestines, but it's often insufficient to control most of your symptoms. Stress can certainly worsen IBS, but it does not cause it.

A fiber deficiency is rarely the problem with IBS. Although getting enough fiber can play a role in gut health, getting too much, or the wrong types, can actually trigger or worsen some of your IBS symptoms. Foods like whole grains, fruits, and vegetables can make your diarrhea worse. They can also have the opposite effect and worsen your constipation.

If you've been diagnosed with IBS, you need to start listening to what your intestines are telling you. The first step to finding relief is to not just try to bandage your diarrhea, pain, or constipation, but to look for the root causes and address them directly. You need to remove the splinter before the wound can heal.

SOME OF THE POSSIBLE CAUSES OF IBS INCLUDE:

- A current gastrointestinal infection from a parasite, bacteria or yeast.
- A past gastrointestinal infection and/or the use of antibiotics that changed your gut flora.
- Increased intestinal permeability (leaky gut).
- One or more food sensitivities (gluten, grains, dairy, soy, fructose, FODMAPs, etc.).
- A gut dysbiosis (imbalance in your gut flora, including overgrowth of bacteria or yeast in your small intestines).

Your IBS symptoms may be due to more than one of these causes. Let's look at each of these different potential problems to help you identify what you need to do to get rid of your digestive symptoms and put yourself on the path to better digestive health.

Gastrointestinal Infections

Microbes like parasites, bacteria, and yeast can cause IBS-like symptoms by disrupting the fragile balance of your gut flora, making your gut lining more permeable, and causing inflammation. These microbes can also damage your intestines on a microscopic level that can't always be seen with regular testing, such as a colonoscopy. One of the first tests to get if you have IBS symptoms is to check if you're infected with any pathogenic (disease-causing) microorganisms. Whether you've had IBS symptoms for a while or not, this is a very wise thing to do and will affect how you should proceed to address your IBS. If you're infected and don't know it, any other approaches you try are likely to be unsuccessful if you don't first take care of the undesirable microbes living in your gut.

How does an infection make its way into your gut? Many people think that only people traveling abroad in third-world countries can get a parasite infection, but this is not the case. People anywhere are at risk of being infected with parasites like *Giardia*, Blastocystis hominis, or Dientamoeba fragilis. The pathogenicity (disease-causing ability) of some of these parasites, especially Blastocystis hominis, is questioned by many doctors. However, it appears that some strains of this parasite can cause symptoms in susceptible individuals. Unfriendly bacteria or yeasts like candida are other critters that can cause an imbalance in your intestines and lead to IBS symptoms.

It can be hard to determine exactly how you were infected, but it can happen more easily than you think, especially if (like most people), you don't have an adequate acid barrier in your stomach as a result of antacid use, stress, or simply aging. With the modern convenience of airplane travel, the world is no longer very large. Getting infected can be as easy as eating the lasagna prepared by a friend who unknowingly caught a parasite while traveling overseas, using a public toilet, or swimming at the local pool.

GI infections can cause bloating, abdominal pain, and diarrhea. Anal itching is also often reported with parasite infections. In addition to the gastrointestinal symptoms associated with a GI infection, it's also possible to experience insomnia, intense cravings and insatiable hunger, headaches, skin rash, depression, brain fog and fatigue.

GETTING TESTED FOR A GI INFECTION

Ready to get tested? Not so fast! If you ask your doctor for a test to see if your IBS is caused by a gastrointestinal infection, make sure to ask for a stool test with a DNA microbial profile. Unless otherwise specified, the traditional (and outdated) test involves trying to grow the microbes in a Petri dish. Most microbes that can infect your intestines are anaerobes: They don't need oxygen to live and actually prefer an environment that's not exposed to air, so our intestines are a perfect environment for them. As you can imagine, trying to grow these kinds of microbes in a Petri dish poses multiple problems, without even considering the many manipulation errors that can affect the reliability and accuracy of the results. If the microbes in your stools don't survive the transport and exposure to oxygen, for example, the technicians at the lab won't be able to make them grow and identify that you have a GI infection. A negative result obtained from these old-fashioned techniques doesn't at all guarantee that you don't have a GI infection.

The DNA testing method is much more accurate and comprehensive and eliminates typical manipulation errors. This technology provides a full profile of your intestinal gut flora by checking for the presence of genetic material from a wide array of microorganisms in your stools. Unfortunately, not many companies use this technology. Metametrix Clinical Laboratory is one of the few, and their tests can be ordered through a licensed healthcare professional. If your doctor is unwilling to help you get the test, you can find a doctor familiar with these tests in the USA through the Metametrix website. BioHealth Laboratory also offers accurate, comprehensive testing panels that can help diagnose a GI infection. If you live in Australia, New Zealand, the UK, Europe, Asia, or South America, the tests can be obtained through one of these international distributors. Check with your health insurance company to find out if the test is covered.

What should you do if the results of your stool analysis suggest that you're infected by a parasite, yeast, or harmful bacteria? Although dealing with a gastrointestinal infection isn't fun, the good news is that you're one step closer to getting your IBS under control! Work with your doctor to decide the right treatment to try to eradicate the microorganisms responsible for your symptoms. If you used a Metametrix test for your stool analysis, the results will also indicate if the microbes are resistant to specific antibiotics, which will help you and your doctor choose the most effective treatment.

Drugs like antibiotics, antiparasitics, and antifungals are usually the treatment of choice for parasite, bacteria, and yeast infections. Combining a pharmaceutical approach with a more natural one that utilizes herbal treatments such as garlic, oregano oil, olive leaf extract, caprylic acid, grapefruit seed extract, black walnut, or goldenseal is another option. Some people choose to follow the natural route alone, as the strong drugs used to treat GI infections can disturb the balance of your gut flora. Whatever option you select, be sure to work closely with your doctor. If you opt for a natural route, consult a qualified health professional, preferably a naturopathic doctor. Herbal antibiotics should only be used under the supervision of qualified experts to make sure you tailor your treatment to the strains of microbes with which you are infected and to your individual situation.

Whatever treatment(s) you choose, it's a good idea to use probiotics during and after the antibiotic treatment to keep your gut flora as healthy as possible (see the chapter on supplements to learn more about probiotics). It's also advisable to take another stool test a few weeks after the treatment to ensure that the infection is gone for good. A second treatment may sometimes be necessary to eradicate it completely.

What if you don't get tested? If you prefer to skip this step for now, you can try implementing the dietary strategies described later in this book. If you're not infected by pathogenic microbes, changing your diet alone should be enough to help you improve your IBS significantly. If you don't see improvements after a few months, however, you should consider getting tested to see if an infection is preventing you from getting your symptoms under control.

POST-INFECTIOUS IBS

Even if your digestive system is free from harmful parasites, bacteria, and fungi (yeast), you might be suffering the consequences of a past GI infection. It's estimated that between four and 32 percent of patients suffering from a GI infection go on to develop post-infectious IBS in the following three to 12 months. The longer lasting and more severe your symptoms, the greater your risk of developing chronic digestive problems later on. If your symptoms started after a bout of gastroenteritis or some other gastrointestinal infection, such as food poisoning or an episode of traveler's diarrhea, you could have post-infectious IBS. This is also true if you recently had a parasite or gastrointestinal infection and are still experiencing symptoms even if a recent stool analysis suggests the microbes are gone.

The diagnostic criteria for post-infectious IBS are very similar to those for IBS. In addition to having to meet the Rome III criteria described in the IBS section, the onset of your symptoms needs to follow an episode of acute gastroenteritis accompanied by at least two of the following:

- Fever (during the gastrointestinal infection), and/or
- Vomiting (during the gastrointestinal infection), and/or
- Diarrhea (during the gastrointestinal infection), and/or
- A positive stool culture test.

Why would you still experience IBS symptoms and digestive problems *after* a gastrointestinal infection? Some parasites and bacteria can actually inflict long-lasting damage to your intestines and gut flora. Research shows that some people with post-infectious IBS seem to experience an ongoing inflammatory reaction in their gut. It's normal to have inflammation in your body when it's under attack. Inflammation is part of your body's normal healing process, like the redness around a wound after you cut yourself or around your irritated nose when you have a cold. The same inflammatory process happens in your gut when you have an infection or an acute illness.

The inflammation is meant to subside once the wound is healed or the infection is gone. With post-infectious IBS, however, the intestines seem unable to recover fully from the infection, and low-grade inflammation levels persist, contributing to bloating, diarrhea, abdominal pain, and other IBS-associated symptoms. Chronic low-level inflammation also prevents your intestines from healing completely, which leaves you stuck in an endless cycle of inflammation and digestive problems.

Your gut flora is another important factor that plays a role in post-infectious IBS. A past GI infection from a parasite, bacteria, or yeast and the use of antibiotics to treat the infection can compromise the balance of the ecosystem in your intestines. Too much of the wrong bacteria and too little of the good kind can interfere with a healthy digestion. Studies have already shown that people with IBS have different and even abnormal gut flora compared to healthy people. It's difficult to know if this gut dysbiosis is due to the infection or the use of antibiotics, but it's most likely a result of both. In any case, the result is the same: bloating, pain, constipation, diarrhea, and gas associated with post-infectious IBS.

The villains responsible for your post-infectious IBS can also compromise the integrity of your intestinal lining, making your gut leaky. The tight junctions between the cells lining your intestines should be close enough to prevent any incompletely digested food particles, toxins, wastes, and bacteria from passing into your bloodstream. If you have a leaky gut as a result of post-infectious IBS, your tight junctions may become loose and allow undesirable substances to enter your body. A leaky gut can cause not just IBS symptoms, but also food sensitivities, headaches, and skin rashes, and can even contribute to or worsen autoimmune conditions such as thyroid disorders, rheumatoid arthritis, and multiple sclerosis.

Some people with post-infectious IBS get better with time, but studies show that the majority (between 57 and 80 percent) still experience symptoms five to six years after onset. These rates could probably be improved by adopting a better approach to address and correct the underlying lingering problems in post-infectious IBS: chronic low-grade inflammation, gut dysbiosis, and a leaky gut. The next chapters will help you better understand and learn how to lower your inflammation, balance your gut flora, and seal a leaky gut to better combat post-infectious IBS.

The Role of Food Sensitivities

Most people with IBS or other digestive problems notice that their symptoms can be influenced by specific foods or food groups. For example, you may have observed that onions and broccoli make you pass gas, that high-fiber breakfast cereals make you constipated, or that dairy triggers your diarrhea. The famous saying that everybody is different is particularly true with IBS. A food that you tolerate can cause symptoms in other individuals and vice versa. It would of course be a lot more straightforward if there were standardized guidelines to follow. Wouldn't it be far easier if broccoli caused gas, bran cereals caused constipation, and yogurt caused diarrhea for everyone with IBS?

"What is food to one man may be fierce poison to others."
— Lucretius

Although it's not entirely clear cut, foods containing specific proteins, carbohydrates, and other ingredients are more likely to be problematic for people suffering with IBS and other similar digestive problems. Eliminating these foods is a good start to your detective work to improve your digestive health.

THE MOST COMMON CULPRITS OF FOOD SENSITIVITIES ARE:

- Gluten (wheat, barley, rye, and many processed foods)
- Grains (with and without gluten, including oats, corn, and rice)
- Dairy (milk, yogurt, cheese, and many processed foods)
- Soy (tofu, protein bars, and many processed foods)
- Legumes (peanut, soy, beans, and lentils)
- Fructose (high-fructose corn syrup, apples, pears, cherries)
- FODMAPs (wheat, high-fructose corn syrup, onion, garlic, lactose, beans)
- Nuts and seeds (almonds, cashews, pepitas, coffee, chocolate)
- Nightshades (tomato, eggplant, bell pepper, hot peppers)
- Natural food chemicals (many fruits, vegetables, nuts)
- Artificial food chemicals (MSG, artificial sweeteners)
- Yeasts and mycotoxins (vinegars, fermented foods, alcoholic beverages)
- Alcohol (beer, wine, hard liquor)

We'll look at each of these food categories to better understand how they can cause digestive problems in the next section and in Chapter 4. Chapter 5 will teach you all about the implementation of an elimination diet protocol to help you determine which one(s) may be contributing to your problems. Remember that everybody is different and while many people with IBS may be sensitive to gluten or dairy, not everyone is. Beware of people claiming they have a cookie-cutter solution to IBS, because one doesn't exist. Following an elimination protocol is the only way to find what works for you.

GLUTEN

Gluten-free breads, flours, and other products used to occupy the small, dusty corner section of the health food store frequented only by people with celiac disease, an autoimmune digestive condition for which a gluten-free diet is the only known medical treatment. Today, the gluten-free market has exploded and these products can be found everywhere, taking up entire aisles at the grocery store and even featured on restaurant menus. Although gluten-free diets are now marketed as a cure for many ailments, they're no fad.

Many people who test negative for celiac disease still find that gluten-containing foods can cause all kinds of health problems, including IBS-like symptoms, headaches, skin problems, and joint pain. It was only in 2011 that a first provocative study showed that gluten can be problematic not only for people with celiac disease but also for non-celiac gluten-sensitive people. Unfortunately, many people who try a gluten-free diet fall into the trap of consuming lots of commercial gluten-free foods, many of which are not REAL food but highly processed food products that could actually be preventing them from getting their digestion under control, as you'll learn in the next chapters.

So what the heck is gluten, anyway? Gluten is simply the term for a type of protein found in grains. Each type of grain has a different type of gluten: Wheat contains glutenin and gliadin, rye contains secalin, barley contains hordein, oats contain avenin, corn contains zein, and rice contains oryzenin. Although not all gluten varieties appear to have the same effect in people with celiac disease or non-celiac gluten sensitivity, they can all be problematic for digestive health.

Gluten proteins can be visualized as a big LEGO construction made of many blocks of different shapes and colors, called amino acids. Each of the different types of gluten molecules contains slightly different combinations of LEGO blocks. For people with celiac disease and gluten intolerance, grains containing gluten with the combination of amino acids in the gliadin family seem to cause the most problems. These are the grains that are blacklisted on a gluten-free diet: wheat and its relatives (triticale, spelt, kamut), barley, rye, and oats. Oats do not contain gluten per se, but they are almost always contaminated with gluten (unless specifically labeled gluten free) since they are usually processed on the same equipment used for wheat and other gluten-containing grains.

GLUTEN-CONTAINING GRAINS

- Wheat and its relatives (triticale, spelt, kamut)
- Barley
- Rye
- Oats (unless labeled gluten free)

These foods are not the only places gluten can lurk in your diet. Most people eat gluten every day, if not at every meal. Wheat is used to produce a variety of food products. Beyond bread, pasta, and breakfast cereals, wheat gluten can hide in deli meats, soy sauce, and even beer. Table 7 shows the many processed foods in your diet that can hide gluten and the following chapters will help you to learn how to avoid it.

Table 7: Where Gluten Hides in Your Diet

Meals	Where Gluten Hides
Breakfast	Breakfast cereals, regular oatmeal, muesli, bagels, muffins, toast, English muffins, croissants, smoothies made with wheat germ, pancakes, waffles
Lunch	Sandwiches (in the bread and possibly the deli meat), pizzas, burgers (in the bread and possibly the meat patty), breaded chicken, salads with croutons, imitation bacon, barley soup, sushi (in the tempura, soy sauce, or imitation crab), dumplings, soups (in the noodles or the thickening agent), seitan, bulgur salad
Dinner	Spaghetti, lasagna, rice and risotto (from the seasoning), noodles, meat pies (from the crust and the sauce in the filling), stuffing, sausages, chicken nuggets, bulgur, couscous, frozen French fries (from the coating)
Desserts	Cookies, cakes, pies, muffins, graham crackers, scones, puddings, some yogurts, baked goods (made from wheat flour or graham flour, or containing other glutenous ingredients), brown rice syrup, candies
Snacks	Granola bars, crackers, nachos, yogurt with granola, pretzels, potato chips (from the flavoring)
Alcohol	Beer, spirits made from grains, many liqueurs and mixes (from thickening agents)
Seasonings	Soy sauce, some tamari sauces, malt vinegar, many salad dressings, sauces and marinades, many seasoning, flavoring, and spice blends, gravies, etc.
Other	Lipstick, vitamin and mineral supplements, medications, communion wafers, cosmetic and personal hygiene products, glue on envelopes and stamps, play dough, etc.

But what exactly is so bad about gluten? Haven't we been eating wheat and other gluten-containing grains for thousands of years? We have, but our ancestors were on a gluten-free (indeed, a grain-free) diet hundreds of thousands of years before they started eating wheat 10,000 years ago. The first agricultural civilizations that introduced grains saw their average height shrink from 5'9" (1.73 meters) to 5'3" (1.58 meters) for men and 5'5" (1.63 meters) to 5' (1.5 meters) for women. Their bone remains also show poor health, providing further evidence that grains may not be the best source of nutrition for humans. Grains have a lower nutrient density (fewer nutrients per calorie) than animal food and vegetables. Grains are also not a source of any essential nutrients that can't be obtained from other foods.

Another important factor to consider is that the wheat we eat today is not the wheat your great-grandparents ate. Since the 1950s, scientists have been trying to increase wheat yields through genetic experimentation. Wheat is not genetically modified (GMO), but it has been extensively genetically engineered using other techniques. While the results of these experiments have helped farmers increase their productivity up to tenfold, it has also affected the composition of wheat. Today's wheat contains a lot more gluten, which some experts believe is contributing to the higher prevalence of gluten-associated health problems. The fact that wheat is so abundant in our food also adds to the problem.

Although we hear mostly about celiac disease, this condition is only one form of gluten sensitivity, and non-celiac gluten sensitivity is actually much more common than celiac disease. The Center for Celiac Research estimates that non-celiac gluten sensitivity affects at least six percent of the population, compared to about one percent for celiac disease—and these estimates may be conservative. Dr. Thomas O'Bryan, a gluten expert and founder of thedr.com, claims that up to 25 to 60 percent of the population could be gluten sensitive. In addition, at least 55 different conditions have been associated with gluten, according to a 2002 study published in The New England Journal of Medicine.

The symptoms of gluten sensitivity and celiac disease can be very similar. Digestive problems like those experienced with IBS are common but do not occur in every case. Apart from bloating, abdominal pain, gas, diarrhea, and constipation, gluten sensitivity can contribute to headaches, migraines, fatigue, anemia, weight gain or loss, skin rash, vitiligo, psoriasis, osteoporosis, depression, attention-deficit hyperactivity disorder (ADHD), schizophrenia, autism, and autoimmune conditions such as rheumatoid arthritis, multiple sclerosis, and some sub-types of thyroid disorders (including Hashimoto's thyroiditis, the most common form of hypothyroidism). And the list goes on! Gluten might not be the cause all of these health problems, but it definitely seems to worsen many of them. If your digestion is not as good as it should be, add gluten to your list of suspects.

There may be other conditions for which gluten is a factor but of which we are currently unaware. What we know for sure is that gluten can affect almost any part of your body if you are sensitive to it, depending on your individual genetic susceptibility.

Testing can help you determine if your gluten intolerance is due to celiac disease, but it's unfortunately not 100 percent accurate. A celiac diagnosis can usually be made with a simple blood test to check for special antibodies called anti-tissue transglutaminase antibodies. However, there are a few practical problems with this test. The first is that your levels will only be high enough to diagnose celiac disease if you have an almost complete atrophy of the villi of your intestinal cells (see Figure 6), the most advanced stage of gut damage with celiac disease. The doctor won't be able to diagnose you if your intestines are only partially damaged. This is why many people with celiac disease or gluten sensitivity may go undiagnosed for many years.

Figure 6

the villi lining the inside of your intestines

a. normal villi
(brand-new carpet)

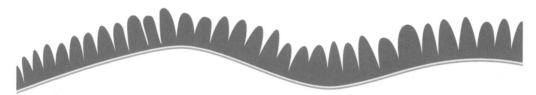

b. mildly atrophied villi
(used carpet)

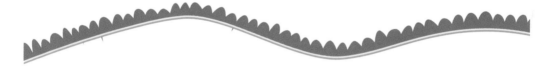

c. completely atrophied villi
(worn-out carpet)

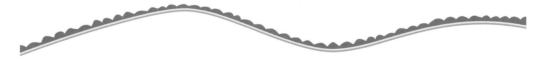

a. Healthy villi (microvilli) line the inside of your gut and allow you to digest and absorb nutrients properly.

b. Mildly atrophied villi show that your intestines are damaged, but not enough to be diagnosed with celiac disease. Digestion and absorption can be compromised.

c. Completely atrophied villi indicate a diagnosis of celiac disease and result in serious malabsorption problems.

Fortunately, a positive result for these antibodies indicates without any doubt that you have celiac disease. Some doctors also ask for an intestinal biopsy either to confirm a positive blood test or when a blood test is negative but celiac disease is still suspected. In any case, some gluten experts like Dr. Stephen Wangen, founder of the IBS Treatment Center, and Dr. O'Bryan, believe that the intestinal biopsy is unreliable and unnecessary. Many potential errors can affect the outcome of this test, and only a completely worn-out intestinal carpet (complete villous atrophy) can be detected with this procedure. Therefore, a negative result for celiac disease does not in any way exclude celiac disease, nor does it exclude non-celiac gluten sensitivity.

Another big flaw with current testing methods is that the usual test for gluten sensitivity only checks for a reaction to gliadin, one of the many possibly problematic combinations of LEGO blocks that form the gluten protein—but not all people with celiac disease are sensitive to gliadin. Some react to other gluten peptides that correspond to different combinations of LEGO blocks comprising the gluten protein. Gluten is so large that it is made of at least 60 different peptides that can all be responsible for celiac disease and non-celiac gluten sensitivity.

Some labs can now check antibody levels for not only anti-tissue transglutaminase, but other gluten peptides, as well. The Array 3 test from Cyrex Labs is a good example, as it measures antibodies for 10 of the most problematic gluten peptides. This test is unfortunately only available in the USA at the time of writing this book. Other tests look for IgG antibodies in your blood only, while other labs, such as those done by Enterolab, look for IgA antibodies in your blood or in your stools. IgA antibodies in your stools are thought to be a better marker of gluten sensitivity than the antibodies in your blood.

What if you're already on a gluten-free diet? Unfortunately, the tests for celiac disease and gluten sensitivity are only valid if you're currently eating gluten, and a good amount of it. Many people try going on a gluten-free diet once they start suspecting gluten intolerance, which is totally understandable if they have been feeling sick and are trying to feel better. There is no problem with finding a solution to your digestion problems by making changes such as removing gluten, but keep in mind that the celiac test results will not be valid if you are on a gluten-free diet since your body won't be producing gluten antibodies.

Many doctors, however, are unfortunately unaware of this factor. If you want to get tested and make sure your celiac test is as accurate as possible, experts recommend consuming the equivalent of four slices of wheat-based bread or two cups of pasta per day for at least six to eight weeks prior to the test. This is why some doctors make their patients go back to eating gluten for several weeks before testing them for celiac disease.

But do you really need to go back to eating gluten? What do you have to prove? You've probably heard the story of the man who goes to his doctor complaining that his arm hurts when he stretches it over his head, so the doctor tells the patient, "Well, don't do it, then!" Why should this be different with gluten? The practice of going back to eating gluten for weeks simply to be tested is unnecessary and dangerous. If you're sensitive to gluten, whether due to celiac disease or non-celiac gluten sensitivity, reintroducing gluten just to please your doctor could have a very negative effect on your health. Gluten is not an essential nutrient. Nobody needs gluten. If you feel better without it, why would you continue eating it? Just as you don't need a diabetes diagnosis to stop eating sugar, you don't need a celiac diagnosis to quit gluten.

Testing someone who's following a gluten-free diet for celiac disease is not only a waste of money, it can also make you believe falsely that you don't have celiac disease or aren't sensitive to gluten. Such invalid results are called "false negatives." Such a misdiagnosis can be dangerous for your health, since reintroducing gluten if you're unknowingly sensitive to it could damage your health, even if you don't experience any symptoms. This is especially true since eight out of nine people with a gluten sensitivity don't experience any of the typical digestive symptoms.

It can take years for some of the serious health consequences associated with a gluten sensitivity to develop and it's unfortunate that diagnostic tools aren't available to detect gluten sensitivity earlier and more accurately. Another study even showed that one out of four people who reintroduce gluten after not eating it for a while can develop an autoimmune disease such as rheumatoid arthritis, type 1 diabetes, or multiple sclerosis, within three years.

If you've already adopted a gluten-free diet and don't intend to go back to eating gluten, great! Most health professionals will warn you that you shouldn't go on a gluten-free diet before you're first tested for celiac disease. If you are still eating gluten, you should definitely take the test because a positive result may give you the motivation you need to switch to a gluten-free diet. On the other hand, if you're already feeling better on a gluten-free diet, suffering for six to eight weeks by adding gluten back into your diet is probably not worth it if you already know that gluten is contributing to your symptoms.

As long as you stick to a 100-percent gluten-free diet, you should be able to control your symptoms and stay healthy, whether or not your gluten sensitivity is due to celiac disease and whether it was diagnosed with a medical test or by going on a gluten-free diet. Remember: there are no risks to adopting a gluten-free diet, and most people have a lot more to gain than lose by ditching gluten grains.

Although there are still many unanswered questions regarding the mechanisms behind non-celiac gluten sensitivity, you don't have to wait until the researchers have all the answers to try a gluten-free diet. If your symptoms improve as a result of going gluten free, the improvements in your digestion and health will be enough to make you forget your love of bread and pasta.

If your symptoms don't improve, it may seem gluten isn't a major factor in your digestive problems. However, even if gluten does not appear to affect your IBS, you may still consider sticking to a gluten-free and even grain-free diet to optimize your digestive health and facilitate gut healing by removing these irritating, hard-to-digest foods, as explained in the next chapters. But the choice is ultimately yours.

***Warning: It's very easy to consume small amounts of gluten mistakenly or contaminate your food with traces of gluten. The equivalent of a crumb of bread, about one eighth of a teaspoon of flour or 10 milligrams of gluten, can be enough to compromise the success of a gluten-free diet. Follow the elimination diet protocol described in Chapter 5 to make sure your gluten-free experiment is successful.

Elimination diets are the gold standard to diagnose food intolerances and sensitivities. They cost nothing, and if done properly, can be very accurate and informative. Of course, you will have some work to do and you may miss some of your favorite foods at first, but I promise you will soon find new favorite foods, especially when you start feeling a lot better with your new way of eating. Table 8 shows you all of the ingredients that indicate the presence of gluten, and the next chapters will help you adopt a foolproof gluten-elimination protocol.

Table 8: Ingredients that Contain Gluten

Gluten-Containing Ingredients	Ingredients that May Contain Gluten
Abyssinian Hard (Wheat triticum durum), Alcohol (Spirits—Specific Types), Amp-Isostearoyl Hydrolyzed Wheat Protein, Atta Flour, Barley Grass, Barley Hordeum vulgare, Barley Malt, Beer (if made from barley or wheat), Bleached Flour, Bran, Bread Flour, Brewer's Yeast, Brown Flour, Bulgur (Bulgur Wheat/Nuts), Bulgur Wheat, Cereal Binding, Chilton, Club Wheat (Triticum aestivum subspecies, compactum), Common Wheat (Triticum aestivum), Cookie Crumbs, Cookie Dough, Cookie Dough Pieces, Couscous, Crisped Rice, Dinkle (Spelt), Disodium Wheatgermamido Peg-2 Sulfosuccinate, Durum wheat (Triticum durum), Edible Coatings, Edible Films, Edible Starch, Einkorn (Triticum monococcum), Emmer (Triticum dicoccon), Enriched Bleached Flour, Enriched Bleached Wheat Flour, Enriched Flour, Farina, Farina Graham, Farro, Filler, Flour, Fu (dried wheat gluten), Germ, Graham Flour, Granary Flour, Groats (barley, wheat), Hard Wheat, Heeng, Hing, Hordeum Vulgare Extract, Hydrolyzed Wheat Gluten, Hydrolyzed Wheat Protein, Hydrolyzed Wheat Protein Pg-Propyl, Silanetriol, Hydrolyzed Wheat Starch, Hydroxypropyltrimonium Hydrolyzed Wheat Protein, Kamut (pasta wheat), Kecap Manis (Soy Sauce), Ketjap Manis (Soy Sauce), Kluski Pasta, Maida (Indian wheat flour), Malt, Malted Barley Flour, Malted Milk, Malt Extract, Malt Syrup, Malt Flavoring, Malt Vinegar, Macha Wheat (Triticum aestivum), Matza, Matzah, Matzo, Matzo Semolina, Meringue, Meripro 711, Mir, Nishasta, Oriental Wheat (Triticum turanicum), Orzo Pasta, Pasta, Pearl Barley, Persian Wheat (Triticum carthlicum), Perungayam, Poulard Wheat (Triticum turgidum), Polish Wheat (Triticum polonicum), Rice Malt (if barley or Koji are used), Roux, Rusk, Rye, Seitan, Semolina, Semolina Triticum, Shot Wheat (Triticum aestivum), Small Spelt, Spirits (Specific Types), Spelt (Triticum spelta), Sprouted Wheat or Barley, Stearyldimoniumhydroxypropyl Hydrolyzed, Wheat Protein, Strong Flour, Suet in Packets, Tabbouleh, Tabouli, Teriyaki Sauce, Timopheevi Wheat (Triticum timopheevii), Triticale X triticosecale, Triticum, Vulgare (Wheat) Flour Lipids, Triticum Vulgare (Wheat) Germ Extract, Triticum Vulgare (Wheat) Germ Oil, Udon (wheat noodles), Unbleached Flour, Vavilovi Wheat (Triticum aestivum), Vital Wheat Gluten, Abyssinian Hard (Wheat triticum durum), Wheat amino acids, Wheat Bran Extract, Wheat Bulgur, Wheat Durum Triticum, Wheat berries, Wheat Germ Extract, Wheat Germ Glycerides, Wheat Germ Oil, Wheat Germamidopropyldimonium, Hydroxypropyl Hydrolyzed Wheat Protein, Wheat Grass (can contain seeds), Wheat Nuts, Wheat Protein, Wheat Triticum aestivum, Wheat Triticum Monococcum, Wheat (Triticum Vulgare) Bran Extract, Whole-meal Flour, Wild Einkorn (Triticum boeotictim), Wild Emmer (Triticum dicoccoides)	Artificial Color, Baking Powder, Caramel Color, Caramel Flavoring, Clarifying Agents, Coloring, Dextrins, Dextrimaltose, Dry Roasted Nuts, Emulsifiers, Enzymes, Fat Replacer, Flavoring, Food Starch, Food Starch Modified, Glucose Syrup, Gravy Cubes, Ground Spices/Spice Blends, HPP, HVP, Hydrolyzed Plant Protein, Hydrolyzed Protein, Hydrolyzed Vegetable Protein, Hydrogenated Starch Hydrolysate, Hydroxypropylated Starch, Maltose, Miso, Mixed Tocopherols, Modified Food Starch, Modified Starch, Natural Flavoring, Natural Flavors, Natural Juices, Non-dairy Creamer, Pregelatinized Starch, Protein Hydrolysates, Seafood Analogs, Seasonings, Sirimi, Smoke Flavoring, Soba Noodles, Soy Sauce, Soy Sauce Solids, Stabilizers, Starch, Stock Cubes, Tocopherols, Vegetable Broth, Vegetable Gum, Vegetable Protein, Vegetable Starch Vitamins, Wheatgrass juice, Wheat Starch

Dairy

Dairy can be another problematic food for people with IBS. You're probably aware of lactose intolerance, a common source of digestive problems, but lactose is only one of the many compounds in milk that can be problematic for your intestines. The topic of lactose intolerance will be discussed in the FODMAP section, but for now we will focus on the protein part of dairy. The main protein found in almost all dairy products, whether they contain lactose or not, is called casein (whey, the other type of protein in dairy, is present in smaller amounts). Like gluten, casein can be hard to digest, and if it's not broken down properly you can react to it. Like all food intolerances, casein sensitivity can manifest in many ways, including IBS symptoms and other digestive problems. Although most people may not realize it, casein intolerance is common for people with digestive disorders and autoimmune conditions, especially if a leaky gut is part of the picture.

A sensitivity to dairy is different from a true dairy allergy. A food allergy involves a dramatic response from your immune system, generally involving the rapid onset of severe symptoms. In some cases, it can cause an anaphylactic reaction, or severe breathing difficulties resulting from the swelling of the mouth and throat that can ultimately lead to death. Other symptoms associated with food allergies include skin rash, nausea, abdominal pain, vomiting, and diarrhea. The symptoms associated with a food sensitivity can be very similar, with the exception of anaphylaxis. Table 9 can help you better understand the difference between food allergies and food sensitivities.

Table 9: Food Allergies vs. Food Intolerances

Characteristics	Food Allergy	Food Intolerance
Symptoms	More limited and predictable: • Tingling or itching in the mouth • Hives, itching, or eczema • Swelling of the lips, face, tongue, and throat, or other parts of the body • Wheezing, nasal congestion, or trouble breathing • Abdominal pain, diarrhea, nausea, or vomiting • Dizziness, lightheadedness, or fainting • Anaphylaxis (breathing difficulties that can lead to death)	Wide range of symptoms and more than one symptom is usually experienced at the same time: • Abdominal pain • Aches and pains • Acid reflux • Asthma and wheezing • Arthritis • Bed wetting • Behavioral problems (autism, ADHD, etc.) • Bloating • Constipation and/or diarrhea • Fatigue • IBS • Headaches and migraines • Nausea • Heart palpitations (or increased heart rate) • Skin problems (rashes, urticaria, eczema, and hives) • Rhinitis • Sinusitis
Onset	Immediately to up to two hours after eating a food	As quick as 30 minutes, but usually after a few hours to up to a few days (48 hours or more in some cases) after eating a food
Tolerance	None (even a tiny bit will trigger an allergic reaction)	Severity of symptoms depends on the amount consumed (dose response)
Mechanism	Response mediated by the immune system (most often with IgE antibodies)	Unclear and may depend on the food and individual; not always mediated by the immune system (but can involve IgG or IgA antibodies)
Prevalence	About 1-4% of adults and 6-8% of children	Much more common than food allergies, but statistics are currently unavailable due to the difficulty of accurate diagnosis
Diagnosis	Skin-prick test and blood test to check for IgE antibodies to specific foods	• Elimination diets are the gold standard • Other tests (including blood and stool tests for IgG and IgA antibodies) are unreliable according to latest scientific evidence and not yet validated

*If you have a true allergy to a food, never reintroduce it into your diet.

Unfortunately, current testing methods for food sensitivities aren't foolproof. The skin-prick test, as well as blood tests, only check for specific antibodies (IgE) that your body may release in presence of an offending protein (such as casein), but most forms of food intolerance are either mediated by other types of antibodies (IgG or IgA) or don't involve the immune system at all.

Can you guess the best way to determine if casein is contributing to your digestive problems? An elimination diet protocol! Eliminate casein-containing dairy products for a few weeks before reintroducing them. If your symptoms return upon reintroducing casein, you'll know that your body can't handle it. If nothing changes when you start eating casein again, you'll know that it doesn't seem to be problematic for you.

Casein is found in varying amounts in almost all dairy products, with the exception of ghee (clarified butter). Although butter and cream contain only trace amounts, these levels can be enough to cause problems if you're very sensitive to casein. Cheese, yogurt, ice cream, and milk are all very high in casein. Casein can also hide in milk chocolate, sauces, margarine, muffins, breads, and other baked goods, as well as in seasonings, non-dairy creamer, and many other processed foods. Table 10 lists ingredients that contain dairy. The next chapters will help you identify the casein-containing foods in your diet so you can attempt your own dairy-elimination challenge.

Table 10: Ingredients Containing Dairy

Dairy-Containing Ingredients	May Contain Dairy
Butter (butter fat, butter oil, butter solids)	Chocolate
Buttermilk and buttermilk powder	Flavorings
Buttermilk solids	
Casein	High-protein flour
Caseinate (calcium caseinate, sodium caseinate, etc.)	Hot dogs
Cheese	
Condensed milk	Luncheon and deli meats
Cream	
Curds	Margarine
Custard	Sausages
Dry milk powder	
Dry milk solids	Starter distillate
Evaporated milk	
Half & half	
Kefir	
Goat's milk	
Lactalbumin	
Lactose	
Lactoferrin	
Lactoglobulin	
Malted milk	
Milk in any form (milk powder, milk protein, nonfat milk, skim milk, and milk solids)	
Natural butter flavor	
Nougat	
Paneer	
Pudding	
Sour cream	
Yogurt	
Whey in any form (whey powder, whey protein concentrate, whey protein hydrolysate, delactosed whey, whey solids, etc.)	

Tip: The kosher labeling Parve or Pareve (the letter "U" in a circle, with no other letters) is certified dairy free.

Soy

Soy, like dairy and grains, contains proteins to which you may be sensitive. Even if you don't think you eat a lot of soy, you may be surprised to find that soy has snuck into many food products beyond tofu and soy milk. Soy is everywhere, especially in processed foods and those labeled as "healthy." Pick up any packaged food at the grocery store and the ingredient list is likely to reveal the presence of soy in one form or another, whether as soy lecithin, monoglycerides, diglycerides, soy protein, or monosodium glutamate. Soy-derived ingredients are often added to breakfast cereals, margarines, mayonnaise, chocolate, muffins, protein powders, soy beverages, granola bars, sauces, vegetarian burgers, soy sauces, frozen entrées, gravies, smoothies, bouillon cubes, and even as a filler in meat patties and sausages.

What's more, almost all the soy available in North America is genetically engineered (GMO). The long-term health consequences of consuming GMO soy are unknown and some experts believe that the protein of GMO soy may cause even more food sensitivities and allergies. Table 11 lists some of the ingredients that can indicate the presence of soy.

Table 11: Ingredients that Contain Soy

Other Names for Soy	Soy-Containing Ingredients	Ingredients Likely to Contain Soy
Bean curd	Hydrolyzed soy protein	Bouillon cubes
Bean sprouts	Mono- and di-glycerides	Bulking agent
Edamame	MSG (monosodium glutamate)	Hydrolyzed plant protein (HPP)
Kinako	Soy	Hydrolyzed vegetable protein (HVP)
Miso	Soy albumin	Flavorings
Natto	Soy flour	Gum arabic
Niname	Soy grits	Guar gum
Okara	Soy lecithin	Lecithin
Shoyu	Soy nuts	Mixed tocopherols
Soy sauce	Soy protein	Natural flavoring (may be soy-based)
Soya/Soja	Soybean oil	Stabilizer
Soybean	Teriyaki sauce	Thickener
Tamari	Textured vegetable protein (TVP)	Vegetable broth
Tempeh		Vegetable gum
Tofu		Vegetable starch
Yuba		Vegetable shortening
		Vegetable oil
		Vitamin E (often contains soybean oil)

Soy protein is one of the many ingredients found in processed food that can bother people with IBS or other similar digestive problems. The best way to whether soy may be problematic for you is—you guessed it—an elimination diet.

Although you might be wondering what will be left to eat on your elimination diet with gluten, dairy, and soy out of the picture, don't worry. By ensuring your diet contains only REAL foods, you won't starve. As an added bonus, you'll be getting all the nutrition you need to help heal your gut, and you won't have to read food labels! It has become very difficult to know what is in the food we eat, especially if we eat the processed "foods" engineered by the food industry. That's why the approach proposed in this book is based on REAL food. Eating REAL food takes the guesswork out of your digestive problems and increases your chance of success.

Short-Chain Fermentable Carbohydrates (FODMAPs)

Besides the proteins found in grains, dairy, and soy, some types of carbohydrates known as fermentable oligo-, di-, and mono-saccharides, and polyols (FODMAPs) or short-chain fermentable carbohydrates can also contribute to digestive problems. Although the association between these carbohydrates and digestive disorders has been known for over a century, this fact may come as a surprise for many IBS sufferers. It is only recently that the concept has resurfaced, thanks to the work of a team of researchers from Monash University in Melbourne, Australia. The results of their studies show that certain kinds of carbohydrates can cause or worsen bloating, abdominal pain, diarrhea, constipation, and gas. The studies were conducted mostly on people with IBS and Crohn's disease, but the same phenomenon can occur with digestive disorders such as celiac disease, ulcerative colitis, and GERD. Beyond digestive problems, foods rich in these problematic carbohydrates are also associated with fatigue, lethargy, nausea, heartburn, and acid reflux in people with IBS and similar disorders. Restricting foods containing these problematic carbohydrates could be a factor in relieving your digestive symptoms.

The substances classified as FODMAPs (see Table 12) represent specific types of carbohydrates that can be fermented excessively and draw too much water inside your intestines. You are probably already familiar with at least two FODMAPs: lactose and fructose. For most healthy people, FODMAPs do not cause any problems, but in susceptible individuals they can wreak havoc on digestion and health.

Table 12: FODMAPs

Acronym		Synonym		Examples
F	Fermentable	Short-chain fermentable and osmotically active carbohydrates	Oligosaccharides	• Fructans
O	Oligosaccharides			• Galactans
D	Disaccharides		Disaccharides	• Lactose
M	Monosaccharides		Monosaccharides	• Fructose
A	And		Polyols	• Polyols (sorbitol, mannitol)
Ps	Polyols			

Why would you react to FODMAPs? In some cases, it can be due to a malabsorption problem, whether you lack specific enzymes (for lactose, for example) or a have problem with transporters responsible for the absorption of certain nutrients (with fructose, for example). Gut dysbiosis, which can result from having the wrong kind of bacteria or too much of certain bacteria, can also be linked to short-chain fermentable carbohydrates.

LACTOSE

Milk's natural sugar is responsible for one of the most common food intolerances in the world, affecting about 70 percent of people worldwide. Lactose is a disaccharide that is made of two molecules of sugar: one glucose and one galactose. In order to absorb lactose, it has to be broken down into single units of glucose and galactose by the enzyme lactase, which is produced by the cells lining your intestines. Unfortunately, many people lose the ability to produce this enzyme, often because of the elimination of dairy products from their diet or the normal aging process. Damage to the lining of your intestines caused by repeated episodes of diarrhea, gluten exposure, or other food intolerances can also decrease your intestines' ability to produce lactase and can ultimately result in lactose intolerance.

If you're unable to absorb lactose well, it can turn into a short-chain fermentable carbohydrate and be fermented in your intestines. Abdominal cramps, gas, bloating, and diarrhea are the most common symptoms of this food intolerance. Although diarrhea is more frequent, lactose intolerance can also cause constipation in some people.

The lactose content of different dairy products varies from none (ghee) to a lot (milk). As with other FODMAPs, your personal tolerance threshold may vary. In addition, the effect of lactose is cumulative, so the more you consume in a certain period of time (within a few hours to a couple of days), the more severe your symptoms may be.

Milk has the highest amount of lactose per serving. Cheese, cream, butter, ghee, are almost all fat and contain only traces of the lactose, while yogurt and ice cream fall in between. People with lactose intolerance are usually able to tolerate three to four grams of lactose at once (about one third of a cup or 80 ml of milk), but very sensitive people may react to even the small amounts of lactose found in cheese or heavy cream. Table 13 shows the lactose content of different dairy products. Keep in mind that the lactose found in raw milk, raw cheeses, and fermented dairy products (such as yogurt and kefir) is usually better tolerated because these products contain probiotic bacteria that help break down the lactose. However, many dairy products contain both lactose and casein, making it hard to know what's causing the problem: lactose, casein, or both. The elimination diet protocol will help you make the distinction to determine what your digestive system can tolerate.

Table 13: Lactose Content of Dairy Products

Category	Food	Serving	Lactose Content
High	Milk	1 cup / 250 ml	12 g
Moderate	Yogurt (commercial)	¾ cup / 175 ml	5-9 g
	Ice cream	½ cup / 125 ml	6
	Parmesan	1 oz / 30 g	1 g
	Cheddar	1 oz / 30 g	less than 0.05 g
Low	Yogurt (homemade, fermented 24 hours)	¾ cup / 175 ml	Trace
	Cream	1 tbsp / 15 ml	0.6 g
	Butter	1 tbsp / 15 ml	Trace
	Ghee	1 tbsp / 15 ml	Almost none

Lactose intolerance can usually be diagnosed easily by trial and error, but a simple breath test is also available. This test involves taking a dose of 20 to 25 grams of pure lactose then blowing into a bag every 15 to 30 minutes for up to two to three hours. The lab will then analyze the amount of hydrogen and methane gas present in the bags. High levels of either gas may indicate that you haven't absorbed all the lactose and that part or all of it was fermented inside your intestines, suggesting a diagnosis of lactose intolerance.

Following a low-lactose diet is usually sufficient to manage lactose intolerance if a lactase deficiency is your only problem. For most people, though, lactose intolerance is only part of the problem, so reducing or eliminating lactose may not be sufficient to get rid of your digestive problems. Looking at other FODMAPs in your diet may help your gut get greater relief.

FRUCTOSE

Fructose is another FODMAP that is often responsible for triggering IBS symptoms. Fructose malabsorption is the term used to refer to the inability to absorb fructose, which can result in its fermentation by the bacteria in your intestines. As with other FODMAP intolerances, the symptoms of fructose malabsorption are similar to those of IBS.

If you have fructose malabsorption, you may be able to handle small amounts of fructose. It is only if you exceed your individual tolerance threshold that fructose may start causing problems. Other than the digestive problems commonly associated with IBS, fructose malabsorption can also contribute to certain nutrient deficiencies and depression.

Fructose malabsorption is different from hereditary fructose intolerance, a rare genetic disorder that causes convulsions, irritability, jaundice, and vomiting and warrants the strict elimination of all forms of fructose and sugar.

Fructose malabsorption is also associated with depression. Why would this be the case? It may have something to do with feeling like your bowels are controlling your life, but it's not all in your head. Well, it is—but it's not your fault. Studies done in Austria show that fructose malabsorption induces physiological changes that alter your brain chemistry, making you feel down. These findings show higher depression scores in people with fructose malabsorption, especially women, which are attributed to their lower levels of tryptophan compared to other people with similar gastrointestinal issues without fructose malabsorption. Tryptophan is an amino acid required for the biosynthesis of serotonin, an important neurotransmitter (brain messenger) that helps you feel calm and happy. Serotonin is a natural anti-depressant that your body can usually produce in sufficient amounts from tryptophan, which is found in protein-rich foods like poultry, meat, fish, and eggs. People with fructose malabsorption don't have enough tryptophan, even if they eat enough of it, and therefore can't produce enough serotonin to feel good.

The good news is that, according to the same team of researchers, a low-fructose and low-sorbitol diet (sorbitol is another FODMAP) can help improve not only IBS symptoms but symptoms of depression; in their study, reducing dietary fructose resulted in a 65-percent improvement in depression score in only four weeks. The exact mechanism is not completely understood and more studies are needed, but these results suggest reducing fructose can be a positive step toward gut health and overall well-being.

But why exactly wouldn't you be able to absorb fructose properly? One of the receptors that allow you to absorb fructose from your intestines into your bloodstream is called GLUT5. GLUT5 functioning is impaired in people with fructose malabsorption. It's unclear if this is due to a genetic defect or damage to the intestinal lining. Some people may also experience symptoms from fructose-rich foods even if their GLUT5 receptor works fine. In that case, fructose malabsorption would be due to an overgrowth of intestinal bacteria that get their hands on the fructose you eat before you have a chance to absorb it yourself. In either case, the result is the same: the unabsorbed fructose is fermented and draws a lot of water inside your intestines. Just as with lactose intolerance, the intestinal fermentation of fructose may cause gas, bloating, cramping, and changes in the frequency and consistency of your bowel movements.

Fructose malabsorption can be diagnosed with a breath test, similarly to lactose intolerance. The only difference is that you will be given a fructose-sweetened drink instead of lactose at the start of the test, then asked to breathe into a bag every 15 to 30 minutes. High levels of hydrogen, methane, or both in your breath indicate fructose malabsorption.

Although fructose is one of the main sugars found naturally in fruit, fruit is not the major source of dietary fructose for most people. Most fructose in the Western diet comes from added sugar, in various forms. Table sugar, or sucrose, is half glucose and half fructose. If you eat a bowl of breakfast cereal containing 18 grams of table sugar, at least half of it is very likely fructose.

Foods and beverages sweetened with high-fructose corn syrup (HFCS) are even higher in fructose, since this sweetener is made of at least 55-percent fructose and 45-percent glucose. If your bowl of cereal in the example above had been sweetened with HFCS, a serving would provide about 10 grams of fructose. A recent study even revealed that although many food manufacturers claim that the HFCS in their products is 55-percent fructose, the actual fructose content is sometimes closer to 65 percent. HFCS is now routinely added to many processed foods, making it very easy to consume more fructose than you think.

Agave nectar, also called agave syrup, is even worse than HFCS, since it consists of 90 percent fructose and 10 percent glucose. Your bowl of cereal would contain over 16 grams of fructose if sweetened with agave! Agave syrup is often added to so-called "health" foods because it's believed to be more "natural," but don't be fooled: Agave is a heavily processed ingredient.

The good news is that a diet based on REAL food is naturally lower in fructose and can help you improve your digestion if you have fructose malabsorption. What's more, many researchers, including Dr. Robert Lustig of the University of California San Francisco, now believe that the recent increase in our fructose consumption (due to increased sugar intake and consumption of processed foods) is largely responsible for rising rates of obesity, high blood pressure, elevated triglycerides, heart diseases, fatty liver disease, diabetes, polycystic ovary syndrome (PCOS), cancer, gout, urticaria, and accelerated aging. Lowering your fructose intake could help you improve your digestion and avoid these chronic diseases of civilization.

Foods that contain a high fructose-to-glucose ratio (more than 0.5 grams of fructose in excess of glucose per 100-gram serving or more than three grams of fructose per serving) are considered FODMAPs. Table 14 lists those foods that are more likely to cause symptoms in people with fructose malabsorption.

Table 14: High-Fructose Foods

Food Groups	High-Fructose Foods
Fruits	Apple, boysenberries, cherries, figs, grapes, mango, pear, tamarillo, watermelon, dried fruits, canned fruits, fruit bars
Vegetables	Artichoke, asparagus, sugar snap peas, tomato juice, tomato sauces, tomato paste
Sweeteners	Agave syrup, honey, high-fructose corn syrup (HFCS), corn syrup solids
Drinks	Fruit juices, fruit punches, soft drinks, energy drinks, sweeter wines, port wines, some ciders

Most people with fructose malabsorption will experience digestive symptoms when they eat too much fructose at once, but your symptoms could also be the cumulative effect of the fructose you've eaten over the course of a few hours or even a day or two. It can be difficult to know for sure since symptoms can take a few hours to up to 48 hours to manifest.

Foods that contain equal amounts of fructose and glucose or more glucose than fructose are usually better tolerated. This is because fructose can also be absorbed by another receptor, GLUT2. The GLUT2 receptor is activated by the presence of glucose and can help you better absorb some of the fructose you eat. Even if your GLUT5 receptors are impaired, your GLUT2 receptors may save you from experiencing severe digestive symptoms. As an example, blueberries and table sugar don't usually cause problems for fructose malabsorbers because about half of their sugars consist of glucose and the other half fructose, so the glucose portion of these foods enhances the absorption of the fructose they contain.

Some fructose malabsorbers are also told to add dextrose powder, which is 100-percent glucose, to high-fructose foods to enhance their fructose absorption (by activating the GLUT2 receptor) and decrease the severity of the digestive side effects caused by fructose. This trick only works as long as your total fructose intake does not exceed your personal fructose tolerance threshold, which is highly individual and may range between five and 25 grams of fructose. And it won't work at all if you have SIBO or a yeast (candida) overgrowth. Adding pure glucose to your food can actually worsen your symptoms in these cases by feeding the excess bacteria or fungi in your body.

In general, adding dextrose may help in some cases in the short term, but you will still need to address the root causes (intestinal damage and gut flora imbalance) of your digestive problems if you truly want to improve your food tolerance. No one ultimately benefits from adding sugar to their diet, whatever the form, especially if their digestive health is impaired. Sugar doesn't provide any necessary nutrients and can weaken your immune system, worsen imbalances in your gut flora, and compromise gut healing by negatively affecting your blood sugar levels. Dextrose doesn't fit in the REAL food category and your health is much better off without it.

Table 15 lists the factors that can facilitate or inhibit fructose absorption.

Table 15: Factors that Affect Fructose Absorption

Facilitate Fructose Absorption	Decrease Fructose Absorption
• Foods with more glucose than fructose	• Sorbitol and other FODMAPs
• Foods with equal amounts of glucose and fructose	• Foods with more fructose than glucose
• Adding extra glucose (dextrose powder)	• Consuming too much fructose within a certain period of time (within a few hours to up to within 2 days)
• Spreading your fructose and FODMAP intake over the day	• Small intestinal bacterial overgrowth (SIBO)
	• Yeast or candida overgrowth

Foods containing more fructose than glucose are the worst offenders for people with fructose malabsorption, but remember that excessive fructose, even if balanced with equal amounts of glucose, can also trigger symptoms. For most people, 25 grams of fructose is the most that can be tolerated at once, but this number can vary. Table sugar and blueberries may have a good fructose-to-glucose ratio, but eating too much (two tablespoons/30 milliliters of table sugar, or two cups/500 milliliters of blueberries) at once can still be more than your intestines can handle.

If you're diagnosed with fructose malabsorption, you'll most likely be given a list of foods to avoid for the rest of your life. Avoiding fructose, if fructose malabsorption is the only cause of your IBS, can help you feel better, but it doesn't address the underlying causes. It's like putting a bandage on an infected wound. If you want to eat apple, asparagus, mango, honey, or watermelon again without suffering the consequences, you will need to first heal your gut and re-balance your gut flora. It's probably a good idea to stay away from HFCS or the processed foods to which it's often added, whether or not you have fructose malabsorption. But you should be able to treat yourself to fresh fruits once in a while, Mother Nature's own candies that are packaged with water, fiber, vitamins, minerals, and antioxidants. Chapter 3 will guide you through this healing process to increase the likelihood of improving your food tolerance.

FRUCTANS

Fructans are another class of FODMAPs that can cause an unhappy tummy and trigger symptoms similar to IBS. As an oligosaccharide (a type of carbohydrate made of between three and 10 molecules of sugars), fructans are actually made of a few molecules of fructose attached to each other. Even though no one can actually digest or absorb fructans, these FODMAPs only cause digestive trouble in people with abnormal intestinal sensitivity or gut dysbiosis. Similarly to other FODMAPs, fructans can trigger symptoms only if they are fermented excessively by the bacteria in your intestines and draw too much water inside your digestive system.

Wheat is by far the largest source of fructans in the standard Western diet, accounting for about 70 percent of your daily fructan intake (unless you already eat gluten free or wheat free). It is therefore possible that you react to wheat not because of its gluten but because of its fructans. You may also react to both gluten and fructans, which can explain severe symptoms when eating wheat-based foods.

Onions and garlic are also a large source of fructans for many people. They are common ingredients many sauces, soups, marinades, commercial broths, salad dressings, and seasoning blends, which makes them difficult to avoid if you eat out or consume commercially prepared products often. Just removing the onions from a dish doesn't work since the fructans are water soluble and can be present in the sauce or liquid in the dish. Even onion powder, garlic powder, or soups, stews, and broths prepared with these high-fructan aromatic vegetables can trigger your IBS symptoms. Reading food labels won't guarantee an onion- and garlic-free diet; the labeling of these ingredients is not compulsory since they are not allergens. They can hide under the names of vegetable salt, chicken salt, vegetable powder, and dehydrated vegetables. You may need to contact the company directly to know whether their products contain any forms of onion or garlic instead of relying on ingredient lists. As with any food intolerance, it is more prudent to cook your own food at home to avoid GI disturbances.

A fructan content of more than 0.2 grams per serving is considered high. Table 16 lists other high-fructan foods.

Table 16: High-Fructan Foods

Food Category	High-Fructan Foods
Grains	Wheat, rye, and barley (bread, pasta, couscous, gnocchi, muesli, wheat bran, and other foods derived from these grains), sweet corn
Vegetables	Onions (all types, including brown onions, white onions, Spanish onions, red onions, shallots, leeks, and the white part of green onions), garlic, artichokes, asparagus, Jerusalem artichokes, beetroot, broccoli, Brussels sprouts, dandelion leaves, fennel, butternut squash, green peas, snow peas, cabbage, okra
Fruits	Custard apples, nectarines, peaches, persimmons, pomegranate, rambutan, tamarillo, watermelons
Nuts and Seeds	Pistachios, cashews, almonds, hazelnuts, flaxseeds
Seasonings	Onion powder, onion salt, garlic powder, garlic salt, bouillon cubes, broths, stocks, chicken salt, vegetable salt, vegetable powders, dehydrated vegetables, gravies, soups, marinades, sauces, spices, and seasonings (often contain some form of onion or garlic)
Sweeteners	Coconut sugar (also called coconut nectar or coconut crystals)
Other	Inulin, chicory root, fructooligosaccharides (FOS), prebiotics

PREBIOTICS

"Health" food products are often enriched with fiber or prebiotics such as inulin, chicory root, or fructooligosaccharides (FOS). All these ingredients contain fructans and can induce IBS symptoms. Probiotic supplements also sometimes include some of these ingredients because of their prebiotic effect. The term prebiotic means "food for bacteria." In people with a healthy digestive system, prebiotics can help feed and maintain a healthy gut flora. If you have IBS or a gut dysbiosis problem, though, adding prebiotics to your intestines can make things worse! Carefully read the labels of everything you put in your mouth, including supplements. You may be surprised to find FODMAPs or other ingredients that could be perpetuating your symptoms. The elimination diet protocol outlined in Chapter 5 shows you how to determine the foods to which you may be sensitive and create a diet that is optimal for you.

POLYOLS

"Polyol" is a synonym of sugar alcohol. Sugar alcohols are often used by food manufacturers in sugar-free products such as gums, candies, ice cream, cookies, chocolate, and even some medications and supplements. Sugar alcohols supply fewer calories and sugar than regular sweeteners because they are incompletely absorbed. Some vegetables and fruits also contain sorbitol and mannitol, two of the most common polyols. A food is considered high in FODMAPs if it contains over 0.3 grams of any individual polyol or a total of 0.5 grams of polyols per serving. Table 17 lists the foods with a high polyol content.

Table 17: High-Polyol Foods

Food Category	High-Sorbitol foods	High-Mannitol foods
Vegetables	-	Cauliflower, celery, mushrooms, snow peas, sweet potatoes, butternut squash, pumpkins
Fruits	Apple, apricot, avocado, blackberries, cherries, longan, lychee, nectarines, pears, plums, prunes, and juices from these fruits	Peaches, watermelons
Sweeteners	Sugar alcohols, such as sorbitol, mannitol, maltitol, xylitol, and isomalt	
Other	Gums, candies, and other sugar-free items with sugar-alcohol sweeteners	Some beers and some wines

GALACTANS

Galactans, also known as galactooligosaccharides, are the last class of short-chain fermentable carbohydrates in the FODMAP family and include the carbohydrates raffinose and stachyose. Although lesser known, these FODMAPs, which include beans and lentils, are some of the most well-known gas-producing FODMAPs. No human has the ability to digest galactans, but they appear to cause more distressing symptoms in people with IBS and an altered gut flora. Table 18 lists foods that are considered FODMAPs because of their high galactan content.

Table 18: High-Galactan Foods

Food Category	High-Galactan Foods
Legumes	Legumes, beans (chickpeas, red kidney beans), lentils, hummus, soy-based products (especially if made with whole soy beans or soy protein)
Vegetarian Foods	Soy-based products like tempeh, soy burgers, and soy yogurt (especially if made with whole soy beans or soy protein)
Beverages	Soy milk (especially if made from whole soy beans)
Vegetables	Broccoli, Brussels sprouts, cabbage, butternut squash, pumpkin, edamame

FODMAP TESTING

Only three of the FODMAPs can be tested: lactose, fructose, and sorbitol. For the other FODMAPs (fructans, mannitol, and galactans), an elimination diet protocol is recommended. An elimination diet can actually be used to identify if you have problems with any one of the FODMAP groups. Supervision by a qualified dietitian or health professional is also helpful to minimize errors and confusion and optimize results. Or follow the protocol in Chapter 5 to better understand how to design your elimination diet and determine which FODMAPs are problematic for you. Some people may be sensitive to only one or two types of FODMAPs, while others could react to none or all of them.

Breath testing is the only way to measure if your digestive problems are due to FODMAPs being fermented excessively by the bacteria in your intestines. The main gases produced by this fermentation are hydrogen and methane. Humans don't produce these gases, so high levels of hydrogen or methane in your breath can only be caused by the fermentation the FODMAPs fructose, lactose, or sorbitol. Many doctors and GI specialists are unfortunately unfamiliar with FODMAPs, apart from lactose, and even less so with the different breath tests available. You may want to ask your doctor about this testing option, especially if you need a referral to take the test (some labs, but not all, require you to go through a healthcare practitioner).

You can find info about these tests in the USA on siboinfo.com. In Australia, check out Gastrolab and Stream Diagnostics. In the UK, Biolab and the London Gastroenterology Partnership offer these tests. In Canada, breath tests can be obtained from some American companies, such as Metabolic Solutions and Commonwealth Laboratories. Make sure to ask about the diet that you should follow in the days prior to the tests, as it could affect the accuracy of the results.

Is it necessary to be tested for all the different FODMAPs? If you don't have health insurance or if your plan does not cover these tests, it is probably best to skip them. The breath tests for lactose, fructose, and sorbitol can easily add up to hundreds of dollars, and you would still need to experiment with your diet to see if you react to fructans, mannitol, and galactans, as well as determine your personal threshold for all the different FODMAP-containing foods. Skipping these breath tests and embarking on a well-designed elimination diet can help you not only save a lot of money but also feel better faster and help you design a diet that works for you more quickly. It is important to be aware that these tests are not 100-percent accurate, either.

SIBO AS A CAUSE OF FODMAP INTOLERANCE

If you think that taking a breath test would help you feel more motivated to begin your elimination diet, the SIBO breath test using the sugars lactulose and glucose may be your best option. A study published in 2005 by a team of Italian researchers showed that positive breath tests for fructose, lactose, or sorbitol may actually reveal the presence of SIBO, an overgrowth of bacteria in your small intestines. The symptoms of SIBO are the same as the ones associated with IBS: fructose malabsorption and excessive FODMAP fermentation. In other words, your breath test will more likely show that you do not tolerate lactose, fructose, or sorbitol if you have SIBO, an excess of bacteria living in your small intestines (you'll learn more about SIBO in the next pages). In many cases, fructose malabsorption and an intolerance to FODMAPs can actually be due to SIBO, so correcting SIBO can help improve your tolerance to FODMAPs and other foods over time.

ELIMINATION DIET

Elimination diets can be a great tool to diagnose intolerances to FODMAPs and other food groups that could trigger and worsen gastrointestinal problems. Since it is impossible to test for every possible substance you could be sensitive to, adopting an elimination diet protocol can help you address many foods all at once. It requires patience and effort, but it can help you establish a list of foods that you can eat safely while keeping your symptoms under control. And it won't cost anything. Wouldn't it be wonderful to know, at last, what you can and can't eat to reach optimal digestive health?

Now that you better understand what FODMAPs are and where you can find them, it is time to better understand how these carbohydrates can worsen your digestive problems.

HOW FODMAPS AFFECT YOUR DIGESTION

The symptoms associated with FODMAPs are the result of both osmosis and excessive fermentation inside your intestines. The simple presence of undigested FODMAPs in your intestines, especially fructose, lactose, and polyols, can have an osmotic effect. The simplest way to think of osmosis is what happens when you put a dry sponge in a bucket of water. The water will move from the area most concentrated in water (the bucket) to the least concentrated area (the dry sponge) until the water concentrations of the bucket and sponge more or less even out. Similarly, if you have too much unabsorbed sugar in your intestines, your body will try to dilute them by drawing water from other parts of your body. The pressure of extra water in your intestines can induce bloating, discomfort, and abdominal pain. In some cases, you can even feel and hear the extra water floating around in your belly. You may also experience a form of diarrhea called osmotic or watery diarrhea, as if a sponge filled with water was squeezed inside your intestines to drain them of the excess. This is one of the things that can cause your stools to look like type 7 on the poop chart (page 24).

Another problem with FODMAPs, in addition to potential osmotic diarrhea, is that they can become food for the bacteria in your colon. How do bacteria eat? By fermenting! The fermentation process they use to feed off fructose and other FODMAPs produces a lot of gas. According to Elaine Gottschall, biochemist and creator of the Specific Carbohydrate Diet (more on this diet later), the amount of lactose found in as little as one ounce (30 milliliters) of milk can produce more than one gallon (five liters) of gas in your intestines if you are lactose intolerant. If you drink more than one ounce of milk or eat a lot of FODMAPs like onions, pears, and a HFCS-sweetened beverage at the same time, the bacteria in your intestines will take advantage of this free buffet. You may experience a swollen belly from this extra gas in your intestines. For some, it may also cause belching and flatulence. For others, the extra pressure of the gas trapped in your intestines can cause discomfort, pain, and even cramping.

Figure 7

fructose malabsorption & FODMAP intolerance

a. normal digestion and normal gut flora

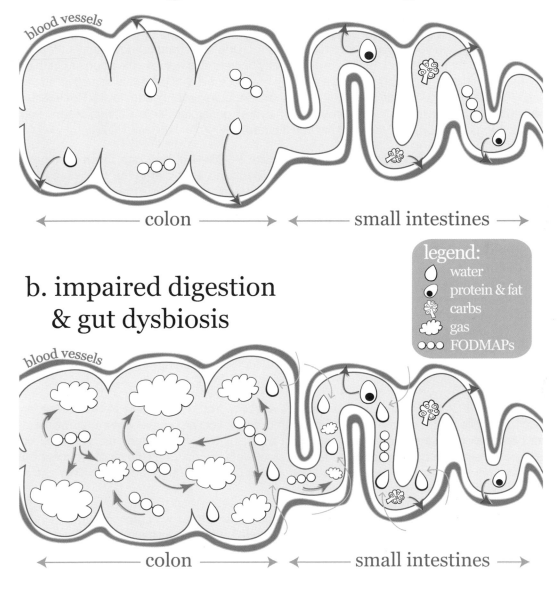

legend:
- water
- protein & fat
- carbs
- gas
- FODMAPs

b. impaired digestion & gut dysbiosis

a. With a normal digestion and balanced gut flora, protein, fats, and carbohydrates are absorbed from the small intestines and water is absorbed from the colon into the bloodstream. FODMAPs like lactose and fructose are also absorbed in the small intestines, while unabsorbed polyols, fructans, and galactans don't cause any problems.

b. With fructose malabsorption and FODMAP intolerance, the presence of unabsorbed FODMAPs in the small intestines can draw a lot of water from other parts of your body into your intestines through a process called osmosis, which can result in bloating and watery diarrhea. In your colon, FODMAPs are fermented excessively by your gut flora, creating a lot of gas. The pressure from this abnormal amount of gas inside your colon can cause bloating, abdominal pain, flatulence, diarrhea, or constipation.

There are three ways these gases can be expelled from your body. They can move up your gastrointestinal tract as a burp or take the other way and exit the back door as flatulence. Most of the gas, however, is absorbed into your bloodstream and expelled by your lungs in your breath. Some people can perceive a change in the smell of their breath after eating FODMAPs and foods that cause excessive gut fermentation. The diffusion of the gas produced in your intestines can take many hours; this is why you can feel bloated for up to one or two days after the start of your food reaction.

Some of the gas produced by FODMAP fermentation can also affect the motility (movement) of your intestines. Depending on the types of gas produced by the bacteria in your gut, you may be more prone to either diarrhea or constipation. Hydrogen gas tends to speed up the movement of stools through your intestines, preventing you from completely digesting what you eat and leading to stools that look like types 5, 6, or even 7 on the poop chart (page 28).

On the other hand, if your gut bacteria are producing primarily methane, the opposite can also happen and you could be skipping a few days with your bowel movements, strain on the toilet, and produce stools that look like types 1 or 2. Although many people think that constipation is due to lazy bowels, it is actually the opposite in this case! People with constipation due to methane-producing bacteria actually have bowels that are twice as active as those in healthy people, according to some studies. The problem is that methane induces reverse peristalsis. Peristalsis is the normal movement of the intestines to help move things through, but reverse peristalsis means things are moving in the wrong direction! The result: things back up and you become constipated.

It doesn't really matter what symptoms your experience with FODMAPs. Any one of these digestive problems indicates that there is something wrong with your digestion. Modifying your diet is the best place to start to try to improve your digestion, lessen your symptoms, start feeling better, and eventually broaden your food tolerance.

DELAYED RESPONSE AND CUMULATIVE EFFECT

One of the reasons food intolerances are difficult to figure out is that we rarely eat foods in isolation. Another problem is that a reaction may not be immediate. With fructose malabsorption and FODMAP intolerance, most of the mechanisms triggering your symptoms occur in your colon (provided that you don't have SIBO). For most people, it can take a couple of hours to up to 48 hours before symptoms manifest themselves, and even longer with severe constipation. It would be normal for you to blame the polyols in the cauliflower and mushrooms you ate at the last meal if you start to feel bloated within a few hours, but you could actually be reacting to the fructans in the slice of bread you ate two days ago!

To add to the confusion, FODMAPs also have a cumulative effect. You may be able to tolerate an apple (fructose and sorbitol) once in a while, but it may not go down as smoothly if you also have watermelon (fructose, mannitol, and fructans) and broccoli (fructans and galactans) within a day or two. In other words, you may not experience unpleasant side effects from just eating an apple, a few slices of watermelon, or a little bit of broccoli… but all of them at the same time or within a certain period of time can be a ticking time bomb for your IBS. This can also make the interpretation of your symptoms that much more difficult.

If the last FODMAP-containing food you ate before experiencing symptoms was broccoli, you may think broccoli is a problematic food for you when it may have been fine if you hadn't had eaten other FODMAPs earlier in the day or the day before, making you exceed your personal tolerance threshold. Trying to make sense of the foods that could be worsening your digestive symptoms can seem like an impossible task if you don't know how to proceed.

Eliminating all of these potentially problematic foods and reintroducing them in a systematic way can help you clear the confusion. The elimination diet will allow you to reset your body by removing the foods to which you might be intolerant, especially those that feed the bacteria in your gut and lead to excessive fermentation in your intestines. It's like pushing a reset button for your intestines, removing the factors confounding the analysis of your situation and helping you feel better as quickly as possible. Only then will you be able to see a clearer picture of what is truly affecting your digestive health.

Figure 8

your personal tolerance threshold

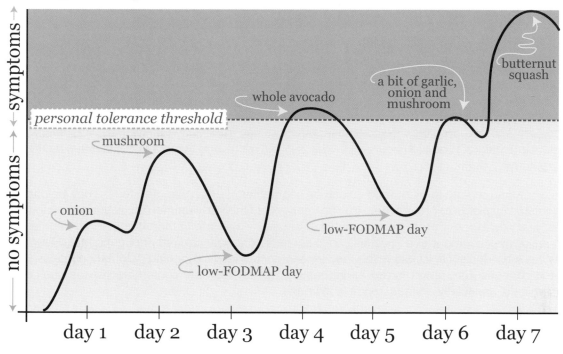

Your symptoms only appear once you exceed your personal tolerance threshold by eating too much of the foods to which you are sensitive within a certain period of time. In this example, you might think only avocado and butternut squash are problematic for you when in fact, the onions, mushroom, and garlic are also contributing to putting you above your tolerance threshold and the triggering of your symptoms. The blame is not always on what you ate last!

ARE FRUCTOSE MALABSORPTION AND FODMAP INTOLERANCE FOR LIFE?

Unlike gluten sensitivity, which warrants a gluten-free diet for the rest of your life, other food intolerances can improve over time. Unless you have a true food allergy, you may even be able to tolerate some gluten-free grains or soy again after your digestive system has healed fully. Whether these foods are worth reintroducing is another matter, though (which will be addressed in the next chapters), considering that most of them are processed extensively, contain anti-nutrients, and do not provide any particular benefits to your health.

On the other hand, most FODMAPs are not necessarily bad for your health, unless you have a gut dysbiosis or damaged intestines. Many of the FODMAPs are found in REAL foods, including nutrient-dense vegetables, tubers, fruits, some dairy products, and nuts. If you'd like to be able to bite into an apple, enjoy some yogurt, or treat yourself to antioxidant-rich cabbage, broccoli, or Brussels sprouts again, balancing your gut flora and correcting bacterial overgrowth in your small intestines could help you better tolerate these foods. It may take some time—months or even years in more severe cases—so be patient.

In any case, the best way to improve your tolerance to these foods also happens to be the best way to manage your IBS and digestive symptoms, so it is definitely worth a shot. Whether or not your food tolerance improves, modifying your diet will allow you to better control your symptoms, which may be all you're looking for at this point, anyway.

Besides gluten, casein, soy, and FODMAPs, other foods can also play a role in your digestive problems. Learning more about them will give you more dietary strategies to adopt and build your own REAL-food-based diet.

Natural Food Chemicals

Non-allergic intolerance to food chemicals appears to be less common than gluten sensitivity, fructose malabsorption, or FODMAP intolerance, but it could still be partly responsible for your digestive problems. As with FODMAPs, most of the research and clinical experience regarding natural food chemicals and GI disorders originates from Australia. Most of the North American-based research in these areas seems unfortunately to focus primarily on pharmaceuticals and drugs.

What are natural food chemicals? Though the term food chemicals may evoke images of laboratories and man-made ingredients, most food chemicals, such as salicylates, glutamate, and amines, occur naturally in food. Some of these compounds either contain histamine or trigger your body to release histamine, potentially interfering with the normal functioning of your digestive system, as well as resulting in skin rashes, hives, eczema, asthma, fatigue, behavioral problems, mood problems, headaches, and migraines in sensitive individuals. It is almost impossible to completely eliminate natural food chemicals from your diet, but reducing your intake could make a difference in some of your GI symptoms.

Salicylates are found mainly in plant foods, such as vegetables, fruits, nuts, and teas. They belong to a family of chemicals produced by plants to protect them from the dangers of their environment by acting as natural antibacterials, preservatives, and pesticides. For this reason, most of the salicylates are in the outer layer of vegetables and fruits. Peeling high-salicylate cucumber and zucchini can lower their salicylate content enough to make them well tolerated even by sensitive individuals. Salicylate levels also tend to decrease with ripening. A tomato contains less salicylates as it ripens and changes from green to red. Unfortunately, as the salicylate content decreases, the concentration of other food chemicals, especially amines, tends to increase.

Amines, also called biogenic amines, include tyramine, histamine, and glutamate. All amines are formed by the breakdown of protein in food as they age. The amine content is therefore very high in aged meats and cheeses, as well as ripe bananas, tomatoes, and avocados. Other strong-tasting foods such as soy sauce, meat extracts, chocolate, sauerkraut, and other fermented foods are also rich in amines. The protein in fish has the particularity of being broken down very quickly and even one-or-two-day-old fish can be too high in amines for sensitive people. The browning of meat, fish, and chicken skin on the grill also results in the formation of amines.

Table 19 shows you the different foods rich in these naturally occurring food chemicals.

Table 19: Foods that Contain Salicylates and Amines

Food Groups	Salicylates	Amines
Vegetables	Avocado, bell pepper (capsicum), broccoli, cauliflower, cucumber with peel, eggplant, mushrooms, nori, olives, onion, pickled vegetables, pumpkin, radicchio, radish, sauerkraut, spinach, spring onion, tomato, vegetable juice, soups, vegetable soups and stocks, zucchini with peel	Avocado, broccoli, cauliflower, eggplant, olives, mushrooms, nori, pickled vegetables, radicchio, sauerkraut, spinach, tomato, vegetable soups and stocks
Fruits	Berries, cherries, citrus, dates, dried fruit, fruit juices, grapes, kiwifruit, mango, passion fruit, pineapple, plum, pomegranate, rhubarb, ripe banana, strawberry, watermelon	Berries, cherries, citrus, dates, dried fruit, fruit juices, grape, just-ripe banana, kiwi, mango, passion fruit, pineapple, plum
Sweets	Chewing gums, honey, jams and jellies, licorice, mints, raw sugar	Chocolate, jams and jellies
Seasonings	Commercial gravies, sauces, stocks, herbs, spices, mustard, tomato sauce, ketchup, tomato paste, spices (cinnamon, anise, cloves), vinegar (balsamic, red wine, etc.)	Commercial gravy, sauces, stocks, fish sauce, mustard, tomato sauce, ketchup, tomato paste, soy sauce, spices (cinnamon, anise, cloves), vinegar (balsamic, red wine...)
Animal Protein	Beef (aged, corned, smoked, cured), commercial gravies, fish sauces, meat pies, sausages, stocks	Anchovies, beef (aged, corned, smoked, cured), bacon, canned salmon, canned sardines, canned tuna, chicken skin, commercial gravies, fish fingers, fish sauce, game meat, ham, liver, meat pies, pork, turkey, sausages, shrimp, smoked fish, surimi (fake crab), stock
Legumes	Beans, falafel, hummus, textured vegetable protein (TVP)	Beans, falafel, hummus, textured vegetable protein (TVP)
Nuts and Seeds	Almonds, Brazil nuts, chestnuts, coconut, hazelnuts, macadamia, peanuts, pecans, pine nuts, pistachios, walnuts, and butters from these nuts, flaxseeds, pumpkin seeds, sesame seeds, sunflower seeds	Almonds, Brazil nuts, chestnuts, coconut, hazelnuts, macadamia, peanuts, pecans, pine nuts, pistachios, walnuts, and butters from these nuts, flaxseeds, pumpkin seeds, sesame seeds, sunflower seeds
Fat	Almond oil, avocado oil, extra-virgin and regular olive oil, sesame oil, walnut oil, oils with added antioxidants, commercial marinades, salad dressings and mayonnaise, coconut milk, coconut cream, coconut oil, suet	Almond oil, avocado oil, extra-virgin and regular olive oil, sesame oil, walnut oil, oils with added antioxidants, commercial marinades, salad dressings and mayonnaise, coconut milk, coconut cream, coconut oil, suet
Grains and Starchy Foods	Breads (containing corn, dried fruit, nuts, coconut, vinegar, and preservatives), breakfast cereals (containing corn, cocoa, coconut, dried fruit, honey, nuts, artificial colors and flavors), potato chips, corn, French fries, muesli, nachos, pasta, polenta, rice cakes, rice crackers	Breads (containing corn, dried fruit, nuts, coconut, vinegar, and preservatives), breakfast cereals (containing corn, cocoa, coconut, dried fruit, honey, nut, artificial colors and flavors), potato chips, French fries, muesli, rice cakes, rice crackers
Dairy	Flavored milk (chocolate, etc.), fruit-flavored yogurt	Flavored milk (chocolate, etc.), fruit-flavored yogurt, mild cheeses (cheddar, Swiss, feta, halloumi), strong cheeses (Brie, camembert, Parmesan, etc.)
Beverages	Coffee (regular and decaffeinated), teas, herbal teas, chai spiced tea, soft drinks	Chai spiced tea, soft drinks
Alcohol	Beer, champagne, cider, spirits, liqueurs, wines	Beer, champagne, cider, spirits, liqueurs, wines
Other	Fermented foods, nutritional yeast, aspirin (acetylsalicylic acid), natural flavorings, perfumes, botanical oils, liquid medications	Cocoa powder, fermented foods

Artificial food chemicals can induce the same problems in sensitive people. Artificial sweeteners, colorings, flavorings, MSG (monosodium glutamate), sulfites, and preservatives are some of the many ingredients to watch for if you have digestive problems or other side effects after eating certain foods. MSG, in particular, is added to many processed foods to "enhance" their flavors.

Some people certainly notice a connection between these ingredients and their IBS symptoms. Although the food industry says MSG is safe, it often hides MSG under the ingredient "spices," making it difficult to detect when reading an ingredient list. Since this book is all about using REAL foods to improve your digestion, fortunately, you won't have to worry too much about MSG and other problematic chemicals. You won't even have to decipher complicated ingredient lists at all!

Tolerance to food chemicals, like everything else, is highly individual. Some people may react only to salicylates, while others may have problems with almost all types of natural food chemicals. The amount you can tolerate before experiencing symptoms can also vary between individuals since reactions to food chemicals are dose dependent. If you are sensitive to one of the food chemicals, you could start experiencing symptoms as soon as one hour to up to several hours, even days, after eating tomato, avocado, balsamic vinegar, bacon, or MSG. Like FODMAPs, food chemicals have a cumulative effect, which can complicate the interpretation of what foods cause your digestive symptoms.

An elimination diet approach is also the gold-standard approach to determine the role food chemicals play in your diet. Although intolerance to natural food chemicals is a lot less common than gluten sensitivity, FODMAP intolerance, and bacterial overgrowth (SIBO), it is important that you be aware of these compounds in case you notice a pattern between intake of these foods and symptoms when journaling in later weeks. The more you know about specific food compounds that could be problematic, the easier it will be for you to create your personal optimal diet.

SIBO

SIBO has already been mentioned a few times as a potential cause of bloating, abdominal pain, and other IBS-associated problems. But why is SIBO bad? Isn't it good to have plenty of gut flora to help optimize your digestion? Unfortunately, too much of a good thing can be just as bad as not enough.

It's perfectly normal to have lots of bacteria in your intestines. You might remember from the first chapter that your body holds over 100 trillion bacteria, which is 10 times more than the number of cells in your body. However, the majority of these bacteria should be located in your colon. Even though your small intestines contain a respectable amount of bacteria (up to 500,000 cells per teaspoon), your colon holds 100,000 to 1,000,000 times more bacteria per teaspoon! Table 20 shows you the number of bacteria found in different parts of the body.

Table 20: Bacteria in the Body

Bacteria Cells in Your Body	The (Big) Numbers
Entire body	100,000,000,000,000
Colon	10,000,000,000 to 100,000,000,000/ml
Small Intestines (normal)	< 100,000/ml
Small Intestines (with SIBO)	> 100,000/ml

*One ml is equivalent to about ¼ of one teaspoon; one teaspoon is equivalent to ~five ml.

If, for some reason, large numbers of bacteria decide to move to your small intestines to settle and raise their ever-growing families, you digestion could suffer. Although people often talk about the health benefits of supplementing with probiotics, an overgrowth of bacteria in your small intestines can cause a lot of problems, not just for your digestion, but for your overall health, too.

SIBO can be defined as a chronic infection of the small intestines. The excess of bacteria that take up residence there are not necessarily bad in the way of those that can cause food poisoning or a bout of gastroenteritis. It's just that these bacteria are not where they should be. If too many of them move from the urban center (colon) to the rural area (small intestines), the small intestines don't have the infrastructure to handle all of these newcomers. The bacteria will make use of their new real estate to build lots of microbreweries. How will all these new factories affect your digestive health? Considerably! To produce the energy cocktail they like, bacteria use the nutrients from the foods you eat, especially sugars and starches, and ferment them. The fermentation process in these millions of microbreweries creates a lot of gas, which can lead to many digestive problems.

Emerging research is now suggesting that many cases of IBS are actually caused by SIBO. Research by Dr. Mark Pimentel, author of "A New IBS Solution," shows that 84 percent of people with IBS have a bacterial overgrowth in their small intestines. If this estimate is right, a large majority of people who complain of bloating, diarrhea, or constipation are likely to have some degree of SIBO.

MECHANISMS OF SIBO

Remember the FODMAP section? What happens when bacteria eat? Fermentation! With FODMAPs, the fermentation occurs mainly in the colon (if you don't have SIBO). In the case of SIBO, the quiet little towns of your small intestines have been overrun by hundreds of thousands of gassy bacteria. The bacteria that have now settled in your small intestines can ferment not only the FODMAPs in the food you eat, but all types of sugars and starches, as well as some kinds of fiber. These fermentable carbohydrates are found in potatoes, fruits, sugars, soft drinks, candies, breads, breakfast cereals, cookies, and anything made with flour or sugar—including whole grains.

The more carbohydrates you eat, the more food the bacteria in your small intestines will have to ferment, creating gas. Unlike excessive gas produced in your colon, which can easily be expelled by passing it, the gas in your small intestines is pretty much stuck there. Result: bloating.

The presence of high concentrations of unabsorbed sugars in your intestines can also result in an osmotic response. Just like FODMAPs, incompletely digested and unabsorbed sugars and starches can draw a lot of water from other parts of your body into your intestines. This extra water floating in your small intestines can also worsen your bloating, cause discomfort and pain, and even trigger watery diarrhea (type 7 on the poop chart).

SYMPTOMS OF SIBO

What happens if the bacteria of your gut flora overcrowd your small intestines? The most common symptoms of SIBO are the same ones as IBS and mainly affect your gastrointestinal system. In addition to uncomfortable and life-disrupting GI symptoms, SIBO sufferers often also experience one or more systemic symptoms that result from having a leaky gut, including joint pain, headaches, depression, eczema, asthma, and behavioral problems. Associated issues, such as autoimmune conditions, are also common because of their connection with a leaky gut. If you have SIBO, you are also very likely to have multiple food sensitivities (gluten, dairy, soy, nuts, eggs, etc.).

Table 21 lists all of the symptoms and conditions associated with SIBO.

It's still unclear exactly how SIBO relates to all of these symptoms and associated conditions. Do these conditions cause SIBO, or is it the other way around? In either case, many people manage to better control both their digestion and overall health once they tackle their SIBO and leaky-gut issues. While researchers figure out the details, though, you can still take action now

Table 21: SIBO: Symptoms and Associated Conditions

Category	Symptoms and Associated Conditions
Gastrointestinal Symptoms	• Abdominal distension or bloating • Excess gas (flatulence and/or belching) • Abdominal discomfort, pain, or cramping • Changes in your bowel movements (diarrhea, constipation, or alternating constipation and diarrhea) • Acid reflux, GERD, or heartburn • Nausea and vomiting
Malnutrition	• Malabsorption and nutrient deficiencies (iron-deficiency anemia, B_{12} deficiency) • Fat-soluble-vitamin deficiencies (vitamins A, D, E, and K) • Fatty stools (steatorrhea) • Carbohydrate and sugar cravings • Involuntary weight loss (not always, but sometimes)
Systemic Symptoms (associated with leaky gut)	• Fatigue • Food sensitivities • Joint pain • Headaches and migraines • Skin problems (hives, eczema, rashes) • Concentration issues (brain fog, fatigue) • Respiratory problems (asthma) • Depression • Autism
Associated Conditions	• Anemia • Leaky gut • Autism • Cystic fibrosis • Fibromyalgia • GERD • Acne rosacea • Hypochlorhydria (low stomach acid) • Autoimmune disorders (celiac disease, Hashimoto's thyroiditis, rheumatoid arthritis, diabetes) • Inflammatory bowel diseases (Crohn's disease, ulcerative colitis) • IBS • Fatty liver disease (non-alcoholic steatohepatitis or NASH) • Diverticulitis • Lyme disease • Interstitial cystitis • Parkinson's disease • *H. pylori* infection • Chronic fatigue syndrome • Obesity • Restless leg syndrome • Scleroderma

Figure 9

SIBO
(small intestinal bacterial overgrowth)

a. normal digestion and normal gut flora

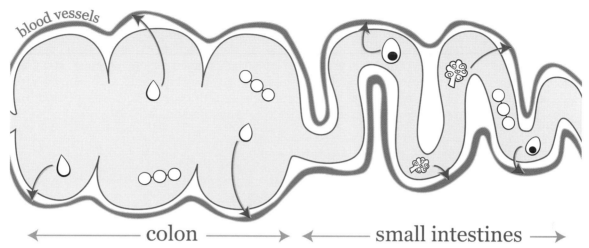

b. SIBO: excessive intestinal carbohydrate fermentation

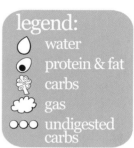

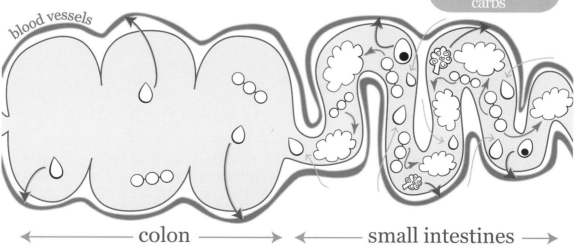

a. With a normal digestion and balanced gut flora, protein, fats, and carbohydrates are absorbed from the small intestines and water is absorbed from the colon into the bloodstream.

b. With SIBO, the excess bacteria in the small intestines results in the fermentation of carbohydrates (FODMAPs, sugars, and starches) before you even get a chance to digest and absorb them. Some of these carbohyrdates can draw a lot of water from the rest of your body into your small intestines through a process called omsosis, which can result in watery diarrhea. The fermentation of the undigested carbs by the bacteria in your small intestines also forms a lot of gas, which is responsible for bloating, abdominal pain, diarrhea, and constipation.

BLOATING

Bloating can be a big problem for many people with IBS, especially if SIBO is involved. It was thought for many years, however, that the bloating associated with IBS was "all in the head." It was only when European researchers invented a special belt to measure abdominal distension throughout the day that bloating was admitted to be a real symptom of IBS. In their study, the waist circumference of IBS sufferers increased more than that of people without IBS, by as much as four to five inches (10 to 12.5 centimeters) over the course of a day.

MOTILITY CHANGES

In addition to the bloating that results from the abnormal amount of gas produced by the fermentation process, gas can also create discomfort and even pain and cramping. It can also affect the motility of your intestines, causing diarrhea or constipation. If the excess bacteria in your small intestines produce mostly methane, you are more likely to be prone to constipation since this gas actually tells your intestines to move backwards, causing the wastes in your intestines to stall or back up. On the other hand, hydrogen-dominant SIBO seems to be associated with diarrhea, although the exact mechanism explaining this association hasn't yet been elucidated fully.

IBS = GAS

All the gas produced by the fermentation process in your intestines has to escape eventually. For years, researchers hypothesized that people with IBS produced more gas, but studies failed to detect a significant difference between the amount of gas they released compared to people without IBS. The researchers believed intestinal gas could only be released through the lower end of the digestive tract, so they just measured the gas released via flatulence (wouldn't you have loved to be part of that research team?). But when they also thought of measuring the gas expelled through the lungs, they finally saw a big difference. People with IBS produce on average five times more gas than those without IBS, demonstrating that there is a lot of fermentation going on in the guts of people with digestive issues. If you don't expel this gas by either farting or belching, your body has to reabsorb the gas into your bloodstream and excrete it through your lungs when you breathe out. This is why breath testing is the best way to identify excessive intestinal fermentation and diagnose SIBO.

> "Bacterial putrefaction is the cause of all disease."
> – Elie Metchnikoff (1908)

Testing for SIBO

The small intestines are a mysterious and largely inaccessible part of your body. An endoscopy can be used to see what is going on inside your gastrointestinal tract by inserting a tiny camera attached to a tube into your mouth, but it only shows the first two feet (60 centimeters) or so of your small intestines. Even with a colonoscopy, another form of endoscopy that goes through the rectum, very little of the other end of the small intestines can be seen.

BREATH TESTING

Breath testing is therefore the best method available to diagnose SIBO. Since most of the methane and hydrogen gas that results from excessive fermentation in your intestines is expelled in your breath (and these gases are not produced by the body), high levels of these gases in your breath automatically indicate excessive bacterial fermentation in the intestines.

As with fructose malabsorption and FODMAP intolerance, breath testing for SIBO is not perfect. Hydrogen breath tests have an estimated diagnostic accuracy of only 54 to 65 percent. There are two different types of sugars that can be used for SIBO breath tests: lactulose or glucose. Each of these tests has its own limitations. The lactulose test can be difficult to interpret, while the glucose test mainly allows the detection of bacterial overgrowth in the first part of your small intestines but not the more distal part closer to your colon. The accuracy of the test can also be affected by the testing time (1.5 vs. three hours) and compliance with the preparatory diet.

As with the lactose intolerance and fructose malabsorption test, you will first be given a drink containing either glucose or lactulose, then asked to blow into a bag every 15 to 30 minutes over the course of 1.5 to three hours. Levels of hydrogen or methane above a certain threshold will point to a SIBO diagnosis. But remember that even a negative result doesn't rule out SIBO completely, since 60 to 69 percent of SIBO cases are not detected with breath testing.

If you still choose to take the breath test, check with your insurance company about coverage, since it can cost over $300. For information on companies offering breath tests in the USA, see siboinfo.com. In Australia, check out Gastrolab and Stream Diagnostics. In the UK, Biolab and the London Gastroenterology Partnership offer these tests. In Canada, breath tests can be obtained from some American companies, such as Metabolic Solutions and Commonwealth Laboratories. All labs recommend you follow a special diet for one to three days before the test. It is also important to remember that if you have already been diagnosed with fructose malabsorption, lactose intolerance, or sorbitol intolerance with a breath test, it's likely you also have SIBO.

URINE ORGANIC ACIDS

A more recent test that measures levels of different organic acids in your urine may also be useful to detect gut dysbiosis, such as bacterial and yeast overgrowth. This test is currently offered by Metametrix Clinical Laboratory in the USA, and looks at the levels of specific organic acids in your urine, which are metabolites (byproducts) that are produced by bacteria and yeast in your intestines. These compounds make their way into your bloodstream before being eliminated by your kidneys in your urine. High levels of the organic acid D-arabinitol indicate a candida overgrowth, while elevated levels of D-lactate can reveal the presence of SIBO derived from the overgrowth of a type of bacteria in the Lactobacillus acidophilus family. Although this test shows promise, its accuracy and precision have yet to be validated fully.

STOOL TESTING

Some stool tests can give you a good idea of what your gut flora looks like, but they cannot be used to diagnose SIBO since they don't tell you where these bacteria are located. You could have SIBO and see completely normal results with a stool test.

ADDITIONAL CLUES

Whether or not you decide to be tested for SIBO, there are a few other hints that can help you determine if SIBO is a cause of your digestive problems. One hint that you have SIBO is improvement in your symptoms after taking antibiotics, because the antibiotics can kill some of the excess bacteria in your small intestines. Unfortunately, symptoms often return within a few weeks to a few months as the bacteria overgrow again if the underlying causes are left unaddressed.

Another common indicator of SIBO is a reaction to all types of carbohydrates, not just FODMAPs. With FODMAP intolerance, the fermentation takes place in your colon and the bacteria in your large intestines take advantage of any leftover carbohydrates (especially fructose, lactose, sorbitol, mannitol, fructans, and galactans) that you are not able to digest and absorb. If you have SIBO, these bacteria are not limited to your leftovers; instead, they have VIP access to all the food you eat.

Most of the nutrients you eat are slowly absorbed as they move through your small intestines and this is why the excess bacteria in your small intestines can get their hands on these nutrients before you even get a chance to absorb them. These bacteria have a sweet tooth, and they will opt mainly for sugars. Sugar is found not only in foods and beverages that taste sweet, such as desserts and sodas, but also in the starches in pasta, rice, potatoes, and other flour-based foods. Every time you eat one of these carbohydrate-containing foods, much of it gets fermented in the microbreweries operated by the bacteria in your small intestines. The result is excess fermentation and gas production, along with bloating, pain, diarrhea, constipation, and so on.

"Prebiotic" is the term used to describe food or ingredients that can feed your gut flora. Examples include soluble fibers, inulin, chicory root, and fructooligosaccharides (FOS). These nutrients are important to maintain a healthy and thriving gut flora, but if you have a bacterial overgrowth, many foods that should be used by your body are instead used by the bacteria in your small intestines. In other words, nutrients that healthy people are able to extract from their food become prebiotics if you have SIBO. Table 22 lists the types of foods that can feed a bacterial overgrowth and induce digestive symptoms through their fermentation in your intestines.

Table 22: Foods that Can Feed a Bacterial Overgrowth

Nutrients	Specific Foods
Starches	• Grains and foods made from their flours: Breakfast cereals, bread, pasta, rice, couscous, granola bars, whole grains, cakes, cookies, baked goods • Legumes: Beans, lentils • Starchy vegetables and tubers: Potatoes, sweet potatoes, yucca, cassava/tapioca, winter squashes
Sugars	• Fruits: All types, including juices, canned fruits, frozen and fresh fruits, etc. • Fructose: High-fructose corn syrup, agave syrup, honey, high-fructose fruits • Lactose: Milk, yogurt, ice cream, and some cheeses • Sugars: Table sugar, dextrose, maple syrup, molasses, brown rice syrup, and all other types of sugars
FODMAPs	• Short-chain fermentable carbohydrates: Fructose, fructans, lactose, galactans, and polyols
Soluble Fiber	• Grains and seeds: Flaxseeds, oats, barley, psyllium, chia seeds, etc. • Thickeners: Guar gum, xanthan gum, arabic gum, mastic gum, locust bean gum, carrageenan, agar agar, pectin • Vegetables: Eggplant, okra, mushrooms

Another hint that you have SIBO is if you experience gastrointestinal symptoms even with carbohydrates that are low in FODMAPs, gluten free, and low in food chemicals. You are more likely to see the effects of these carbohydrates on your symptoms if you are already on a low-allergen diet (free of gluten, soy, and dairy). Table 23 lists the carbohydrate choices that should be tolerated even by sensitive individuals unless they have SIBO. If you feel like you react to any of these carbohydrate-containing foods, there's a good chance you have SIBO.

Table 23: Carbohydrate-Rich Foods that Can Cause a Reaction with SIBO

Carbohydrate Category	Grain-Free, Gluten-Free, Dairy-Free, Soy-Free, Low-FODMAP, and Low-Food-Chemical Carbohydrates
Starches	• Rice (white, brown, any type) • Rice noodles • Plain rice crackers (gluten free) • Puffed rice and rice-based cereals (gluten free) • White potatoes, peeled • Sweet potatoes, peeled (<1/2 cup) • Pumpkins or butternut squash (<1/4 cup) • Rutabaga (swede) • Parsnips • Turnips • Quinoa • Tapioca or cassava • Buckwheat and buckwheat pasta • Gluten-free breads made with rice, potato or buckwheat (no nuts, seeds, fruits, dried fruits, honey, high-fructose corn syrup, oats, or any other ingredients containing FODMAPS, food chemicals, or gluten)
Sweeteners	• Maple syrup • Table sugar • Golden syrup (inverted sugar) • Dextrose (powder or tablets)

*Note that no fruits are low in FODMAPs and food chemicals.

In the next chapters, I will share with you the approach I developed to help you avoid unnecessarily restrictive and ineffective dietary modifications. Chapter 5 will show you how to determine effectively and accurately which foods to eat or avoid to design a diet for optimal gut health.

Health Consequences of SIBO

In addition to causing the common digestive symptoms associated with IBS, SIBO can interfere with your health well beyond your intestines. The symptoms of SIBO can reach almost any part of your body, and living with a chronic bacterial overgrowth for months or even years is not without consequences.

Excess bacteria in your small intestines can rob you of precious nutrients, especially vitamin B_{12} and iron. Some bacteria can also synthesize vitamin B_{12} analogues. These analogues may look like vitamin B_{12}, but they don't perform the same functions as real vitamin B_{12}, such as supporting brain and nervous-system function and the formation of new blood. Some blood tests cannot differentiate between real and analogous vitamin B_{12}, so you may be B_{12} deficient even if blood work shows normal levels.

If you have been diagnosed with iron deficiency but supplementing with iron doesn't seem to be helping, it could be because your iron supplements are being used by the bacteria in your small intestines. Fatigue and anemia are common with SIBO and can be due to a lack of either iron, vitamin B_{12}, or both. Supplementing with iron and vitamin B_{12} may help some, but you will have better success correcting your nutritional deficiencies by addressing the problem at the source.

Fat is an important source of energy, but SIBO could be preventing you from benefiting from it. Bacteria can break down the bile acids produced by your liver by a process called deconjugation. As you know, bile is essential to help you absorb fat and fat-soluble nutrients such as anti-inflammatory omega-3 fatty acids, vitamins A, D, E, and K, CoQ10, and beta-carotene. From a fat-digestion standpoint, having SIBO could be just the same as not having a gallbladder. The fat you are not able to absorb if your bile is deconjugated by SIBO can rob you of this precious source of energy, as well as important fat-soluble nutrients. Inadequate fat absorption resulting from bile deconjugation can also induce diarrhea. You may be malabsorbing fat if you have fatty stools (steatorrhea or subtype a on the poop chart). Fatty stools tend to float, are lighter in color (chalky or light grey), and have a foul stench. They can even be frothy or have a foamy appearance. Remember in this case that your body hasn't lost its ability to tolerate, digest, absorb, and use fat. It's the excess bacteria in your gut that is interfering with your body's normal process. Fixing SIBO will help your body better digest, absorb, and utilize fat.

In addition to not absorbing fat properly, you may also become malnourished and lose weight involuntarily if the surplus of bacteria in your small intestines consumes a big part of the carbohydrates you eat. In some cases, weight loss can be exacerbated by the severity of your symptoms, especially if you experience nausea, vomiting, or changes in appetite. Diarrhea can also worsen malnutrition by not allowing enough time for your body to absorb the nutrients in your food. Some people with SIBO reach a point where they adopt a very restrictive diet or even fear eating because of the awful symptoms they experience, causing even more weight loss and nutritional deficiencies.

But not all people with SIBO lose weight or are underweight. SIBO is also common in overweight and obese people. The inflammation and chronic stress resulting from SIBO can promote high cortisol levels and insulin resistance, metabolic problems associated with weight gain, or an inability to lose weight. More studies are needed on this topic, but anecdotal evidence seems to support this observation. Although body weight is not a reliable indicator to diagnose SIBO, a bacterial overgrowth in your small intestines could be preventing you from maintaining a healthy weight.

Food intolerances are common with SIBO, and one study even showed that SIBO may eventually lead to gluten sensitivity and celiac disease if left untreated. This is probably because SIBO is also associated with increased intestinal permeability (leaky gut). Another study showed that about one third of people with SIBO have antibodies for gluten in their intestines. Although these antibodies did not appear in their blood (yet), this finding indicates that a large number of people suffering from SIBO could be on the path toward celiac disease or non-celiac gluten sensitivity.

It's unclear whether leaky gut occurs as a result of the damage to the gut lining caused by bacteria or because of the inflammation that is associated with SIBO. Remember that healthy intestines should be somewhat permeable to allow good stuff to get into your body, but if your intestines become too permeable, as is the case with leaky gut, incompletely digested food particles, bacteria, and toxins can get inside your body. Remember that the inside of your intestines are actually outside your body from your body's point of view. The harmful substances that should be eliminated in your stools can become problematic for your health if they circulate in your blood. Some of the most common such consequences are food intolerances, headaches, migraines, joint pain, fatigue, brain fog, and autism. Many of these symptoms have been directly associated with bacterial metabolic toxins (toxic compounds produced by bacteria); they include mouth ulcers, depression, eczema, sinusitis, asthma, muscle pain, increased urination, heart palpitations, and sore throat.

It is also thought that a leaky gut precedes the development of various autoimmune conditions. According to the theory, not fixing your leaky gut could, after months, years, or decades, result in your body's attacking itself, leading to conditions such as rheumatoid arthritis, type 1 diabetes, celiac disease, Hashimoto's thyroiditis, or Graves' disease. A leaky gut is a recipe for poor digestion and poor health.

Whether or not you develop an autoimmune condition depends on your individual susceptibility, but the whole cascade of events leading to these health problems is likely to be precipitated by a leaky gut. Note that people with SIBO usually have both gastrointestinal symptoms and systemic symptoms associated with a leaky gut, but not all people with a leaky gut (without SIBO) experience gastrointestinal symptoms. In fact, a large number of people with abnormal intestinal permeability have an apparently healthy digestion, but this doesn't prevent damage from occurring.

The protocol proposed in this book can also benefit people with an autoimmune condition or a leaky gut, whether or not they experience digestive symptoms. Health starts in the gut. You can't go wrong by eliminating potentially problematic foods and basing your diet on REAL nutrient-dense, anti-inflammatory, low-irritant foods.

TREATMENT FOR SIBO

The many negative health consequences and digestive problems associated with SIBO can be corrected by eradicating the bacterial overgrowth in your small intestines. There are three different forms of treatment available to deal with this chronic infection. Even though they use different mechanisms, they share the common goal of eliminating the excess bacteria in your gut. This can be achieved either directly, by killing the bacteria, or indirectly by starving them.

ANTIBIOTICS

If you received antibiotics for a past infection, you may have noticed a temporary improvement in your IBS symptoms. Antibiotics can help control a bacterial overgrowth, at least for a period of time. Dr. Mark Pimentel, one of the main researchers in the field of SIBO, prefers the use of an antibiotic called rifaximin for most of his patients, but often combines it with neomycin in constipation-prone patients.

Unlike other conventional antibiotics that kill bacteria anywhere in your body, rifaximin and neomycin are absorbed poorly into the blood. Almost all of rifaximin (99.6 percent) and neomycin (95 percent) stays in your intestines, compared to less than 10 percent for regular antibiotics. This characteristic of these drugs makes them good options to target a small-intestinal bacterial overgrowth. It also helps reduce the common side effects associated with antibiotics and prevents unbalancing the gut flora elsewhere (such as the skin, urinary tract, and genital area).

The main problem with this treatment option is that these antibiotics are not yet approved for the treatment of IBS and are therefore not always covered by insurance companies. They are also expensive (in the hundreds of dollars), unless you buy generic versions, which appear to be less effective and cause more side effects. Other doctors have developed protocols using different types of antibiotics. Antibiotic treatment for seven to 14 days has been shown to help eradicate SIBO in 70 to 91 percent of cases. Consult your doctor for help choosing the best option for you. Dr. Pimentel also recommends following the antibiotic treatment with medications that help increase the natural cleansing waves in your intestines to prevent SIBO recurrence. You will learn more about these cleansing waves in the section on the underlying causes of SIBO.

If you don't want to use pharmaceutical antibiotics, herbal antibiotics are another option. Although herbal antibiotics have a long history of use for all kinds of infections, only one study supporting this alternative SIBO treatment had been conducted at the time of writing this book. This study used enteric-coated peppermint oil for 20 days with a success rate varying between 25 and 50 percent. Ample anecdotal evidence also shows that a variety of herbal antibiotics can be beneficial for digestive disorders. These include berberine, garlic, oregano, cinnamon, and grapefruit seed extract.

Even though herbal antibiotics are natural, several factors must be considered to ensure their effectiveness. The choice of herbal antibiotic can depend on the types of bacteria in excess in your small intestines. Herbal remedies can also have interactions with other supplements or medications, so don't use them without supervision. Working with a qualified healthcare professional familiar with these herbs, such as a naturopathic doctor, is recommended.

ELEMENTAL DIETS

Elemental diets are another medication-free alternative to antibiotics. Elemental diets are nutritive liquid preparations of pre-digested nutrients. They are what is often given through a tube to hospitalized patients who can't eat, whether due to surgery or an unconscious state. They are similar to liquid meal replacements, with the exception that the nutrients are broken down into smaller particles to bypass digestion and facilitate absorption. In theory, these formulas are nutritionally adequate to support life, which means they could serve as your only food for the rest of your life.

If you decide on this option to treat your SIBO, you will have to replace all of your meals and snacks with an appropriate elemental diet formula for two to three weeks, and shouldn't consume anything else except water. Since the nutrients in an elemental diet formula are predigested, you should be able to easily and quickly absorb them in your small intestines before the bacteria get to them. The principle is simple: starve the bacteria. The success rate is high, ranging between 80 and 85 percent.

The main problems are that these formulas are expensive and not usually covered by health insurance for the treatment of SIBO. Using an elemental diet formula to cover all of your nutritional requirements for a treatment can easily add up to at least US$500 to $1,000 (provided you need roughly 2,000 calories per day). Of course, you should take into account that you will be saving on groceries during that time.

The nutritional quality of most elemental diets is also questionable, since they tend to be made of maltodextrin, modified food starch from corn, soybean oil, and other processed ingredients. The very low-fat and high-carb content of these formulas may leave you feeling hungry and trigger blood sugar swings that can affect your energy levels. They don't fit the REAL food definition at all, but could be a good compromise for some SIBO cases if used briefly to speed up your recovery.

It's important to work in concert with your doctor if you decide to try an elemental diet. You'll need help figuring out which diet formula is right for you and how much of it you need to support your nutritional requirements. You will also need your doctor's approval if you have diabetes, kidney disease, or other health conditions. Note that it is not effective to take antibiotics at the same time since starving bacteria go into hibernation mode before they die, making them immune to antibiotics during that time.

Whether you choose to use antibiotics or an elemental diet formula to treat your SIBO, you will need to follow your treatment with dietary modifications to prevent recurrence. Even though the success rate of these treatments is high, recurrence is unfortunately very common if you return to your previous way of eating and don't correct what led to your SIBO in the first place (more on this in the next section). Eating the right diet is also important to promote the healing of your inflamed and leaky intestines, a process that can take between three and 12 months. What you eat matters and can make an enormous difference for your digestive and overall health.

DIET ONLY

While dietary changes should always be used in conjunction with all the different SIBO treatment options, they can also be used alone to alleviate symptoms and correct your gut dysbiosis. Although no studies have investigated this treatment option to date, many health care practitioners have used diet to treat SIBO successfully for over a century.

The Specific Carbohydrate Diet (SCD) by Elaine Gottschall and the Gut and Psychology Syndrome (GAPS) diet by Dr. Natasha Campbell-McBride, which you will learn more about in the next chapter, are examples of dietary strategies used to control SIBO. Even though the authors of these diets don't specifically use the term SIBO, they knew decades ago that an overgrowth of bacteria could be responsible for many of their patients' digestive problems.

Using diet alone to starve bacteria can take more time and effort than other treatment options. Fortunately, you can start seeing significant improvements in your symptoms in a few weeks by changing your way of eating even though the bacterial overgrowth itself may take longer to resolve. A couple of years on average, but up to five years for some people, is usually necessary to completely correct the gut dysbiosis. This is why many SIBO sufferers choose to jump start their recovery with antibiotics or an elemental diet formula.

The choice is up to you, but you should discuss your options with your doctor before making a decision. Remember that bacteria are not susceptible to antibiotics if they go into hibernation mode, so if you opt for antibiotics, adopting a diet that starves the excess bacteria in your small intestines could be counterproductive.

So, what should you eat? If you want to control your bacterial overgrowth and associated symptoms with diet alone or if you have treated your SIBO successfully with another option and want to prevent recurrence, following a diet that cannot feed these bacteria is the best way to kill them or prevent another overgrowth. The next chapters will discuss such a diet in more details, but if you are eager for a primer, the diet is one low in carbohydrates that eliminates most starches and sugars. And don't worry, it won't be a starvation diet for you—just for the bacteria. You'll be able to eat plenty of tasty fats and protein, as well as non-starchy vegetables. In other words: plenty of delicious REAL food!

Of course, addressing the underlying causes that caused you to develop SIBO in the first place should also be part of your action plan to prevent a bacterial overgrowth from recurring.

Underlying Causes of SIBO

Why do some people develop SIBO? For most people, it is a combination of factors. The most common potential causes identified so far are:

- An anatomical problem in your small intestines
- Insufficient stomach acid
- Impaired cleansing waves

ALTERED SMALL INTESTINAL ANATOMY

Even if you don't know it, your small intestines may have a slightly different anatomy that could promote SIBO. The most common anatomical factors include bowel adhesions following a surgery, a surgical change to your intestinal anatomy, strictures (narrowing of the bowels) associated with Crohn's disease, or endometriosis that extends into your intestines. In all of these cases, the altered anatomy of the small intestines can make it easier for bacteria to accumulate in certain areas of your bowels where they can then overgrow. A defective ileocecal valve, the valve separating your colon from your small intestines, could allow bacteria from your colon to move up into your small intestines, eventually leading to SIBO. There is little you can do if an anatomical problem makes you more susceptible to SIBO. Some chiropractors may be able to make special manipulations to put your ileocecal valve in the right position, but most of these problems are beyond the scope of what you can control. To make sure you prevent SIBO from recurring, you can make at least make sure that you address the two other most common underlying causes: low stomach acid and impaired cleansing waves.

LOW STOMACH ACID

The acid in your stomach plays many important roles, as explained in Chapter 1. Perhaps one of the most important is as a barrier to prevent harmful microorganisms from invading your gastrointestinal system. Stomach acid is one of the first lines of defense to protect your body against infections. Without enough stomach acid, too many bacteria may survive the journey through the stomach and make their way into your small intestines, where they can proliferate and overgrow.

Low stomach acid can also prevent your digestive enzymes from working properly. If you can't digest and absorb your food well or quickly enough, it's more likely to end up feeding bacteria and eventually lead to an overgrowth.

If you have insufficient stomach acid, supplementing with betaine HCl is the most effective way to restore normal levels. If this method is too harsh for your digestive system, you can take digestive bitters or apple cider vinegar or lemon juice mixed with water a few minutes before your meals to stimulate stomach acid production naturally. Stress can also reduce the acidity of your stomach, so make sure you stay calm and relaxed, especially during meal times. Read Chapters 6 and 7 to learn more about other strategies to improve your stomach-acid levels, better manage your stress, improve your digestion, and reduce your risk of developing SIBO.

IMPAIRED CLEANSING WAVES

Your intestines perform many functions related to the digestion and absorption of nutrients. The intestines are not simple tubes through which food passes. Digestion is far from a passive process, and the intestines actually do quite a bit of physical activity to ensure the process runs smoothly. Your bowels have three main movements in their daily exercise routine: peristalsis, bowel movements, and cleansing waves.

Peristalsis is a movement of the intestines that allows food to move through your esophagus and small intestines. Bowel movements have a larger amplitude and occur mainly in your colon to help you evacuate stools. The least-known movement of this fitness program is the cleansing wave, also referred to as the migrating motor complex (MMC), or even "housekeeper of the gut."

These cleansing waves start in your stomach with a contractile motion that sweeps any undigested particles, bacteria, and debris from your stomach through your small intestines into your colon. Your intestines activate these cleansing waves every 90 minutes or so, but only when your body is not digesting food. Most of the cleansing waves therefore occur during night time or a few hours after each of your meals (unless you have a snack!).

Ideally, you should have an average of nine cleansing waves per day. Interestingly, one study showed that more than half of one's cleansing waves seem to occur within about 10 minutes of urination. Eating between meals and grazing throughout the day decrease the number of cleansing waves; stress and some medications can also interfere with them. Gastrointestinal infections can also alter cleansing waves, even after the infection is gone. This is because many of these harmful bacteria secrete toxins that inhibit the cleansing waves to prevent the bacteria from being moved out of the intestines. The effect of these toxins can induce long-term and even permanent changes to your intestinal function.

People with SIBO have about 70 percent fewer cleansing waves than healthy individuals, making it easier for bacteria to take up residence in their small intestines.

One way to increase the regularity of your cleansing waves is by limiting yourself to three meals a day at least four to five hours apart and avoiding snacking. Do not consider this option if you're underweight, malnourished, or have blood-sugar dysregulation issues. You shouldn't skip your usual snacks until after a few weeks of starting the elimination diet to allow your body time to adapt to this new way of eating.

All forms of stress (work, moving, traveling, and financial or health problems) inhibit your body's ability to digest, heal, and stay healthy by interfering with your immune system and your cleansing waves. Properly managing your stress is crucial (see Chapter 7) to allow your body to be in a state conducive to regular intestinal cleansing waves.

Probiotics from supplements and fermented foods can help not only improve your digestion, but also give your small intestines the signal to shake off excess bacteria regularly by activating the cleansing waves.

The simple presence of fat or acid (by themselves, not as part of a mixed meal) in the upper part of your small intestines can also trigger your cleansing waves. You can try taking a spoonful of ghee, coconut oil, or olive oil between your meals or at bedtime to encourage your bowels to do what's necessary. A little apple cider vinegar, some raw sauerkraut juice, or even a twist of lemon or lime juice in a little water can also do the trick.

Sometimes, medications to promote gut motility (such as erythromycin) may be necessary to restore inhibited cleansing waves. Your doctor can help you determine if this is a good option for you. In most cases, taking this type of medication for three months is sufficient, although some people may need to take it on a long-term basis if their cleansing waves do not seem to resume naturally. Table 24 reviews the different factors that can inhibit and promote your inner "gut housekeeper."

Table 24: Factors that Inhibit or Promote Cleansing Waves

Factors that Inhibit Cleansing Waves (Contribute to SIBO)	Factors that Promote Cleansing Waves (Prevent SIBO)
• Eating more than three times per day, regular snacking or grazing	• Spacing meals at least 4-5 hours apart
• Gastrointestinal infection (current or past)	• Relaxation
• Stress	• Probiotics
• Gastroparesis (abnormally slow gastric emptying)	• Eating fat on its own (not as part of a mixed meal)
• Some medications (morphine)	• Taking something acidic on its own (lemon juice, apple cider vinegar, or sauerkraut juice)
	• Some medications (erythromycin)

A gut-flora imbalance, also called gut dysbiosis, can also contribute to an increased risk of developing SIBO. Many factors can influence the health of your gut flora. Being born by cesarean section (C-section), not being breastfed, eating a poor diet, taking antibiotics, and stress can all perturb your gut flora. Overconsumption of carbohydrates, especially from sugars and refined grains found in processed foods and beverages, can also contribute to a gut dysbiosis and the eventual development of SIBO.

Remember that in most cases, more than one cause is usually involved. This is why adopting a holistic approach will give you the best results. You will learn more about how to optimize your digestion and gut flora in the next chapters to help you conquer your SIBO and prevent it from returning. But before that, let's address a few other things that could be responsible for your digestive issues.

Celiac Disease

Awareness of celiac disease has increased rapidly in the past several years. However, it is estimated that it still takes between six and 10 years for people with celiac disease to be diagnosed, while about 95 percent of celiacs are still undiagnosed or misdiagnosed with IBS or other conditions. Some undiagnosed celiac sufferers may not even have any symptoms, even though severe damage is still occurring in their intestines.

Celiac disease is an autoimmune condition known to be provoked by a sensitivity to gluten. Unlike non-celiac gluten sensitivity, untreated celiac disease leads to the destruction of your intestines by the immune system after exposure to gluten. This attack by your body on your intestines causes villous atrophy, in which your intestinal cells lose their hair-like villi (a brand-new carpet) and become completely flat (like a worn out carpet; see Figure 6 on page 45). Atrophied villi can't function properly and lose their ability to absorb nutrients and defend your body against harmful substances. This is why celiac disease sometimes leads to malnutrition and weight loss.

Increased intestinal permeability, or leaky gut, is another hallmark of celiac disease. This autoimmune condition is often accompanied (though not always) by symptoms similar to those seen with IBS: abdominal pain, cramping, bloating, gas, diarrhea, and constipation. Other symptoms include fatigue, joint pain, skin rash, headaches, depression, tingling and numbness in the extremities, mouth sores, irritability, thin bones and osteoporosis, infertility, discolored teeth, and delayed growth or failure to thrive in children and adolescents.

There is no pharmaceutical treatment for celiac disease, although drug companies are working hard on one. The only treatment now available for celiac disease is strict, lifelong adherence to a gluten-free diet. As you know from the section on gluten intolerance, the problematic forms of gluten are found mainly in wheat and its cousins kamut, triticale, and spelt, as well as in barley, rye, and some oats (unless labeled gluten free). These gluten-containing grains are omnipresent in almost all of the staple foods in the standard Westernized diet: bread, breakfast cereals, granola bars, pasta, couscous, cookies, cakes, pies, and so on. Although a celiac diet may seem like deprivation, cutting gluten from your diet is actually one of the best things anyone interested in improving their digestive and overall health can do. Of course, it can be difficult to give up gluten-containing food products at first, but it might become the most important dietary changes you ever make, whether you have celiac or non-celiac gluten sensitivity.

Unfortunately, a gluten-free diet doesn't seem to be enough for at least seven to 30 percent of people with celiac disease. Many who suffer from celiac disease never seem to get better, even after eliminating gluten from their diet. Others may feel better for a few months, only to have their symptoms return despite strict adherence to a gluten-free diet. Another proportion may feel fine, but their blood work shows elevated levels of gluten antibodies even after six to 12 months of no gluten. Elevated antibody levels indicate that their body has not healed and that an autoimmune reaction is still attacking the intestinal lining. So why would a gluten-free diet not be effective for all people with celiac gluten sensitivity?

Gluten-free diets seem to be adorned with a health halo, and "special" gluten-free foods are commonly offered in health food stores or the health sections of grocery stores. But the truth is that these foods, while convenient alternatives to their glutenous cousins, are not necessarily healthy.

In fact, many gluten-free products can have a detrimental effect on your health, especially if you are trying to recover from serious digestive issues. These foods often provide little more than empty calories and a lot of artificial and processed ingredients, many of which can trigger your digestive symptoms. They are poor sources of many of the nutrients your body needs to heal and recover, and they can't help you correct the common nutrient deficiencies associated with celiac disease, nor can they help facilitate the healing of your damaged gut.

In addition, the refined corn, potato flour, rice flour, and other processed ingredients used in gluten-free products are rich in high-glycemic carbohydrates, the perfect substrate to feed a gut dysbiosis like SIBO. If that weren't enough, gluten-free products often also contain ingredients like FODMAPs, gums, and sugars that can cause bloating, abdominal pain, and problems with your bowel movements. If you have celiac disease, going on a gluten-free diet is the first step to getting healthier, but gluten-free food products may get in the way of accomplishing your goal of optimal gut health.

Table 25 shows you a few examples of how processed and devoid of nutrients gluten-free products can be. Their ingredient lists show clearly that gluten-free food products are not REAL food.

Table 25: Ingredients in Various Gluten-Free Products

Gluten-Free Products	Ingredients
Crackers	Corn starch, palm oil, soy flour, invert sugar, sea salt, soy lecithin, cellulose gum, sodium bicarbonate, caramelized sugar, yeast extract, sodium pyrophosphate
Apple and Cinnamon Ring Breakfast Cereals	Corn flour, corn starch, dehydrated cane juice, dried apples, honey, natural apple flavor, canola oil, cinnamon, baking powder, salt
Multigrain Bread	Water, potato starch, canola oil, corn starch, tapioca starch, dried egg whites, rice bran, molasses, cellulose powder, yeast, sugar, inverted sugar, modified cellulose, sugar beet fiber, salt, xanthan gum, calcium sulfate, enzymes
Wild Berry Organic Bars	Organic brown rice syrup, organic rice crisp (organic rice, organic evaporated cane juice, salt, organic brown rice syrup), organic corn flakes (organic corn meal, organic concentrated grape juice, sea salt), organic honey, organic evaporated cane juice, natural wild berry flavor, organic quinoa, organic buckwheat, organic flaxseeds, organic sesame seeds, organic high oleic sunflower oil, organic blueberries (organic wild blueberries, organic cane juice, organic sunflower oil), organic dried strawberries (organic strawberries, organic cane sugar, organic canola oil)
Cookies	Flour blend (tapioca starch, potato starch, corn starch, corn flour, white rice flour, carrageenan, gum arabic), organic palm oil, sugar, brown sugar, chocolate chips (sugar, chocolate liquor, cocoa butter, dextrose anhydrous, soy lecithin, vanilla extract), invert sugar, natural flavors, eggs, sodium bicarbonate, sea salt, egg whites, organic caramel color, soy lecithin

Non-Responsive Celiac Disease

When a celiac sufferer tells his doctor he is still experiencing symptoms or does not feel 100 percent, the doctor will often blame it on non-compliance. Although this is sometimes true, most people with celiac disease are trying hard to recover their health, energy, and quality of life. If your gluten-free diet is failing at getting you healthy, it is probably due to one or more of these three culprits:

- Gluten contamination
- SIBO and gut dysbiosis
- Food intolerances (due to cross-reactivity or a leaky gut)

All of these factors can contribute to inflammation in your intestines and prevent your gut from healing. Stress, lack of sleep, and uncorrected nutritional deficiencies can also compromise your gut health and constitute other important factors to consider if your gluten-free diet is not improving your celiac disease. The next pages and chapters will go over every detail of the plan you should follow, beyond a gluten-free diet, to help move your health in the right direction.

GLUTEN CONTAMINATION

A minuscule amount of gluten—less than even a small breadcrumb—is enough to cause damage to your intestines if you don't tolerate gluten. To be effective, a gluten-free diet needs to be 100-percent free of gluten. A low-gluten diet is not enough. Even if you're trying hard to adhere to a strict gluten-free diet, it's still possible that tiny amounts of gluten are sneaking into your body without your awareness.

A weekly communion wafer at church, a bite of cake on your birthday, or gluten-free bread toasted in the same toaster used for gluten-containing bread can be enough to cause problems. Even lipstick with gluten-derived ingredients or a bun-free burger grilled on the same grill as wheat buns. Small traces of gluten can cause a lot of damage, even if you don't feel anything. Some people with celiac or non-celiac gluten sensitivity will start feeling very sick within a few hours of ingesting gluten, but others don't get this alarm signal from their body. Too often, the internal damage that occurs with celiac disease can be insidious.

What if you are already very strict with your gluten-free diet and never consume gluten knowingly? One difficulty is in remembering the dozens of ingredients that are synonymous with gluten, since gluten-containing ingredients are not always labeled clearly. Many foods have ingredient lists that are long and tough to decipher. Would you guess that malted milk, roux, wild emmer, atta flour, and edible films contain gluten? There are so many gluten-containing ingredients that it's very easy to make mistakes.

Eating gluten free goes beyond avoiding wheat-flour-based products like breads, pasta, and baked goods. It's important to also pay attention when buying foods like frozen French fries, soy sauce, sausages, deli meats, seasonings, spice rubs, marinades, sauces, and salad dressings. Even processed foods made from what seem to be safe ingredients or grains and flours that are known to be gluten free are often contaminated. A pilot study in 2010 showed that over two thirds of foods that are supposed to be naturally free of gluten (such as millet flour, buckwheat flour, sorghum flour, soy flour, and white rice flour) were in fact contaminated with enough gluten to be unsafe for people with celiac disease or gluten sensitivity.

Many people believe that opting for certified gluten-free products can help them avoid gluten and save time reading food labels at the grocery store. However, products labeled gluten-free are not necessarily 100-percent gluten-free; products can contain up to 20 parts per million (ppm) to be labeled as such in the United States. The same level is also used by the World Health Organization. Australian standards are stricter and limit gluten to five ppm, the smallest detectable amount, while some northern European countries allow up to 200 ppm. Although some gluten "experts" claim these small amounts of gluten are not deleterious, it's difficult to find hard data supporting this claim.

Inoffensive amounts of gluten can add up over time. What if you start your day with a large bowl of gluten-free cereal and a few pieces of gluten-free toast, then have a gluten-free pasta and tuna salad for lunch, a gluten-free granola bar in the afternoon, and a gluten-free pizza for dinner with a few gluten-free cookies for dessert? This is not an uncommon scenario for someone on a gluten-free diet, but the traces of gluten in these products can easily add up to over five milligrams of gluten per day, the amount in a small crumb of bread, and enough to perpetuate your health problems.

Could this explain why a gluten-free diet is often inadequate for people with celiac disease? Most experts on gluten believe that it's practically impossible to eat a diet that is completely free of gluten considering the contamination of many grains and other processed foods, including gluten-free grains and food products. A study published in 2007 in the American Journal of Clinical Nutrition was conducted to determine what would constitute a safe amount of gluten for people with celiac disease. The researchers concluded that consuming 10 milligrams of gluten per day for a period of 90 days appeared safe for most people with celiac disease, although it induced symptoms and even a relapse in two of the participants. Even if the daily 10 milligram dose of gluten didn't trigger symptoms in most of the celiac participants, it was enough to prevent the intestinal villi of more than half of them from healing. The longer-term effects of these trace amounts of gluten are still unknown.

> Better safe than sorry is a good rule to live by, especially when your health is at stake.

You can actually drop your gluten exposure to zero by avoiding gluten-free food products and adopting a diet based on REAL food. There has never been and will never be any gluten in vegetables, fruits, tubers, meat, and traditional fats. REAL food is also less likely to be contaminated in the same way as other gluten-free grains and processed foods. The dietary approach proposed in this book will help you keep your gluten intake much lower than what you could achieve on a standard gluten-free diet, which might just be the missing link for you to achieve optimal gut health. Until more solid data is available to determine what a "safe" dose of gluten might be, safer and more nutritious naturally gluten-free foods are a preferable alternative to expensive, nutrient-poor gluten-free products. The next chapters will teach you how to adopt a diet based on REAL foods to help you recover your digestive health and forget you have celiac disease.

Cross contamination is another common source of trace gluten that can damage your intestines. Do you eat out and/or share your kitchen with people who eat gluten? Even if you make the effort to specify that you have celiac disease or tell the waiter you are "allergic to gluten," prepared foods can still become contaminated. Using the same cutting board, knives, and skillets to cook foods with and without gluten can be enough to cause problems. The same cross contamination can occur if your chicken or French fries are cooked in the same fryer used to fry chicken nuggets or breaded chicken, or if the gluten-free bread for your sandwich is toasted in the same toaster as regular wheat bread. There are a thousand ways through which your food may be cross contaminated with gluten. Result: your gut lining can't heal, whether or not you experience the associated digestive symptoms.

Eating a gluten-free diet doesn't mean you have to become a hermit. Just make sure to inquire about food-preparation methods when you eat out. Request that your food be prepared with separate, clean utensils and cooking equipment. If you eat out at a friend's or family member's, explain to them the importance of avoiding gluten cross contamination. If you are still worried, propose to bring a gluten-free dish that you can share with everyone. See more tips on eating out in Chapter 8.

Don't forget that cross contamination can happen at home, too. If any of your family members aren't on a gluten-free diet, be extremely careful when preparing your food. Use separate cutting boards, knives, and skillets for your meals. Bread crumbs can also hide in utensil drawers and cupboards or on the kitchen counter. Keep your utensils, plates, and cooking equipment safe in a separate cupboard and always clean the counter before preparing your food.

What about non-food gluten sources? Food manufacturers have found ways to incorporate gluten-derived ingredients into many everyday non-food products. Lipsticks, makeup, toothpaste, moisturizers, shampoos, and other personal care products often contain gluten, so read ingredient lists carefully! Technically, gluten on your skin shouldn't cause too much harm for your intestinal health, unless you are extremely sensitive or suffer from dermatitis herpetiformis (a skin problem caused by gluten). However, it is impossible not to swallow some of your lipstick or gloss. Shampoo is also risky since it can get in your mouth. Medications and dietary supplements often contain gluten as part of their ingredients, as does the glue of envelopes and stamps. Don't lick them! Use a wet sponge or buy envelopes and stamps with stickers. And make sure you don't eat your Play-Doh, either (both homemade and commercial modeling clays contain gluten). Removing gluten from your diet involves more than just paying attention to the foods you eat.

SIBO AND GUT DYSBIOSIS

If you're still stuck with sub-optimal digestion even after excising all traces of gluten from your diet and environment, it's time to look at other possible causes. If you still suffer from non-responsive celiac disease, place your bets on SIBO. An Italian study published in 2003 in American Journal of Gastroenterology showed that two out of three people with celiac disease unable to control their symptoms on a gluten-free diet have SIBO. Removing gluten is, without a doubt, the first dietary change you need to make if you've been diagnosed with celiac disease. If you also happen to have a bacterial overgrowth in your small intestines, however, the fermentation of every little bit of gluten-free carbohydrate you eat could be contributing to your bloating, pain, gas, diarrhea, constipation, fatigue, food sensitivities, and other unpleasant symptoms.

The same study showing that SIBO is frequent in people with celiac disease demonstrated that treatment with rifaximin, one of the non-systemic antibiotics of choice used to eradicate SIBO, eliminated the refractory symptoms in all celiac individuals affected with SIBO. Other available options to treat SIBO (herbal antibiotics, elemental diet formulas, or diet alone) haven't yet been tested specifically in people with celiac disease, but they may be good alternatives with which to experiment under the supervision of a qualified health care practitioner. Whatever path you choose, modifying your diet is also crucial to prevent SIBO from returning and interfering with your health in the future.

You can first get tested for SIBO with a breath test using glucose or lactulose to confirm the presence of this chronic infection in your small intestines, but remember that breath tests are not 100-percent accurate and a negative result doesn't necessarily rule out SIBO. If you feel like most types of carbohydrates, including gluten-free starches and sugars, seem to trigger your symptoms, you very likely have SIBO. It might also be a good idea to ask your doctor to check for the presence of other gastrointestinal infections to rule out this possible cause of non-responsive celiac disease.

FOOD SENSITIVITIES

Whether or not they have SIBO, people with celiac disease can develop food sensitivities because of their compromised intestinal barrier (leaky gut). If you still experience digestive problems after eliminating gluten, it could be because you now not only react to gluten, but to other foods, too. Cross-reactivity is the term used to describe how gluten can cause your immune system to react to other substances in the foods you eat.

The most common foods identified as having potential for cross-reactivity with gluten are:

- Gluten-free grains (corn, rice, buckwheat, millet, sorghum, quinoa, oats)
- Dairy
- Eggs
- Nuts
- Seeds (chocolate, cocoa, coffee, sunflower seeds, pumpkin seeds, psyllium, flaxseeds, sesame seeds)
- Yeast
- Legumes (soy, peanuts)
- Potatoes and other nightshades (tomato, eggplant, bell pepper, paprika, hot peppers)

As long as your intestines are unhealed and your gut dysbiosis is uncorrected, you're also very likely to be intolerant of:

- Lactose
- FODMAPs

Other carbohydrates, such as sugars and starches, can also be problematic, especially if you have SIBO or a similar type of gut dysbiosis. The next chapters outline the best dietary strategies to optimize your digestive and overall health by helping you identify potential food sensitivities.

Inflammatory Bowel Disorders (IBDs)

Crohn's disease and ulcerative colitis are the two conditions that belong to the family of inflammatory bowel disorders (IBD). They are both characterized by very high levels of inflammation in the intestines and, like celiac disease, are considered to be autoimmune disorders.

These conditions are serious, and it's important to rule them out before assuming you have IBS, especially since the symptoms can be very similar. You can suspect IBD if, in addition to bloating, abdominal pain, and cramping, you suffer from rectal bleeding, fever, nausea, loss of appetite, dehydration, or chronic diarrhea (including bloody diarrhea). Involuntary weight loss and nutrient deficiencies (especially iron-deficiency anemia) are also common. If Crohn's disease and ulcerative colitis go uncontrolled for too long, they can eventually damage your intestines to the point where you will need to have part of your bowels removed or end up with an ileostomy or colostomy (a hole in your abdomen with a pouch attached to collect your stools). The risk of colorectal cancer is also significantly higher in people with IBDs.

The typical treatment for IBDs usually involves the long-term use of steroid medications (also called cortisone or corticosteroids) to lower inflammation. Unfortunately, these medications are associated with serious side effects. With time, the use of these drugs can lead to the weakening of your bones (osteoporosis) and make you prone to bone fractures. They can also increase your blood pressure, blood sugar, and your risk of cataracts, diabetes, and infections; affect your fertility; cause depression; slow healing; and make you gain fat on your belly, face, and the back of your neck. It's important to consult your doctor to weigh the risks and benefits of taking these drugs. They can be very helpful, even essential, in the short term if you have a flare-up, but implementing diet and lifestyle changes to control inflammation in your intestines, regulate your immune system, and correct nutritional deficiencies is the best way to improve your health and prevent relapses in the long term. Make sure to work in concert with a qualified health professional to wean yourself off these medications once you start better managing your symptoms with your new way of eating.

IBDs are characterized by increased intestinal permeability, inflammation, and an excessive and inappropriate immune response. Gut dysbiosis, especially in the form of SIBO, is also frequent and can actually be mistaken for an IBD flare-up, according to a study published in BMC Gastroenterology in 2009. Treatment with antibiotics can be helpful to get rid of bacterial overgrowth and speed up recovery, especially if accompanied with the right dietary changes. Like other gastrointestinal disorders, IBDs can benefit from a diet focused on anti-inflammatory, low-irritant, and easy-to-digest REAL food to calm inflammation and autoimmune reactions while allowing your intestines to heal and normalize their permeability. Such an approach has been shown to help 100 percent of patients with both Crohn's disease and ulcerative colitis to reduce their symptoms and over 80 percent to go off their medications completely, according to the results of a pilot study from the University of Massachusetts published in 2011.

GERD and Acid Reflux

The prevalence of acid reflux and GERD seem to be on the rise, especially in people with IBS. In fact, close to two thirds of people with IBS also have GERD. The frequent association between these two conditions is not a coincidence and indicates that they may share common underlying causes.

As counterintuitive as it sounds, GERD may actually be the result of low stomach acid in over 90 percent of cases, according to Dr. Jonathan Wright, author of "Why Stomach Acid is Good For You." Low stomach acid can also promote the development of an *H. pylori* infection or SIBO, which can both exacerbate GERD.

More often than not, not having enough acid in your stomach is at the source of your acid reflux, but it is so often treated with antacid medications. If you have been diagnosed with heartburn, acid reflux or GERD, have you had your stomach-acid levels tested? For 99 percent of people, the answer, unfortunately, is no.

ACID-SUPPRESSING MEDICATIONS

In most cases, your doctor will write you a prescription for a proton-pump inhibitor (PPI) or other acid-suppressing medication when you complain of a burning sensation in your stomach and esophagus. And in most cases, the treatment will work just fine to relieve your symptoms as long as you keep taking them.

As with many of today's chronic conditions, however, the "treatment" simply involves bandaging a wound from which the splinter hasn't been removed. Did you know that most of these medications specifically mention in their monograph (drug pamphlet) that they are meant only for short-term use (defined as four to eight weeks)? If you've taken these medications, did your doctor ever try to find a way to get you off them? Many people suffering with acid reflux and GERD are given no option than to continue taking these drugs for months, years, or even decades, with unknown long-term consequences on their health.

GERD has been very good business for pharmaceutical companies. If you suffer from acid reflux and tried weaning yourself off these drugs in the past, you probably experienced a terrible acid rebound, a worsening of your GERD symptoms that made you run back to your acid-lowering medication. A study conducted in Denmark actually showed that giving PPIs to healthy volunteers for eight weeks caused more than 40 percent of them to develop GERD symptoms. The authors of this study wondered if the rebound acid reflux symptoms caused by the withdrawal of these drugs could actually make people become dependent on them in the long term. PPIs and the like may be appropriate for short-term relief, but they're not a lifelong solution.

LOW STOMACH ACID?

But how does low stomach acid contribute to GERD? First, it's important to understand that your stomach is meant to be acidic, as explained in Chapter 1. Your stomach cells are naturally able to protect themselves against this acidity, unless you have an ulcer or atrophic gastritis. The burning sensation you feel with acid reflux actually comes from your esophagus, the tube connecting your mouth to your stomach. The esophagus is only supposed to be in contact with the food you just swallowed to deliver it to your stomach and it doesn't consist of the same acid-resistant cells in the stomach. If your stomach's contents back up into the esophagus, they will burn your esophagus—and you'll feel it.

Clear as mud? Didn't we say that the problem with GERD is often due to low stomach acid? The pH of a normal stomach should range between 1 and 3. Stomach acid secretion tends to diminish as we age, yet the prevalence of GERD is higher as we get older and lower in children and adolescents. If you have low stomach acid, your pH may be closer to 4, 5, or even 6. This is not acidic enough for your digestion to work optimally, but it's definitely still too acidic for your esophagus' standards. This is why you can experience the burning sensation associated with GERD and acid reflux even if you have low stomach acid levels.

CAUSES OF GERD: *H. PYLORI*, SIBO, AND FOOD SENSITIVITIES

What then causes GERD then if too much stomach acid is often not the problem? The culprit could actually be your lower esophageal sphincter (LES). This sphincter, or valve, is a muscle that acts as a retractable lid between your esophagus and stomach to let in the food you swallow while preventing your stomach contents from going back up. The LES should stay closed at all times, except when you swallow food, belch, or vomit. The problem with GERD is that your LES can become "lazy" and loose. When this happens, the pressure of your stomach contracting to digest the foods you eat can push some of its acidic contents up into your esophagus, burning and damaging its fragile lining. The problem is not too much acid, but that it ends up in the wrong place.

The exact mechanism that causes the LES to malfunction is unclear (and there might be more than one). But the low-stomach-acid hypothesis postulates that having enough acid in your stomach is necessary for the activation of the LES sphincter. In other words, a certain level of acidity in your stomach is required to tell your LES to keep the door of your stomach shut tight. It is also possible that low stomach-acid levels are associated with GERD because they make you more susceptible to *H. pylori*, SIBO, and food sensitivities.

H. pylori is a type of bacteria that likes to settle in your stomach, a dark and moist environment with lots of nutrients. *H. pylori* thrives in a low-acid environment, and has learned to survive in your stomach by turning down your internal acid production. If you take acid-suppressing medications for GERD, it increases your risk of being infected with *H. pylori* by further lowering your stomach acid levels. In addition to being associated with GERD, this bug is also thought to contribute to other serious gastrointestinal problems such as atrophic gastritis, gastric and duodenal ulcers, and even stomach cancer.

SIBO is another common problem associated with GERD that can also worsen your acid reflux problems. Remember that a bacterial overgrowth produces a lot of hydrogen and methane gas by fermenting some of the carbohydrates and FODMAPs in your food. It turns out that many bad bacteria, including *H. pylori*, love hydrogen and use it as a source of energy, making for a very vicious cycle. It is a good idea to get tested for *H. pylori* if you have GERD. Antibiotics can help you get rid of it, so your body can start producing normal amounts of acid again. It might also get your SIBO under control if low stomach acid is part of your bacterial overgrowth problem.

SIBO can also contribute to GERD in and of itself, even if you don't have an *H. pylori* infection. If there is too much fermentation occurring in your digestive system, the added pressure of the gas produced by the bacteria in your small intestines can cause your LES to malfunction. Undigested carbohydrates (such as lactose, fructose, and other FODMAPs) as well as some other sugars and starches, can feed a bacterial overgrowth in your small intestines. All the gas produced by the microbreweries in your gut can put pressure on your LES door, forcing it open and allowing the acidic contents of your stomach to enter your esophagus and cause GERD symptoms. Low stomach acid is a contributing factor to the development of SIBO. Half of people taking acid-suppressing medications for a year end up developing SIBO and some of its unpleasant digestive symptoms, such as bloating, flatulence, abdominal pain, constipation, and diarrhea. Ask to be tested for SIBO if you suffer from chronic acid reflux and GERD.

In addition to increasing your risk for an *H. pylori* infection and SIBO, low stomach acid also increases your risk for developing food sensitivities. Gluten or other proteins found in grains, dairy, soy, nuts, eggs, or other foods can interfere with the good functioning of your LES, preventing it from keeping the acidic contents of your stomach where they belong. This is yet another reason to follow the elimination diet protocol outlined in this book to identify if some of these foods are impeding the good functioning of your digestive system.

Some cases of GERD can be due to excess stomach acid, but this is rare. If none of the possible causes of GERD described above seems to apply to you, consider having your stomach-acid levels measured with the Heidelberg test. If your stomach is too acidic, antacid medications are the best option to prevent burning and damage to your fragile esophageal lining. If you have to stay on these medications, ask your doctor to test you for common nutritional deficiencies associated with low stomach acid, especially iron, calcium, magnesium, zinc, folic acid, and vitamins B_{12} and D.

Gallstones and Gallbladder Diseases

Your gallbladder plays a very important role in digestion. It's crucial for optimal fat digestion and assists the absorption of healthy fats and fat-soluble nutrients. But like most of the organs of your digestive system, your gallbladder can also be responsible for worsening your tummy issues.

The gallbladder is a small pouch that collects and stores the bile salts produced by your liver. When you eat, especially if you eat fat, your gallbladder receives a signal to empty its bile through the bile duct that connects it to the entrance of your small intestines. Problems occur if the bile salts in your gallbladder form stones (gallstones) that obstruct the bile duct, causing a sharp pain in the center of your upper belly that radiates to your back, especially at night or after meals. Sometimes these symptoms become severe enough that they are treated with a cholecystectomy, the removal of your gallbladder.

This is unfortunate, because changing the way you eat can be all you need to prevent the unnecessary removal of this precious organ. If you have gallstones, ask your doctor about trying different nutritional approaches for two or three months to determine the underlying cause of your problem before going under the scalpel. The problem may lie in one of a few key areas, including low stomach acid (again!), autoimmune disorders, a damaged gut, food sensitivities, or a low-fat diet.

GALLSTONES AND LOW STOMACH ACID

One older study showed that over half of people with gallstones have low levels of stomach acid. Unfortunately, no recent studies have examined this topic, and doctors seldom test stomach-acid levels in their patients. It's not a stretch to think that low stomach acid could be related to gallstones, considering that it is associated with other digestive problems such as SIBO and GERD.

Low levels of stomach acid could be implicated in gallbladder problems because having enough stomach acid is required to activate your gallbladder to release its bile. It's when bile stays too long in your gallbladder that bile salts can form stones. Adequate levels of stomach acid are necessary to prompt the gallbladder to release its bile acids regularly and thus prevent gallstones. Another reason insufficient stomach acid could be associated with gallbladder disease is because of its connection with food sensitivities.

Without enough stomach acid, the food you eat cannot be digested properly and some of the incompletely digested food particles can trigger inflammation or an intolerance response from your immune system. If you keep eating the foods to which you are sensitive, you may irritate and damage your gut lining over time, but what's the link with your gallbladder? Your gut lining needs to be intact and in good shape to be able to send the right signals to your gallbladder once food arrives in your intestines ready to be digested. A damaged gut lining, resulting from an intolerance to gluten, dairy, or other hard-to-digest protein, may not be able to tell your gallbladder when it's time to release its bile. If your gallbladder doesn't regularly empty itself of the bile it collects, you will be at an increased risk for the formation of gallstones.

Ever had soy milk? The calcium that is added to enriched soy milk tends to sink to the bottom and form tiny crystals over time if you don't shake it regularly. The same thing can happen in your gallbladder. If its bile salts aren't used regularly and released into your small intestines, they can stagnate and form small crystals, then eventually gallstones. Inflammation can also lead to the swelling of your bile duct, making it even easier for gallstones to form. Your body will eventually let you know, in a painful way, that things aren't functioning as they should be.

GALLBLADDER ISSUES AND AUTOIMMUNE CONDITIONS

Some gallbladder issues can also have an autoimmune cause. Autoimmune cholangitis is a type of gallbladder problem often found in people with celiac disease or other autoimmune disorders, further demonstrating the link between digestive problems, autoimmune conditions, a damaged gut (resulting from increased intestinal permeability), and food sensitivities. The good news is that although the mechanisms are not yet clearly understood, following an elimination diet, as described later in this book, can be an effective way to control your symptoms in as little as a few weeks and possibly save you having to bid painful adieu to your gallbladder.

THE IMPORTANCE OF FAT IN GALLBLADDER HEALTH

Another potential cause of gallbladder disease is not eating enough fat. Bile is required to digest fat, and your body knows it's a waste to release the bile in your gallbladder if you're eating a low-fat diet. A bowl of breakfast cereal with fresh fruit and skim milk, a turkey sandwich with a fat-free yogurt, and a bowl of whole-grain pasta with vegetarian marinara sauce are considered "healthy" according to mainstream standards, but these kinds of high-carb, low-fat meals can be problematic for your digestive health and gallbladder. The problematic gluten, irritating insoluble fiber, and hard-to-digest proteins found in these foods, combined with their lack of gut-health-supporting nutrients and their low-fat content that fails to properly activate your gallbladder, can be the perfect recipe for tummy trouble in susceptible individuals.

One study even found that 25 percent of people following a calorie-restricted, low-fat diet developed gallstones in as little as eight weeks. Without enough fat in your diet, the bile salts get stuck for too long in your gallbladder, increasing the risk of painful gallstones that can eventually obstruct your bile duct. Gradually increasing your fat intake can help get your bile flowing more regularly to prevent gallstones and gallbladder problems.

Without a gallbladder (or with a gallbladder that doesn't function properly), the fat and fat-soluble nutrients you eat can't be digested and absorbed and are simply flushed down the toilet. This produces fatty stools, or steatorrhea, which can float, have a lighter color and/or a frothy appearance, and emit a very foul smell.

People without a gallbladder are often counseled to adopt a low-fat diet. But dietary fat is not the problem! Fat plays many important roles in a healthy diet, including providing energy, producing hormones, assisting brain function, and enhancing the absorption of fat-soluble nutrients like vitamins A, D, E, and K, omega-3 fats, CoQ10, and other antioxidants. Following the elimination diet protocol can help your digestive system heal and improve your tolerance to dietary fats. In many cases of gallbladder problems, though, supplementing with ox bile might be a necessary adjunct to help you fully digest and absorb the fat and fat-soluble nutrients you eat. Special types of fats rich in medium-chain triglycerides (MCTs) like coconut oil don't require bile to be digested and absorbed, which make them a great fat source if you no longer have your gallbladder. Chapter 5 will help you adjust your dietary protocol to address gallbladder issues.

Gut Issues: Get Tested!

Many things can go wrong in your digestive system. The classic IBS symptoms of bloating, abdominal pain, and bowel-movement changes require you and your doctor to do some work to pin down the underlying causes of your discomfort. If you feel overwhelmed by all the things that can go wrong with your digestion, take a deep breath, keep reading, and make arrangements to get the right testing done (see Table 26) to help you finally put a label on your digestive symptoms.

Celiac disease, inflammatory bowel disorders like Crohn's disease and ulcerative colitis, gastrointestinal infections, and colon cancer (especially if you are over the age of 50) should first be ruled out before undergoing more specialized testing (breath tests and lactulose-mannitol tests). Remember that it is also possible that more than one of the following causes is contributing to your IBS symptoms.

Table 26: Testing Options for Various GI Conditions

Gastrointestinal Conditions		Digestive-Health Tests	
SIBO		• Lactulose and/or glucose breath test • Organic urine acids (not validated) • Elimination diet with reintroduction challenges	
FODMAP Intolerance	Fructose Malabsorption	• Fructose breath test	Elimination diet with reintroduction challenges
	Lactose Intolerance	• Lactose breath test	
	Mannitol/Polyol Intolerance	• Mannitol breath test	
	Fructan Intolerance	• Elimination diet with reintroduction challenges	
	Galactan Intolerance		
Low Stomach Acid (hypochlorhydria)		• Heidelberg test (stomach-acid test) • Baking soda test (not validated)	
IBDs	Crohn's Disease	• Colonoscopy	
	Ulcerative Colitis		
Colon Cancer			
Gastroparesis (slow gastric emptying)		• Gastric emptying study	
GERD		• Upper endoscopy • Heidelberg test (stomach acid test) • *H. pylori* test (antibodies in blood) • Ultrasound to look for hiatal hernia	
Gastrointestinal Infections (bacteria, virus, parasites and yeast, including candida overgrowth)		• DNA stool test • Stool culture tests • Urine organic acids (not validated)	
Celiac Disease		• Anti-gliadin antibodies (IgA and IgG) in the blood or stools • Anti-tissue transglutaminase antibodies • Intestinal biopsy • Wheat/gluten proteome reactivity and autoimmunity (not validated)	
Non-Celiac Gluten Sensitivity		• Wheat/gluten proteome reactivity and autoimmunity (not validated) • Elimination diet with reintroduction challenges	
Gallbladder Diseases and Gallstones		• Abdominal ultrasound	
Bowel Obstructions		• X-rays	
Hiatal Hernia (can be a cause of GERD)		• Other imaging techniques	
Increased Intestinal Permeability (leaky gut)		• Lactulose-mannitol intestinal permeability test	
Candida Overgrowth		• Urine organic acids (not validated) • DNA stool test	
Food sensitivities (including dairy, gluten, soy, grains, eggs, nuts, seeds, etc.)		• Skin prick (only detects food allergies) • IgG testing by ELISA (not always accurate) • Elimination diet with reintroduction challenges	
IBS (irritable bowel syndrome)		• Exclusion of all other conditions	

*Note that none of these tests is 100% accurate, especially the breath tests, anti-gliadin antibodies, and biopsy study. Some of these tests also have yet to be validated.

Elimination Diet

From this table, you can see that the elimination diet constitutes a powerful tool to help determine what factors in your diet are contributing to your IBS symptoms. An elimination diet is the best way to go if you experience any kinds of digestive problems, autoimmune conditions, migraines, or other health problems that could be associated with food sensitivities.

The problem with elimination diets is that many people who try one don't know how to proceed or exactly what foods to eliminate. For example, you may have tried an elimination diet that excluded all FODMAP-containing foods for a month. It might have helped you feel better, but most of the time, people who react to FODMAPs also react to other types of foods. They will then have to undertake another elimination diet to exclude gluten and dairy, for example. You can try a specific elimination diet for every food or food group likely to irritate your intestines and worsen your IBS symptoms! Although you can get a lot of information from an elimination diet, you probably don't want to be on one (or more!) for months. Elimination diets are restrictive and should be only a short-term solution. If you want to get answers without having to start all over again, it's important to do it right the first time.

> If you do your elimination diet right the first time,
> you won't have to do it ever again!

Too often, people (or their doctors or friends) blame their health problems on a single food constituent (such as gluten or lactose), when the problem is often much more complex. Aren't you tired of doctors, nutritionists, or friends telling you that [blank] must be your problem? Isn't that a bit simplistic? How could they know? Everyone is different and foods contain many different compounds and ingredients. As great as it would be to have a clear and simple answer to your digestive issues, one just doesn't exist. It's time to take a more holistic approach, one that asks you to listen to and trust your body.

> An elimination diet followed by food challenges is
> the best way to ask all the questions and get all the
> answers you need directly from the most credible
> source of information you can find: your own body.

The next two chapters will help you learn more about the foods you should avoid and the ones you should prioritize during your elimination diet. You will also learn how to implement an elimination diet protocol to get the answers you need to design an optimal diet that will help you manage your IBS symptoms, heal your intestines, and improve your food tolerance in the long term.

CHAPTER 3: Diet to the Rescue!

Even if doctors have told you that diet doesn't have much to do with your IBS and digestive problems, you may have suspected that there's a connection and realized that some foods made your digestive issues worse even if you couldn't quite pinpoint exactly how, when, or why.

After reading this far, you should be able to appreciate how many foods contain substances that can trigger IBS and similar digestive symptoms. That we rarely eat foods in isolation makes things even more complicated. To add to the confusion, the effects of these different substances can be cumulative, and your response to them can be almost immediate or delayed by hours or even days.

These factors may have caused you to give up on previous attempts to get to the bottom of things. As a result, far too many people, no matter what they eat, still experience symptoms and believe they will just have to learn to live with their faulty digestion. Many health professionals, dietitians and gastroenterologists included, will tell you that a balanced diet with everything in moderation is the best way to go. It's now time to learn about another way.

In this chapter, you'll learn that it didn't always used to be this way. Doctors used to recommend dietary interventions to help their patients resolve various digestive disorders. Before pharmaceutical companies transformed health care into "sick" care, there was a time when doctors knew how to use food as medicine.

A Little History

The first description of celiac disease dates back to the first century. A Greek physician known as Aretaeus of Cappadocia (30-90 AD) used the term "celiac affection," from the word "koelia," meaning abdomen in Greek. In his words: "If the stomach is irretentive of the food and if it passes through undigested and crude, and nothing ascends into the body, we call such persons coeliacs." Until the 1950s, the term "celiac disease" was actually used to refer not only to what is now known as the autoimmune condition associated with gluten sensitivity; it also represented all digestive disorders characterized by abdominal distension, abdominal pain, diarrhea, and malnutrition.

In 1888, the English physician Dr. Samuel Gee (1839-1911) revived interest in "celiac disease" and started studying the condition in more depth. He established new diagnostic criteria and determined that this gastrointestinal disorder was associated with putrefaction and fermentation of the food consumed in the intestines (sound similar to SIBO?). He also knew that diet played a big role, suggesting that "if the patient can be cured at all, it must be by means of diet." He also argued that "cow's milk is the least suited kind of food, that highly starchy food, rice, sago, corn flour are unfit" and that "the allowance of farinaceous food must be small." He also implored the medical community to "never forget that what the patient takes beyond his power of digestion does harm," implying that foods that are not digested will either be fermented or trigger food-sensitivity reactions, causing various unsavory digestive symptoms.

Several other doctors around this time observed how intestinal fermentation problems would lead to chronic digestive symptoms. Drs. Luther E. Holt (1855-1924) and Christian A. Herter (1865-1910) stated in a 1908 paper titled "On Infantilism From Chronic Intestinal Infection" that "[t]emporary relapses are very common in the course of this disease, even when great care is taken to prevent them. The most frequent of such relapses is the attempt to encourage growth [referring to children] by the use of increased amounts of carbohydrates."

Later, in 1921, Dr. John Howland read his text "Prolonged Intolerance to Carbohydrates" to the American Pediatric Society, explaining that "from clinical experience it has been found that, of all the elements of food, carbohydrate is the one which must be excluded rigorously; that with this greatly reduced the other elements are almost always well adjusted even though the absorption of fat may not be so satisfactory as in health." Howland developed a three-stage diet based mainly on protein and fat. Only in the last stage were carbohydrates added back, "very gradually with the most careful observation of the digestive capacity … Bread, cereals and potatoes are the last articles which can be allowed. The treatment is time consuming but these patients will repay the effort expended on them."

Dr. Howland worked with Dr. Sidney Valentine Hass (1870-1964), the father of the Specific Carbohydrate Diet (SCD). Dr. Haas was a well-known New York pediatrician specializing in celiac disease in the first half of the twentieth century. Remember that at that time, the term "celiac disease" was still used to refer not only to what is known as celiac disease today but to a broad range of gastrointestinal conditions associated with abdominal bloating, pain, and diarrhea. Haas also noticed that specific carbohydrates from sugars, as well as complex carbohydrates from starchy vegetables and grains, seemed to be problematic for children dealing with this type of digestive disorder.

Dr. Haas' diet, first described in 1924, included a foundation of protein and fat, along with banana and other fruits and vegetables. He also found that banana flour and plantain meal constituted a good source of carbohydrate that was generally well tolerated by his celiac patients. Dr. Haas recommended patients follow his dietary treatment, often called the "banana diet," for at least one year past no symptoms, which took an average of two to three years for most of his patients. Children on the diet tended to get better more quickly, while those with longer-standing digestive issues needed as long as five to seven years to heal completely. This approach allowed Dr. Haas to "cure" 98.5 percent of his celiac patients, a significant advancement considering that celiac disease had a 50-percent fatality rate prior to the advent of his treatment.

Although it is currently believed that there is no cure for celiac disease, Dr. Haas found his treatment would result in patients who "[demonstrated] excellent nutrition, an adequate and happy personality, complete absence of stool abnormality without even temporary diarrhea over short periods, and who can eat a completely unrestricted diet without any recurrence of symptoms." His diet was well accepted in the medicine world as the best treatment for celiac disease. In 1949, Haas was recognized as one of the greatest American pediatricians by the New York Academy of Medicine. Dr. Haas was able to help over 600 celiac patients with his banana diet over a 25-year period. In 1951, he published his life's research and experience in the medical textbook "The Management of Celiac Disease" with his son, Dr. Merrill P. Haas.

Unfortunately, all of Dr. Haas' work sank into oblivion overnight when a research paper about the discovery of the role of gluten in celiac disease was published in the *Lancet* journal less than one year later. The study, based on a small sample of only 10 children, dismissed years of research showing associations between digestive problems and excessive fermentation of specific carbohydrates by attributing the cause of celiac disease only to the gluten protein found in wheat.

Although this discovery was important in better understanding celiac disease, it discarded the role of other dietary factors in most digestive disorders.

From that point on, the diagnosis of celiac disease was reserved for patients showing an atrophy of their intestinal villi, as shown by a biopsy. One of the problems with this new definition of celiac disease was that the majority of the people suffering from gastrointestinal disorders previously diagnosed as celiac disease did not meet the new criteria to "maintain" a celiac diagnosis. As a result, many of them have since been stranded without a diagnosis, or labeled with "IBS" and given very little specific guidance to manage their condition.

As for the people now categorized as having the gluten-sensitive form of celiac disease, the adoption of a gluten-free diet by replacing wheat with gluten-free corn-, rice-, and potato-based breads and baked goods became the primary treatment. Although the simple elimination of gluten may be helpful for some celiac patients, many of them still have villous atrophy after months or years on a 100-percent gluten-free diet. Of course, most doctors attribute this lack of improvement to non-compliance.

Could it be that gluten isn't the only problem in people with celiac disease? Might this condition require a more holistic approach? Beyond the elimination of gluten, should we remove foods that can feed a gut dysbiosis and incorporate foods that promote gut healing? You already know the answers to these important questions—but keep reading to learn more.

The Specific Carbohydrate Diet (SCD)

It was no one else than a mother desperate to help her child who helped rescue the SCD from obscurity. When her eight-year-old daughter Judy, severely affected with ulcerative colitis, was facing the prospect of colon removal, Elaine Gottschall (1921-2005) came upon a last-chance opportunity to visit then-92-year-old Dr. Haas and learn about his dietary approach.

Judy was severely malnourished, suffering from chronic diarrhea and constipation, seizures, and failure to thrive. Within days on the SCD diet, Judy started feeling better and continued to improve until she was completely symptom free after about a year. Not knowing how long she should continue Judy's treatment, since Dr. Haas passed away shortly after Judy started the diet, Gottschall kept Judy on it for seven years. After that, Judy was able to eat almost anything she wanted (with the exception of rice, which she didn't seem to tolerate), and led a normal and healthy life.

This revelation pushed Gottschall to return to school at the age of 47 to study the effects of food on the functioning of the digestive tract. She became a biochemist and obtained a master's degree at the University of Western Ontario in Canada. She published her first book about the SCD in 1987, titled "Food and the Gut Reaction," which was revised several times in the following years and republished as "Breaking the Vicious Cycle: Intestinal Health Through Diet." The vicious cycle Gottschall refers to is the gut dysbiosis that ferments carbohydrates in the intestines and damages the gut lining. This digestive problem impairs carbohydrate digestion and absorption, further feeds the gut dysbiosis and bacterial overgrowth, worsens digestive symptoms, and degrades overall health.

Gottschall modified Dr. Haas' diet and through her book made it available worldwide to people with ulcerative colitis, Crohn's disease, IBS, and even autism. The diet avoids specific carbohydrates like di- and poly-saccharides, mainly found in sugars, starchy and mucilaginous vegetables, and grains, on the basis that people with a damaged gut do not have the ability to secrete the brush border enzymes (secreted by the cells lining your intestines) required to digest these carbohydrates. Undigested and unabsorbed carbohydrates then become food for the bacteria and can contribute to a bacterial overgrowth, worsening all kinds of digestive problems.

Although the term SIBO didn't exist at the time, Gottschall seemed to be aware of the gut-dysbiosis problem that appears to be at the source of many digestive issues. Besides protein and fat, the SCD also allows monosaccharides, a type of carbohydrate that does not require any digestion in order to be absorbed, so your body can thus usually easily absorb them before the bacteria in your intestines start fermenting them. For this reason, the SCD includes carbohydrates from most vegetables, squashes, avocado, ripe fruits, some beans, lactose-free dairy, honey, and even nuts, according to individual tolerance.

The ultimate goal is to slowly starve the overgrowth of bacteria with the intent of positively changing the gut flora and allowing the intestines to heal. The diet includes different stages and a long list of allowed and unpermitted foods based on Gottschall's research. Many SCD-legal cookbooks have been published, including recipes using nut flours and honey to make pancakes, breads, muffins, and other baked goods without any of the problematic carbohydrates. Gottschall was also a big proponent of homemade fermented yogurt as a vehicle for high-quality probiotics. She developed recipes using a 24-hour fermentation period to allow the probiotic bacteria in the yogurt to completely digest the lactose in the milk (since lactose is a disaccharide that should be avoided on the SCD diet).

Table 27 shows an example of a typical menu on the SCD:

Table 27: Typical SCD Menu

Meals	Typical SCD Menu
Breakfast	• Dry curd cottage cheese (to which no milk is added after fermentation) moistened with homemade yogurt • Eggs (boiled, poached, or scrambled) • Pressed grape juice diluted with water • Homemade gelatin made with grape juice, unflavored gelatin, and sweetener (honey or saccharine)
Lunch	• Homemade chicken soup • Broiled beef patty or broiled fish • Cheesecake (homemade from a mixture of eggs, honey, homemade yogurt, dry curd cottage cheese, and vanilla extract) • Homemade gelatin made with juice, unflavored gelatin, and sweetener (honey or saccharine)
Dinner	• Any variation of the breakfast/lunch menu

The doctors behind the SCD believed that "fanatical adherence" was required for the diet to be effective. As Dr. Howland said, "halfway measures are quite unavailing and cause only loss of time" while Dr. Hass argued that "the strictness of this diet cannot be overemphasized nor should the difficulty of adhering to it be minimized." Like her predecessors, Gottschall preached the same dietary strictness: "Infringements will seriously delay recovery and it is unwise to undertake this regimen unless you are willing to follow it with fanatical adherence."

The Gut and Psychology Syndrome (GAPS) Diet

A few decades later, another mother was compelled to research a dietary approach to help her three-year-old son, newly diagnosed with autism. Already a medical doctor, neurologist, and neurosurgeon trained in Russia, Dr. Natasha Campbell-McBride decided to pursue studies in the field of nutrition and autism and completed a second postgraduate degree in human nutrition in the UK. The theories she developed allowed her not only to cure her son of autism but also helped hundreds of her patients suffering with learning disabilities, mental disorders, and other health problems at the Cambridge Nutrition Clinic she founded in 2000. She first published her approach in a book titled "Gut and Psychology Syndrome: Natural Treatment Of Autism, ADHD, Dyslexia, Dyspraxia, Depression and Schizophrenia" in 2004.

The Gut and Psychology Syndrome (GAPS) diet is based on the SCD, but is designed especially for autism and behavioral, cognitive, and mood disorders. Dr. Campbell-McBride's main theory is that a leaky gut is at the source of all these disorders. In addition to avoiding the same carbohydrates as the SCD, the GAPS diet promotes the consumption of raw egg yolk, butter, or ghee, protein from high-quality free-range and pastured animals, and unprocessed, home-cooked foods to heal and seal the gut.

Her dietary approach also includes various supplements (probiotics, cod liver oil, and digestive enzymes) and detoxification methods (juicing and Epsom salt baths). The use of homemade bone broth is also emphasized to promote normal permeability of the gut lining.

Dr. Campbell-McBride is more cautious with dairy than Gottschall and recommends avoiding it completely at first then reintroducing it after six weeks if tolerated. She promotes fermented vegetables, such as sauerkraut and fermented pickles, as a dairy-free alternative to yogurt to correct gut dysbiosis by incorporating gut-friendly bacteria.

The GAPS diet includes an introductory stage followed by six progressive stages before reaching the "full GAPS diet." Campbell-McBride recommends patients stick with her protocol and keep starches and sugars out of their diet for two years before reintroducing more carbohydrates back into their diet. Table 28 shows a typical day on the GAPS diet:

Table 28: Typical GAPS Diet Menu

Meals	Typical GAPS Diet Menu
Breakfast	• Eggs cooked to personal liking • Sausages (with only pure, full-fat minced meat, salt, and pepper) and/or meat, fish, shellfish • Vegetables (cooked or fresh as a salad) • Avocado • Plenty of cold-pressed olive oil as a dressing for the salad and eggs • Cup of warm meat stock as a drink with food • Pancakes made with ground nuts (served with butter and/or honey) • Weak tea with lemon, ginger tea, or mint tea
Lunch	• Homemade vegetable soup or stew in a homemade meat stock • Avocado with meat, fish, shellfish, and raw and/or cooked vegetables, drizzled with olive oil and lemon juice • Cup of warm homemade meat stock as a drink
Dinner	• Any variations of the breakfast/lunch menu

Dr. Campbell-McBride recommends that "about 85% of everything your patient eats daily should be made out of meats, fish, eggs, fermented dairy" and warns that "baking and fruit should be kept out of the diet for a few weeks, and then be limited to snacks between meals and should not replace the main meals. Homemade meat stock, soups, stews and natural fats are not optional - they should be your patient's staples." Unlike with the SCD, however, Dr. Campbell-McBride does not promote fanatical adherence, but rather recommends that her patients adapt the diet to their personal tolerance.

One of the main reasons some people are unsuccessful with SCD or GAPS is that they move too quickly through the different stages of either diet. In addition, some people may not understand how to use the guidelines of these diets to develop their personal diet. Many of those who embark on the SCD or GAPS plan also find these diets very restrictive.

However, it gets easier to find the motivation to stick to a grain-free, starch-free, sugar-free way of eating once your symptoms and your health start improving. Carefully combining the principles of these approaches with the elimination diet protocol described in this book will help you build an optimal diet to manage your symptoms and improve your digestive health.

Ancestral Diets

More recently, a movement built around the adoption of ancestral diets to optimize health has been gaining momentum. Ancestral diets are thought to not only be more optimal for human health, but also more ethical and better for the environment. Examples of ancestral and traditional diets include the Paleo (or Primal, caveman, or Stone Age) diet, as well as the Weston A. Price Foundation (WAPF) diet. Although these diets are not exactly the same as the SCD or the GAPS diet, they are similar in that they are based on REAL foods like animal protein, fats, vegetables, fruits and tubers while eliminating processed foods like grains, soy, sugar, and artificial ingredients.

The Paleo diet is 100-percent free of grains, gluten, legumes, and dairy and is based on:

- Protein from properly raised animals (grass-fed meat, wild-caught fish, and free-range fowl and their eggs).
- Carbohydrates from organic and local vegetables, fruits and tubers.
- Traditional fats from ghee, coconut oil, avocado, olive oil, and nuts and their butters.

The Primal diet is similar to the Paleo diet, though slightly less strict in that it allows the consumption of dairy products. The WAPF diet is similar to both diets but also includes raw and unpasteurized dairy as well as traditionally prepared (soaked and fermented) grains and legumes. The main goal of these diets is to learn from the nutritional wisdom of our ancestors, before the advent of processed foods, to adopt a way of eating that allows us to live a life free from the chronic diseases of civilization like obesity, cardiovascular disease, stroke, diabetes, and cancer.

Many of the principles behind these ancestral diets can also be beneficial to digestive health, especially if combined with the carbohydrate-restricted approach of the SCD and GAPS diets. It's hard to go wrong when eating REAL food that is unprocessed, easy to digest, low in irritants and allergens, and rich in gut-healing and -nourishing nutrients. Indeed, ancestral diets make a lot of sense from a digestive-health standpoint. They can help starve bacterial overgrowth by cutting down on sugar and processed-carb intake while helping you avoid foods that can damage your gut. These ways of eating also prioritize foods that are easier to digest and that provide important nutrients to promote gut healing.

Although many people see their IBS symptoms improve greatly on ancestral diets, this isn't always enough for some people. Despite eliminating gluten, grains, dairy, and legumes, the Paleo diet still allows high-FODMAP foods and carb-rich tubers and fruits that can feed a bacterial overgrowth, as well as hard-to-digest nuts and raw vegetables. Similarly, the WAPF includes some grains, high-FODMAP foods, and dairy products that can trigger digestive symptoms in sensitive people. Using principles of these different dietary plans and combining them with an elimination diet can help you design a diet to optimize both your digestive and overall health.

Why aren't ancestral diets recommended more widely? Unfortunately, most doctors prioritize drugs over dietary changes. Consider that the average doctor visit now lasts less than 10 minutes, and most nutritionists unfortunately follow the dietary guidelines formulated by agencies that are influenced by powerful lobbying groups like grain producers and the processed-foods industry. And who finances the conferences and continuing-education sessions for health professionals? Pharmaceutical companies and the food industry. A little bias in the information provided is thus, regrettably, to be expected. Money rules the world, and diets and REAL food can't be patented.

Hopefully, the general public will come to a point where it becomes sick and tired of being sick and tired and starts looking for answers elsewhere. That's probably exactly where you're standing right now. The good news is that it doesn't cost anything to give REAL food a try. There are no dangerous side effects associated with REAL food, making it exactly what your body needs to regain its natural health and vitality.

Following a strict elimination diet based on REAL food is not necessarily easy. Explaining the principles of this way of eating and convincing people to try it is not easy either, and maybe that's why many doctors don't bother. But people suffering from IBS and other digestive disorders should at least be given the opportunity to learn about this alternative option. You have a lot more to gain than to lose by applying these principles.

The problem is that most doctors and dietitians aren't even aware of these approaches, they think their patients won't be able to make the required dietary changes, or they simply dismiss these approaches because of a lack of clinical evidence.

Despite hundreds of reports of people who have managed their digestive symptoms successfully with the SCD, the GAPS diet, or another similar approach, there is unfortunately a lack of scientific evidence evaluating these dietary approaches.

This is why the Crohn's and Colitis Foundation of America, in an article titled "The Specific Carbohydrate Diet: Does It Work?" does not recommend the SCD: "We're not ruling out the possibility that it works, but you need more than a few successes to establish proof. In the absence of that, it's hard to recommend this or any diet." But just because we don't have a lot of rigorous scientific studies backing up these diets doesn't mean they don't work! And the simple fact that these diets don't come with dangerous side effects (unlike drugs) and don't cost anything (besides the cost of food) makes them a worthy element in your arsenal against digestive problems.

The few studies that have examined the efficacy of the SCD actually showed very promising results. One of them, published by Nieves and Jackson in *Tennessee Medicine* in 2004, reported two case studies of a 51-year-old woman with ulcerative colitis and a 24-year-old woman with Crohn's disease who saw significant relief from their digestive disorders within one month of adopting the SCD. They were also able to manage their conditions with diet alone and go off their medications entirely.

The results of a pilot study conducted by the University of Massachusetts, presented at the "Clinical and Translational Science Research Retreat" in 2011 also showed great potential for an anti-inflammatory dietary approach based on the SCD. The study included 11 participants aged between 19 and 70 and suffering from either Crohn's disease or ulcerative colitis for periods ranging between one and 24 years. Over a period of six to 10 months, 100 percent of the patients experienced significant improvements in their symptoms and nine out of the 11 patients were able stop taking their anti-inflammatory medications.

Unfortunately, that's all the published data available to date. There are not many randomized clinical trials looking at these diets and there may never be. Researchers can get a lot more money from pharmaceutical companies and food manufacturers than they can launching a study on a REAL-food-based diet.

Make Your Own Experiment

What are your choices, then? You can either wait patiently for these studies to be conducted with no guarantee that they will, or you can decide to conduct your own experiment. The latter option will help you determine the most important piece of information, after all: the approach that works *for you*.

What's the best way to find out? Give it a try! What do you have to lose? Of course, it is best to explore this new dietary approach in concert with your health care provider, especially if you are on medications or affected by any health conditions. But using food, especially REAL food, to try to improve your digestive health is a very safe thing to do. The worst-case scenario is you don't see any improvements and have to give up some of your favorite foods for a month or two. Sounds worth a try, doesn't it?

Many health care practitioners have forgotten about elimination diets since they believe their patients aren't ready to do the work needed to benefit from them, but elimination diets have been considered the gold standard in identifying food intolerances for decades. It's time to use this under-utilized approach to your advantage. Are you ready to start your own diet experiment?

DESIGNING YOUR OPTIMAL DIET

Before learning about how to proceed with an elimination diet protocol, you first need to know what food groups you should eat and which you should eliminate. There are seven important factors that go into crafting your personal elimination diet protocol:

The 7 Factors to Design Your Optimal Diet
1. REAL, Unprocessed Food
2. Easy to Digest
3. Low in Irritants and Allergens
4. Anti Inflammatory
5. Nutrient Dense
6. Carb Restricted
7. Customized

REAL, Unprocessed Food: The food you eat should be REAL food, not processed. REAL food is more nourishing and makes it easier to figure out how your body reacts to the food you eat by minimizing the number of variables in the equation. If you react poorly to a slice of bread that contains 10 ingredients, how do you know if it's the wheat, the high-fructose corn syrup, the yeast, the inulin, or the dairy? Perhaps the culprit is the polysorbate 60, tartaric acid, or potassium acid tartrate. You can imagine how this problem would grow exponentially if you eat many multi-ingredient processed foods like this at breakfast, lunch, and dinner, and for snacks. Stick to REAL food to keep things simpler and healthier.

Easy to Digest: You need to be able to digest and absorb the food you eat not only to get the nutrition your body needs to be heal and be healthy, but also to prevent fermentation in your intestines. Incompletely digested foods can feed a bacterial overgrowth (especially carbohydrates) or trigger food-sensitivity reactions (especially proteins).

Low in Irritants and Allergens, Anti Inflammatory, and Nutrient Dense: Food can either make you worse or better. You need to avoid foods that can damage your gut and replace them with foods that promote health. Avoiding irritating, allergenic, and inflammatory foods is the first step to steer your digestive health in the right direction. Replacing problematic foods with anti-inflammatory, nutrient-dense ones to lower inflammation and nourish your body will help promote both intestinal healing and overall health.

Carb Restriction will help you control your gut dysbiosis. You may not need to follow a carb-restricted diet forever, but limiting refined starches and sugar is important to prevent excessive fermentation in your intestines and correct any gut-flora imbalance.

Customization is probably the most important factor. There is no one-size-fits-all approach with diet. Whether you want to lose weight, manage your diabetes, or improve your athletic performance, you need to find what works *for you*. Eating to optimize your digestive health is no exception.

A lot of foods you might be eating on a daily basis don't meet all of the seven criteria needed to construct your own optimal diet and improve your digestive health. These non-optimal foods include:

- Grains (with and without gluten)
- Dairy
- Legumes
- Sugar
- Starches
- Some fruits
- Nuts
- Seeds
- Some vegetables
- Processed foods

But don't worry. This doesn't mean that you won't be able to eat these foods for the rest of your life—just that you'll do better without them for a little while, at least during the elimination phase of the protocol, which lasts about one month. There will still be plenty of foods left for you to eat, and you should be able to add back many of the "non-optimal" foods eventually, depending on your individual tolerance.

Table 29 gives you an overview of what foods you should avoid or prioritize during your elimination diet to help you see the quickest improvement in your digestive health and gather as much information as you can.

Table 29: Foods to Avoid or Prioritize in the Elimination Diet

Food Groups	Potentially Problematic	Generally Well Tolerated
Protein	• Soy • Legumes (beans, lentils, peanuts, peanut butter) • Nuts*, seeds, and their butters • Dairy products (with the exception of ghee)* • Eggs*	• Animal protein (poultry, meat, fish, seafood)
Fats	• Refined oils (soybean oils, canola oil, corn oil, cottonseed oil, sunflower oil, margarine) • Hydrogenated fats (shortening and trans fat) • Commercial salad dressings and mayonnaise	• Ghee (clarified butter) • Cold-pressed oils (coconut oil, extra-virgin olive oil, macadamia nut oil, avocado oil) • Animal fats (tallow, lard, duck fat)
Grains	• All grains (with or without gluten, including pseudo-grains)	• None
Vegetables	• High-FODMAP vegetables* • Nightshades* • Cruciferous vegetables* • Starchy vegetables* • Raw vegetables*	• Cooked low-FODMAP vegetables (with the exception of the nightshade and cruciferous families)
Fruits	• All fruits*	• None
Sweets	• Sugars of all kinds (HFCS, maple syrup*, honey*, table sugar, dextrose, sugar alcohols, etc.)	• None
Beverages	• Alcohol (with and without gluten) • Caffeine (coffee, chocolate, energy drinks and black tea) • Sugary drinks (soft drinks, juices, punches and caffeinated drinks)	• Water (regular, sparkling, and/or with lemon/lime juice) • Rooibos tea • Green tea • Homemade bone broth
Other	• Artificial ingredients (MSG, flavorings, guar gum, xanthan gums, etc.) • Yeast*	• Unrefined salt • Apple cider vinegar • Chives • Fresh herbs and spices

*Eliminate these foods during the first part of the elimination diet. You will likely be able to bring back some of them during the reintroduction phase.

The goal of all these dietary changes is to correct the root causes of your digestive problems. Potentially problematic ingredients can worsen your gut dysbiosis, leaky gut, inflammation, and food sensitivities, as depicted in Figure 10.

Figure 10

root causes
of your digestive symptoms

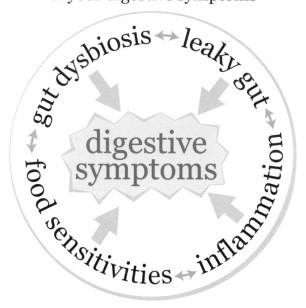

REAL food that meets the seven factors to build your optimal diet will help you stop this vicious cycle so you can improve your gut flora, seal your leaky gut, and decrease your food sensitivities. The elimination diet protocol (Chapter 5), in conjunction with stress management (Chapter 6) and appropriate supplementation (Chapter 7), will help you follow the four steps to optimizing your digestion and overall health (see Figure 11).

Figure 11

the 4 steps
{to better digestion and health}

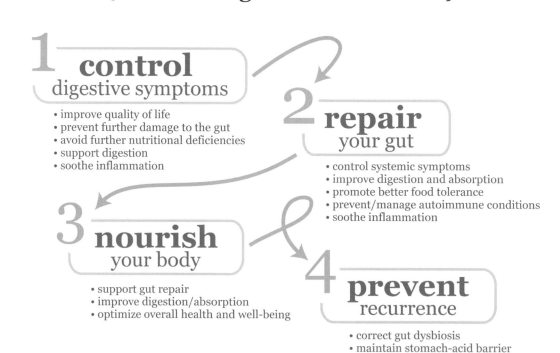

1 control digestive symptoms
- improve quality of life
- prevent further damage to the gut
- avoid further nutritional deficiencies
- support digestion
- soothe inflammation

2 repair your gut
- control systemic symptoms
- improve digestion and absorption
- promote better food tolerance
- prevent/manage autoimmune conditions
- soothe inflammation

3 nourish your body
- support gut repair
- improve digestion/absorption
- optimize overall health and well-being

4 prevent recurrence
- correct gut dysbiosis
- maintain stomach-acid barrier
- promote regular cleansing waves
- strengthen your immune system

Eliminating Potentially Problematic Foods

Many of the foods that may be contributing to your digestive problems should be avoided in the first phase of your elimination diet since they may contain substances that can irritate your intestines, promote inflammation, provoke food sensitivities, or result in excessive fermentation in your digestive tract. After a few weeks, you should be able to follow the reintroduction protocol and bring back some of these foods, to determine whether or not they still cause problems for you. Adopting a stricter approach at the beginning of your elimination diet should help you get your digestive symptoms under control more quickly so you can then move on to the next phase.

GRAINS

Grains have been at the foundation of the food pyramid for decades and now occupy a large quarter of the USDA's "MyPlate," released in 2011 to replace the former "MyPyramid." But are grains really healthy for you? If you suffer from IBS or other digestive disorders resulting in similar digestive symptoms, it is likely that your doctor recommended you eat more fiber from "healthy" whole grains. In many cases, however, grains only contribute to worsening your symptoms. Whether you react to the gluten, fructans (FODMAPs), insoluble fiber, or starches, food products made from grains (such as breads, pasta, and baked goods) are loaded with potentially problematic ingredients.

PROCESSED (*UNREAL*) FOODS

Most grains and grain products are *not* REAL food. REAL food is food that you can obtain or prepare yourself in your kitchen. Meat, eggs, fish, vegetables, fruits, nuts, and tubers are good examples of REAL food. REAL foods are those for which you know the source and could even find yourself in nature with the right skills. All you should need to do before putting REAL food on your plate is cook and season it—and even these steps may be optional.

Grain products, on the other hand, need to be processed extensively before they become edible. Yes, even whole grains. You won't find a bread loaf or puffed-rice breakfast cereal growing in a field. Grains need to be dehulled and processed into flour before being shaped it into your favorite breakfast cereals, pasta, or baked goods. Many other processed ingredients are usually added to the mix to produce variety in the final products and make them shelf stable.

If you tried to make grain-based foods yourself at home, you would expend a lot of time and energy for very little food. All the cultivating, harvesting, dehulling, and grinding of grains would produce just a few cups of flour at the end of a whole summer of hard labor—probably enough for only three or four loaves of bread!

CARBOHYDRATES, GLYCEMIC INDEX, AND GLYCEMIC LOAD

In addition to being processed, food products made from grains are also very high in carbohydrates. All carbohydrates, whether in the form of starches or sugars, are broken down into single molecules of sugars (mainly glucose) during the digestion process. Once the sugars derived from carbohydrates enter your bloodstream, they elevate your blood-sugar levels. If you consume a lot of grains, it is very likely that your blood-sugar levels fluctuate quite widely throughout the day, affecting your energy levels similarly (see Figure 12).

This concept is known as the glycemic index (GI) and glycemic load (GL). The large blood-sugar swings associated with high-GI and -GL foods can predispose you to heart disease, obesity, PCOS, type 2 diabetes, and even cancer. Foods with the lowest GI and GL values belong mainly to the REAL, unprocessed food category (meat, fish, eggs, vegetables, fruits, nuts, and healthy fats) and are therefore more protective for your health.

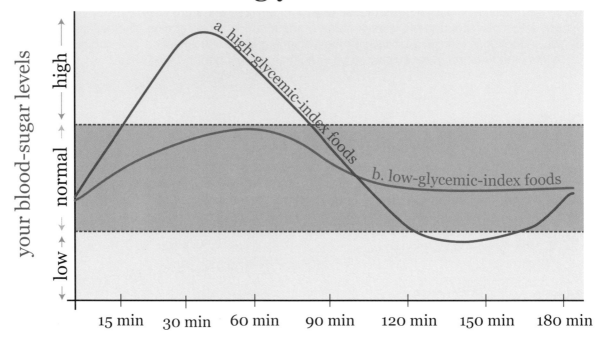

Figure 12

the glycemic index

a. Foods with a high glycemic index (GI), such as bread, breakfast cereals, and rice, cause a quick rise in your blood-sugar levels followed by a quick crash. The fluctuations in blood-sugar levels associated with high-GI foods result in unstable energy levels and an increased risk for many chronic diseases (diabetes, obesity, heart disease).

b. Foods with a low glycemic index, such as vegetables, fruits, animal protein, nuts, and fats, keep your blood-sugar levels more stable.

Foods with a GI value above 70 are considered high GI, while a value between 56 and 69 is considered medium GI (see Table 30). High-GI and -GL foods can send your blood-sugar levels on a roller coaster. Many breads, breakfast cereals, rice, baked goods, and other grain-based products fall into this category.

Table 30: Glycemic Index and Glycemic Load Scales

Categories	Glycemic Index (carb quality)	Glycemic Load* (carb quality + quantity)	
		Per serving of food	Per day
Low (healthier)	55 or less	Below 10	80 or less
Medium	56 to 69	11-19	81-119
High (less healthy)	70 and more	20 and more	120 and more

*Unlike the GI, which only represents the quality of the carbohydrates in a food, the GL also takes into consideration the quantity. The GL values of the foods you eat throughout the day can be added to obtain your daily dietary GL.

What about whole and unrefined grains? It's commonly believed that whole grains are nutritionally superior to refined grains, since whole grains are less processed and contain more of their natural nutrients. Some researchers have hypothesized that preserving the fiber of the bran of whole grains could slow down the rise in blood sugar after a meal—but it does *not* seem to work that way. Data actually show that multigrain bread, sugar-free breakfast cereal, and brown rice all have GI and GL values similar to those of many refined grains (see Table 31).

Table 31: GI and GL Values of Various Foods

	Foods	Serving Size	GI	GL*	↑↓
Grains	White bread	2 slices (2 oz or 60 g)	70-75	20-26	
	Multigrain bread	2 slices (2 oz or 60 g)	53-80	14-18	
	Gluten-free multigrain bread	2 slices (2 oz or 60 g)	79	20	↑↑↑ Medium to High GI/GL ↑↑↑
	Sugar-Free Breakfast Cereals (corn flakes, puffed rice, or oat rings)	1 oz (30 g)	74-93	19-23	
	Donuts	1 donut	75-76	15-17	
	Muffins (wild blueberry and 10-grain)	1 muffin	57	22	
	Pretzels	1 oz (30 g)	81	18	
	Rice cakes	2	82	12	
	Rice, white	1 cup	91	41	
	Rice, brown	1 cup	66-87	27-36	
	Spaghetti, white	1 cup	42-50	18-22	
	Spaghetti, whole wheat	1 cup	45	15	
	Spaghetti, gluten free	1 cup	51	23	
REAL Food	Most fruits	1 medium	24-52	4-8	↑ Low GI/GL ↓
	Non-starchy vegetables	1 cup	Less than 15	Below 1-2	
	Sweet potatoes	1 medium	44-46	10	
	Meat, poultry, fish, and eggs	3 oz.	0	0	
	Coconut oil, olive oil, or ghee	1 tbsp.	0	0	
	Nuts	1 oz (30 g)	Below 15	Below 1-2	

*The glycemic index (GI) only represents the quality of the carbohydrates, while the glycemic load (GL) concept considers both the quality and quantity of carbohydrates consumed. Unlike GI values, GL values are additive for each of your meals consumed throughout the day.

The large amounts of starches, and sometimes added sugars, found in grain products can also feed a bacterial overgrowth (SIBO), as well as other types of gastrointestinal infections and gut-dysbiosis problems, especially if your digestion is impaired and you are not able to absorb carbohydrates before your bacteria do.

GLUTEN AND FRUCTANS

Another problem with many grains is the gluten they contain. Even if your test for celiac disease comes back negative, you can't really rule out gluten sensitivity. As discussed extensively in Chapter 2, non-celiac gluten sensitivity is much more widespread than celiac disease, especially in people with digestive disorders. Unfortunately, most available testing methods are far from 100-percent accurate. The gold standard to determine whether gluten is contributing to your symptoms is to follow an elimination diet as described in the next chapters. Table 32 reminds you where grains (both with and without gluten) can be found.

Table 32: Gluten and Gluten-Free Grains

Categories		Grains
With Gluten		Wheat, barley, rye, spelt, regular oats, kamut, triticale
Gluten Free	Grains	Gluten-free oats, rice, sorghum, corn, millet, wild rice
	Pseudo-grains	Quinoa, amaranth, buckwheat, chia, teff

Besides their potentially problematic gluten, wheat, barley and rye are the largest source of fructans, a type of FODMAP that is known to trigger various gastrointestinal side effects. Many grain products contain additional problematic ingredients such as chicory root, inulin, and psyllium, as well as thickeners and gums that can be fermented excessively in your intestines. And you already understand what happens when the food you eat is fermented in your gut!

GLUTEN-FREE GRAINS

Although gluten-free and "pseudo" grains do not contain the same potentially problematic protein for people with gluten sensitivity, they contain other forms of gluten and other hard-to-digest compounds that can irritate a damaged digestive system.

Some studies have shown that people with celiac disease and gluten sensitivity can still react to gluten-free grains like quinoa, corn, rice, and gluten-free breads. Plus, most gluten-free products actually contain more carbohydrates and less fiber, and have a higher glycemic index and glycemic load, than their gluten-containing versions. These factors could be very problematic if you have SIBO, a gut dysbiosis, or blood-sugar issues, or are overweight. On top of that, manufacturers of gluten-free products almost always add other potentially problematic substances such as gums, thickeners, chicory root, inulin and FODMAP-containing ingredients.

Many gluten-free grains, especially corn, often come from genetically modified crops (at least in North America). The Environmental Protection Agency claims that the *Bacillus thuringiensis* toxins found in genetically modified corn is destroyed during the digestion process, but a Canadian study published in 2011 showed detectable levels of these toxins in the blood of women who had consumed GM corn. These results show clearly that some of these toxins resist digestion and can be absorbed into the body. The long-term consequences of consuming these GM foods are unknown, but we know that there *are* potentially serious health consequences that could affect your risk of allergies or food sensitivities, fertility, and even infant mortality. Digestive health is also on the list of potential problems associated with GM foods like corn. Another recent European study from 2012 showed that the consumption of GM corn was associated with increased intestinal permeability (leaky gut), a good reason in and of itself to avoid all grains and grain-based foods.

NUTRITIONAL DEFICIENCIES

If you have been struggling with digestive problems, you are at risk of developing nutrient deficiencies. If your digestion is not working properly, your body can have difficulty absorbing the nutrients in the food you eat, especially if your intestines are damaged, irritated, and inflamed. Some of these deficiencies can also be due to a gut dysbiosis since bacteria and other microbes can steal nutrients from you.

Eating grains can contribute further to the problem, not only because of the potential to damage your gut and worsen a bacterial overgrowth, but also because of the anti-nutrients they contain. Anti-nutrients are substances that do the opposite of what nutrients do. Instead of nourishing you, anti-nutrients deprive you of the important nutrients your body needs. Anti-nutrients in grains can bind easily to the minerals calcium, iron, magnesium, and zinc, making them impossible to absorb. This might explain, for example, why your iron-enriched breakfast cereals and granola bars may not do much in helping you overcome your iron-deficiency anemia. Removing grains can help you correct nutrient deficiencies by making the minerals in your diet easier to absorb instead of flushing them down the toilet.

NUTRIENT DENSITY

If you have nutritional deficiencies as a result of your digestive issues, it is important to consume nutrient-dense foods. Nutrient density refers to the amount of nutrients per unit of food. While whole grains are more nutrient dense than refined grains, they are still far behind meat, fish, eggs, vegetables, fruits, and even healthy fats like avocado, ghee, and extra-virgin olive oil.

The next table shows you the nutrient density of various food groups. The higher the number, the more nutrients the food group provides per calorie. Vegetables are the clear winners, followed by seafood, lean meats, and fruits. It is important to remember that nutrient bioavailability has not been taken into account in this calculation, and it would be very difficult to do so since we still don't yet know enough about it. But we do know that the bioavailability of many nutrients (such as iron, vitamin A, and omega-3 fats) found in animal products such as meats and seafood is often higher than that of the nutrients in whole grains, which means that their scores should actually be a bit higher.

Table 33: Nutrient Density Scores of Various Foods

Nuts & seeds	Refined grains	Whole grains	Whole milk	Fruits	Lean meats	Seafood	Vegetables
38	Less than 44	44	44	48	50	65	81

*Adapted from Cordain L, et al. **Origins and Evolution of the Western Diet: Health Implications for the 21st Century.** *Am J Clin Nutr.* 2005. 81: 341-354.

Also, because diets rich in whole grains tend to be lower in fat, they can make it more difficult for your body to absorb fat-soluble nutrients (vitamins A, D, E, and K, omega-3 fatty acids, CoQ10, and various antioxidants). Grains can also displace nutrient-denser foods such as vegetables, seafood, and lean meats, preventing you from getting the nutrients you need. You can see a good depiction of this phenomenon in the next table. Skipping the bread in your sandwich in favor of more protein-rich foods, vegetables, and healthy fats could help you get more nutrients with the same number of calories.

Table 34: Nutritional Comparison of Grain-Filled and Grain-Free Meal

Nutrient Comparison		Typical Lunch		Grain-Free Lunch	
Menu		Sandwich: • 2 slices whole-wheat bread • 3 oz. beef sirloin • 1 tbsp. light mayonnaise Salad: • 1 cup lettuce • ½ cup cherry tomatoes • 1 tbsp. fat-free ranch dressing Dessert: • 1 small low-fat bran muffin • 1 medium apple		Salad: • 1 cup lettuce • 1 cup spinach • 2 tbsp. grated carrots • ½ cup cherry tomatoes • ½ cup steamed broccoli • 6 oz. beef sirloin • 1 tbsp. olive oil • ¼ avocado • Balsamic vinegar Dessert: • 1 medium apple	
Nutrition	Calories	571 calories		566 calories	
	Carbs	87 g (56% of calories)		36 g (23% of calories)	
	Fiber	16 g (64% of DRI*)		12 g (48% of DRI*)	
	Protein	32 g (22% of calories)		43 g (31% of calories)	
	Fat	14 g (22% of calories)		30 g (46% of calories)	
Vitamins	Vitamin A	3,399 IU	25%*	10,059 IU	74%*
	Vitamin C	22.5 mg	30%*	95 mg	127%*
	Vitamin E	2.5 IU	11%*	9.4 IU	42%*
	Vitamin B1	0.49 mg	45%*	0.31 mg	28%*
	Vitamin B2	0.43 mg	39%*	0.5 mg	46%*
	Vitamin B3	10.9 mg	78%*	14 mg	100%*
	Vitamin B5	1.5 mg	31%*	2.5 mg	51%*
	Vitamin B6	0.87 mg	67%*	1.6 mg	121%*
	Vitamin B12	0.98 mcg	41%*	1.9 mcg	77%*
Minerals	Calcium	195 mg	20%*	148 mg	15%*
	Iron	5.2 mg	29%*	5.2 mg	29%**
	Zinc	5.4 mg	67%*	8.0 mg	100%*
	Magnesium	123 mg	40%*	116 mg	37%*
	Potassium	1,010 mg	21%*	1,677 mg	35%*

*The % of DRI corresponds to the percentage of each of your daily nutrient requirements provided by each meal. **Although both meals contain the same amount of iron, its bioavailability is higher in the grain-free meal (because more of it is in the heme form and there is more vitamin C to enhance its absorption); using United States Department of Agriculture USDA National Nutrient Database Food Search for Windows, Version 1.0, Database Version SR23.

In this table, both meals provide about the same number of calories, but the grain-free lunch is clearly nutritionally superior. In fact, it provides more of 10 out of 14 nutrients than the typical lunch based on whole grains. Who said you need grains to meet your daily nutritional requirements?

WHAT ABOUT FIBER?

Are you worried that you won't be able to get enough fiber in your diet without eating grains? First, it is important to know that grains are not the only dietary source of fiber. You can actually find a lot more fiber (per calorie) in vegetables. Fruits, tubers, nuts, and seeds are also excellent sources. Refer to Table 35 below to see how much fiber is found in these REAL foods. As a bonus, these foods provide a lot more minerals, vitamins, antioxidants, and other important nutrients than even whole grains.

Table 35: Fiber Content of Various Foods

Food Group	REAL Food	Serving Size	Fiber (g)*
Vegetables	Broccoli, cooked	1 cup	5.1
	Leafy greens, cooked	1 cup	4.3-5.1
	Brussels sprouts, cooked	1 cup	4.1
	Squash (spaghetti, butternut)	1 cup	2.2-6.6
	Onions, cooked	1 cup	2.9
	Cauliflower, cooked	1 cup	2.9
	Eggplant, cooked	1 cup	2.5
	Carrots, raw or cooked	1 cup	2.3
	Cabbage, raw or cooked	1 cup	1.8-2.8
	Leafy greens, raw	2 cups	1.3-2.1
	Sauerkraut, raw	¼ cup	0.9
Tubers	Sweet potatoes, cooked (without skin)	1 cup	8.2
	Plantain, cooked	1 cup	3.5-4.6
	Potatoes, cooked (without skin)	1 cup	3.1
Fruits	Berries	1 cup	3.6-8.0
	Pear	1 medium	5.5
	Mango	1 medium	5.4
	Apple	1 medium	4.4
	Dried figs	5	4.1
	Banana	1 medium	3.1
	Orange	1 medium	2.3
Nuts	Nuts	1 oz	1.9-3.5
	Nut butter	2 tbsp	3.2
	Almond flour	2 tbsp	1.5
	Coconut (unsweetened, dried)	2 tbsp	4.6
	Coconut flour	2 tbsp	6-10
Fats	Avocado	1 medium	13.5
	Olives	5 jumbo	1

*United States Department of Agriculture. **USDA National Nutrient Database Food Search for Windows**, Version 1.0, Database Version SR23.

During the first phase of the elimination diet, you'll be obtaining your dietary fiber exclusively from vegetables, but you should be able, over time and according to your tolerance, to introduce other fiber-rich foods like fruits, tubers, nuts, nut butters, and nut flours. In fact, it's on purpose that the first phase of your elimination diet is a bit lower in fiber. Getting too much fiber, especially the insoluble kind found in whole grains, is a bad idea if your intestines are already irritated and inflamed. If you've experimented with a higher-fiber diet in the past for your IBS and digestive problems, per your doctor's recommendations, you may have noticed that more fiber usually means more symptoms. Insoluble fiber is found mostly in the bran of grains, which means that wheat bran, high-fiber cereals, and other "healthy" whole grains could be worsening your digestion. Insoluble fiber is not digested at all and moves intact through your whole digestive tract. If your intestines are damaged, eating insoluble fiber from grains is a bit like rubbing a scrub brush on an open wound. Give your intestines a break and decrease your insoluble fiber intake by going grain free.

Food quality matters!

GRAINS, FIBER, AND CONSTIPATION

If you're worried about becoming constipated not eating grains, you'll be relieved to know that fiber is not the only—or even the most important—factor in regular bowel movements, despite what doctors and dietitians insist.

When Arctic explorers visited the Inuit for years at a time to study their way of life in the early twentieth century, they had no choice but to adopt the Nordic ancestral (fiber-free) diet of wild meat and fatty fish. These explorers inspired researchers at the Bellevue Hospital in New York to conduct a small experiment with two of the explorers to observe the impact on their health of eating an all-meat and -fat diet for a period of over one year. The results, published in 1930, showed undisturbed bowel elimination throughout the study. As the doctor in charge of the study reported: "The stools were smaller than usual, well formed, and had an inoffensive, slightly pungent odor. No flatus was noted." Bottom line: you don't need fiber to poop.

The bulk (75 percent) of your stools is actually *not* fiber, as most people believe, but dead bacteria. What you really require for an easy daily number two is a healthy gut flora. Probiotics and fermented foods can help (more on this topic later). In addition to gut-friendly bacteria, adequate fat intake can help you stay regular since fat and the bile it releases can promote colon motility (the movement of your intestines). The grain-free, sugar-free elimination diet described in the next pages is higher in fat than the standard American diet, which should help keep things moving inside your intestines.

LOW-RESIDUE DIETS

Some doctors and gastroenterologists recommend the opposite of a high-fiber diet and advise their patients to go on a low-residue diet to avoid the irritating insoluble fibers in whole grains. A low-residue diet basically eliminates whole grains, fibrous vegetables, and fruits with seeds, skins, or membranes. One example is the BRAT diet, which is based on bland, low-fiber foods like bananas, rice, apple sauce, and toast. The problem is that refined grains (white breads, sugary cereals, crackers, cakes, and cookies), sweets, sugary beverages, starchy vegetables, and processed foods are all *allowed* on a low-residue diet.

While a low-residue diet may help to alleviate some irritation by taking insoluble fiber out of the mix, it still includes many problematic ingredients like gluten, sugar, and other refined ingredients that can promote inflammation and induce GI problems. Processed low-residue foods also include a lot of carbohydrates that could feed a bacterial overgrowth or another form of gut dysbiosis. If that weren't enough, a low-residue diet tends to lack the nutritional density required to provide your intestines with all the important nutrients they needs to repair themselves. You need all the nutrients you can get your hands on to recover your optimal digestive health. Only REAL food fits the bill.

BOTTOM LINE

There are NO good reasons to keep grains in your diet. The gluten they contain, as well as their high glycemic carbohydrates, fructans, poor nutrient density, and extensive processing make them unworthy of the title of REAL food. Although some people can *tolerate* grains, no one really benefits from eating them—especially people with digestive issues. Adopting a grain-free diet can be a scary change, but what do you really have to lose? The *worst* that can happen is that you miss your favorite foods for a few weeks. Give it a try for a month or two to see how your body responds. This will likely be all the motivation you need to stick to a grain-free diet for the long term.

Dairy

Dairy is also a staple for most people, and this food group, like grains, occupies a predominant place in the pyramid of recommended foods. But is dairy a good choice for optimal digestive health? Is it a REAL food? The answer is it depends on what type of dairy we're talking about!

Most of the dairy products people eat on a daily basis should indeed be considered processed foods. The skim and pasteurized milk, fruit-flavored low-fat yogurt, and American cheese you find at the grocery store come from cows raised in confinement and fed an unnatural diet of grains instead of grass, making their milk less nutritious. The milk from grain-fed cows is lower in vitamins A, D, E, and K_2, conjugated linoleic acid (CLA, an anti-cancer compound), and omega-3 fats. Cows are not meant to eat grains, but a grain-based diet causes them to produce more milk and thus more profits for the dairy industry. Despite labels that depict cows grazing in the meadows, the majority of dairy cattle don't ever get to see pastures or even natural sunlight.

On top of that, most dairy is now pasteurized, homogenized, and supplemented with sugar, additives, flavorings, and other processed ingredients. These processing steps denature milk and further decrease its nutritional value, which is already reduced by the cows' grain-based diet.

UNPASTEURIZED AND PASTURED IS BEST

To be considered REAL food, dairy products should come from pastured, grass-fed animals. Don't confuse *pastured* with *pasteurized*!

- *Pastured* cows are allowed access to meadows where they can graze and ruminate, eating their natural diet of 100-percent grass, free to walk around and enjoy the warming rays of the sun.
- *Pasteurized*, on the other hand, refers to the process of heating milk to sterilize it with the goal of killing any potentially harmful bacteria that could be present in the milk.

But the risks of getting sick with raw (unpasteurized) milk are unfortunately greatly exaggerated. You are actually more likely to get food poisoning by eating deli meat or even *pasteurized* milk than by drinking raw milk, according to a report published by the Center for Food Safety and Applied Nutrition of the FDA and the Food Safety and Inspection Service of the USDA (2003).

Raw milk from pastured cows is safe, especially if you know the farmer who raised them and have visited the farm. It's also more ethical for the animals, better for the environment, and more nutritious for you. Fermented dairy products, such as yogurt, kefir and cheese, as well as cream, butter, and ghee, produced from the milk of grass-fed cows (or other ruminants) would all be considered REAL food. But even if you choose the highest-quality dairy products, they may still not a good option for *you* if you are dealing with digestive problems.

CASEIN

Both the protein and carbohydrate parts of dairy can contribute to your IBS symptoms. The protein casein is hard to digest and can trigger a food sensitivity reaction in some people, especially if you have a leaky gut.

Casein is found in all dairy products, with the exception of ghee (clarified butter), which is supposed to be 100-percent (or almost) casein free. Butter and cream contain only traces of casein, but it can be enough to trigger a reaction in sensitive people. Milk, cheese, and yogurt have the highest casein content and should be avoided, at least during the initial phase of your elimination diet.

You may have heard of A2 milk, a type of milk produced by Jersey cows, goats, buffalo, camels, and a few other ancestral ruminant species. There are two different types of casein: A1 and A2. Most of the dairy products available in grocery stores come from Holstein cows and contain predominantly the A1 type of casein. Some people believe that A2 casein is easier on the digestive system. No studies have been done to validate this observation, but it is something to keep in mind if you decide to reintroduce dairy into your diet. If you don't tolerate regular dairy products, you might be able to better tolerate A2 milk and dairy products made from this milk. Being aware of these little differences is really important to help you understand how foods affect you so you can design an optimal diet customized just for you (as explained in Chapter 5).

Casein is the most abundant protein in dairy, corresponding to about 80 percent of the protein in dairy. Although casein is more likely to be problematic, whey is another dairy protein that can also cause food-sensitivity reactions in some people. Going dairy free will help you avoid both casein and whey, but beware of dairy-derived casein-free products. Whey protein, for example, is free of casein but can still trigger food reactions in sensitive people.

LACTOSE

The natural carbohydrate found in milk and many other dairy products is lactose. Lactose is a short-chain fermentable carbohydrate and therefore belongs to the FODMAP family. Lactose content is highest in milk, followed by yogurt, ice cream, and fresh cheese. Aged cheese and cream have very little lactose, while butter and ghee have practically none.

Lactose intolerance is a common source of GI upset, especially in people with digestive problems. Many adults seem to lose the ability to digest lactose as they age. Lactase, the enzyme required to digest lactose, is secreted by the cells lining your intestines. If your intestines are damaged and inflamed, your ability to produce lactase and break down lactose will be reduced. Lactose is a disaccharide, a carbohydrate made of the two sugars glucose and galactose, and it is *impossible* for your body to absorb lactose if it isn't first broken down into glucose and galactose. Unabsorbed lactose will be fermented in your intestines, either by the bacteria in your small intestines (if you have SIBO) or those in your colon.

Primary lactase deficiency is thought to be the most common form of lactose intolerance. People with this deficiency lack the specific gene to maintain their intestines' ability to produce lactase as they age. This type of lactose intolerance is permanent. Many people with gut inflammation and intestinal damage can temporarily lose the ability to produce lactase and suffer from *transient lactose intolerance*. This type of lactose intolerance may resolve once your intestines heal.

GOING DAIRY FREE

After going dairy free for at least one month as part of the first phase of the elimination diet protocol, your body will be able to tell you whether it can handle this food so you can decide if you want to reintroduce it. If you find that dairy is a problem, you may be reacting to casein, lactose, or both. Chapter 5 will help you determine which components of dairy are problematic for you.

Almost everyone seems to tolerate ghee, which is free of casein and lactose. Butter is also well tolerated by most people. You might be able to tolerate fermented dairy, especially if you make your own yogurt and let it ferment for 24 hours. Store-bought commercial yogurts are usually fermented an average of only four to 10 hours, making them relatively high in lactose. By fermenting your yogurt longer, you allow the probiotic bacteria in the yogurt to digest all the lactose, so the fermentation process happens in the yogurt container instead of your intestines.

If you have a leaky gut or severe digestive symptoms, though, you might find that you do better by keeping your diet 100-percent dairy free (perhaps with the exception of butter and ghee). And remember that if you don't tolerate dairy on your first try, it doesn't mean you won't be able to eat it later on. With time, as your intestines heal, your tolerance may change to allow you to enjoy yogurt, milk, or cheese again. If so, be sure to stick to high-quality dairy from happy, pastured cows and avoid the commercially processed low-fat and sugar-added varieties that don't belong in a REAL food diet.

WHAT ABOUT CALCIUM?

Isn't it dangerous for your bone health to give up dairy for any period of time? Calcium is definitely important for your bones, but there are three more important factors to consider:

- Dairy isn't the only potential source of calcium in your diet
- If your intestines stay inflamed and damaged as a result of consuming dairy, you won't be able to absorb the calcium in your food.
- Calcium isn't the only factor that contributes to bone health

Let's expand a little on the topic of calcium to help you feel better about experimenting with a dairy-free diet. First, although dairy is a good source of calcium, you can find this mineral in other dairy-free foods. There are several examples of tribes and ethnic groups, such as the Inuit and Japanese, who have very healthy bones without eating any dairy. You can get all the calcium you need from homemade bone broth, sardines, leafy greens, broccoli, and almonds. Table 36 compares the calcium content of different foods to help you find suitable non-dairy sources of calcium.

Table 36: Calcium Content of Various Foods

Food Groups	Food	Serving Size	Calcium Content*
Dairy	Milk	1 cup	352 mg
	Yogurt	½ cup	173 to 191 mg
	Cheese	1 oz	143 to 204 mg
Dairy Free	Homemade bone broth	1 cup	Unknown but highly bioavailable
	Sardines, canned with bones	3 oz	325 mg
	Collard greens, cooked	1 cup	266 mg
	Spinach, cooked	1 cup	245 mg
	Salmon, canned with bones	3 oz	203 to 249 mg
	Broccoli, cooked	2 cups	125 mg
	Almond butter	2 tbsp	111 mg
	Rhubarb	1 cup	105 mg
	Shrimp	4 oz	103 mg
	Chards, cooked	1 cup	102 mg
	Kale, cooked	1 cup	94 mg
	Almonds	1 oz (23 almonds)	75 mg
	Orange	1 large	74 mg
	Eggs	2	56 mg
	Dried figs	3	41 mg

*United States Department of Agriculture. **USDA National Nutrient Database Food Search for Windows**, Version 1.0, Database Version SR23.

Second, as long as you continue to have digestive symptoms, you can assume that your intestines are damaged. One of the main roles of your intestines is to absorb the nutrients your body needs, and damaged intestines can't do that very well. This is why people with digestive disorders often end up with nutrient deficiencies. No matter how nutritious your diet, if your digestion isn't optimal, the nutrients you consume will stay in your gut, unabsorbed, and will later be excreted in your stools without making it into your bloodstream. If dairy seems to be contributing to your digestive problems, take it out of your diet to allow your digestive system to repair itself and regain its ability to absorb nutrients properly.

Third, calcium isn't the only factor that can influence your bone health. A meta-analysis published in 2007 in *American Journal of Clinical Nutrition* and another published in 2011 in *Journal of Bone and Mineral Research* even showed that neither milk nor calcium intake are associated with one's risk of a bone fracture. This is probably why many people can achieve strong, healthy bones despite not eating any dairy.

This is also probably why Americans also have the highest rates of osteoporosis despite one of the highest calcium intakes in the world. A *nutrient-dense* diet is required to build healthy bones and calcium is *not* the only factor. Consuming a meal of processed foods with a glass of milk or popping a calcium supplement just won't do it. Other nutrients like magnesium, phosphorus, and vitamins K_2 and D_3 play a big role when it comes to building bones. Weight-bearing exercises, like walking and lifting weights, also contribute. Rest assured that your bones will be fine on a dairy-free diet, as long as you include plenty of nutrient-dense and mineral-rich REAL foods.

Legumes

Legumes are a family of plant that includes beans, lentils, soy, and peanuts. Most people are aware that beans and lentils can be pretty hard to digest. Some of the indigestible carbohydrates they contain can be fermented in your digestive tract, leading to bloating and flatulence. You can make them slightly more digestible by soaking them properly and boiling them long enough, but it might be best to avoid them completely while you are trying to recover from your digestive issues.

In addition to the FODMAPs they contain (specifically, galactooligosaccharides, GOS, or galactans), beans and lentils are also rich in starches that can feed a bacterial overgrowth (if you have SIBO). Their high fiber content can also further irritate your already damaged intestines.

And don't worry. You won't be missing out on any nutrients by avoiding beans and lentils since you can get the fiber and antioxidants you need from vegetables. Although legumes are frequently used by vegetarians as an animal-free source of protein, their protein is incomplete and inferior to that of animal protein. You need each bite of food to contain as many high-quality nutrients as possible to get healthy and legumes simply don't fit the bill. Fortunately, not many people are too sad to give them up!

WHAT ABOUT SOY?

Soy also belongs to the legume family, but its nutritional value is quite different from that of beans or lentils. Nevertheless, soy is far from the angel "health" food it's often portrayed to be, *especially* when it comes to your digestive health. First of all, soy contains protein with some of the highest allergenic potential. Even if you're not allergic to soy, you can still be sensitive to it. Food sensitivities can show up in different ways, but IBS and similar digestive symptoms are a frequent manifestation. Moreover, many soy-based foods contain other highly processed ingredients that can bother your intestines. Tofu, soy milk, vegetarian "meat" alternatives, soy cheese, and soybean oil should not be on your plate if you want to recover your digestive health.

NEED MORE REASONS TO SKIP SOY? HERE ARE SIX:

- Soy is one of the foods with the **highest concentration of goitrogens**, a compound that interferes with thyroid function. Soy could therefore make you feel worse if you suffer from hypothyroidism.
- Soy has often been shown to be **contaminated with high levels of aluminum**, which can be toxic over time.
- Soy, like grains, **contains anti-nutrients** that can inhibit the absorption of some of the precious nutrients your body needs.
- The **protein in soy is incomplete** and inferior to animal protein.

- The **phytoestrogens in soy can disrupt your hormones** and potentially contribute to infertility, PCOS, and hormone-related cancers such as breast cancer. There is controversy around this issue, though. Some researchers believe that phytoestrogens have a protective effect, while others are more cautious and even think they may be deleterious for your health. If you don't want to gamble with your health, abstinence is probably safest. Especially if you don't want to be forced into *sexual* abstinence. Soy has been used historically by Zen monks to decrease their libido. Japanese wives also used to sneak soy into the meals of their cheating husbands with the same intention.
- Soy tends to be **processed heavily** to make soybean oil, hydrolyzed soy protein, textured vegetable protein, vegetable gum, thickener, stabilizer, and flavoring. The ingredient lists of soy burgers, soy milk, and soy-filled breakfast cereals make them look like anything but REAL food.

WHAT ABOUT PEANUTS?

Most people think of peanuts as nuts, but they actually belong to the legume family. Why does this matter? The protein in peanuts is a common source of food sensitivities, which can trigger all sorts of unpleasant symptoms, including GI distress. Peanuts' high levels of potentially irritating insoluble fiber and inflammation-promoting omega-6 fats make for a good combination to keep you feeling miserable. Things are even worse with MSG-enhanced BBQ peanuts or peanut butter with sugar and trans fats from hydrogenated oils.

Peanuts probably don't qualify as a health food, anyway, even if they don't cause you any digestive problems. For one, they are often contaminated with aflatoxins, toxic compounds produced by fungi that appear on the list of known carcinogens. Besides cancer, aflatoxins are also associated with gastrointestinal problems in some people. The government checks peanuts to make sure they don't exceed a certain aflatoxin limit, but they always contain small amounts. Eating peanuts once a month probably wouldn't pose a big risk, but many people can't live without their daily spoonful of peanut butter. It is very possible that you might be consuming enough aflatoxin to affect your GI tract. Do you want to take that risk?

Peanuts also contain a special type of lectin, very creatively called peanut lectin. This lectin has been shown to have significant atherogenic potential, meaning it can increase your risk of developing heart disease. Peanut lectins are found in all peanut foods, including peanut butter and peanut oil. It might be best to stay away from peanuts if you don't want to take any chances with your health.

Nuts and Seeds

Although true nuts and seeds don't have the harmful aflatoxins and lectins found in peanuts, they can still be hard to digest if your digestive system has been damaged. Pistachios, cashews, almonds, and hazelnuts are also very high in FODMAPs, which can be fermented in your intestines and promote bloating and other GI symptoms.

Many nuts are also high in omega-6 fatty acids, a type of fat that can induce inflammation in your body, especially if eaten in excess of omega-3 fatty acids. Brazil nuts, cashews, almonds, pecans, sunflower seeds, sesame seeds, and pumpkin seeds contain a lot more omega-6 than omega-3, which can promote low-grade inflammation in your intestines and prevent healing. The types of protein found in nuts and seeds can also be responsible for a food-sensitivity reaction, just like eggs, soy, or dairy. Nuts and seeds are also implicated in the most common food allergies. Note that coffee and cacao are actually considered seeds and many people with gluten sensitivity also react to the proteins found in these foods. This is a phenomenon called cross-reactivity. If you are sensitive to a specific protein (such as gluten), you are also more likely to be sensitive to other proteins with a similar makeup (like dairy, corn, eggs, coffee, or chocolate). You are also more likely to have food sensitivities if you have increased intestinal permeability (leaky gut). Table 37 lists many common varieties of nuts and seeds that might be present in your diet.

Table 37: Nuts and Seeds

Nuts	Seeds
• Almonds • Walnuts • Cashews • Chestnuts • Macadamias • Hazelnuts • Pecans • Brazil nuts • Pistachios • Pine nuts • Shea nuts	• Coffee • Cacao • Flaxseeds (linseeds) • Chia seeds • Hemp seeds • Psyllium • Sunflower seeds (including sunbutter) • Pumpkin seeds (pepitas) • Sesame seeds (including sesame oil and tahini) • Nutmeg • Anise seeds • Black caraway seeds (regular caraway seed should be fine) • Celery seeds • Cumin seeds • Dill seeds • Fennel seeds • Fenugreek • Mustard seeds (including mustard powder, prepared mustards, mustard oil, and mustard leaves) • Poppy seeds

Although coconut has the word "nut" in its name, it doesn't belong to the tree-nut family. Coconuts come from the palm tree, which is actually an herb, botanically speaking, making coconut a *drupe*. While it is possible to be allergic to coconut, people with tree-nut sensitivity are not necessarily sensitive to coconut. Fortunately, coconut has the advantage of rarely causing anaphylactic allergic reactions.

You might be able to add some nuts or seeds back into your diet once your digestive tract has healed, as explained in Chapter 5. Special preparation methods for nuts, like soaking and blanching to remove the skin, can also make them easier to digest and tolerate.

Refined Oils

The vegetable oils and margarines promoted in recent decades as healthy-fat alternatives are just like wolves in sheep's clothing. Most people replace healthy, satisfying butter and animal fats with canola oil, soybean oil, peanut oil, cottonseed oil, corn oil, sunflower oil, and other processed foods containing these refined oils thinking they are making a healthier choice.

How do you think food manufacturers manage to extract oils from corn, soybean, or canola plants? With a LOT of complex processing steps involving many different chemical products. Refined oils are often acquired using hexane, a chemical solvent related to gasoline, as well as other chemical compounds to bleach, distill, degum, and deodorize these oils.

Recent advances in food-processing technology and the subsidizing of these crops have made possible the production of these oils, which wouldn't have been possible just a few decades ago. They are now produced in such quantities that they show up in all sorts of foods: margarines, salad dressings, mayonnaises, sauces, chips, popcorn, frozen entrées, baked goods, and just about any kind of processed food.

The high-heat process used to extract oils from these seeds damage the delicate polyunsaturated fats and nutrients they contain. Their fats are usually rancid by the time they hit the shelf of your grocery store. Consuming oxidized refined oils can do a lot of damage inside your body, as well as deplete your body's antioxidants (the helpful compounds needed to fight aging-promoting inflammatory compounds and disease-promoting free radicals). Refined oils and foods containing them are decidedly *not* REAL food.

OMEGAS AND THE IMPORTANT RATIO

The polyunsaturated omega-6 fat linoleic acid found in corn oil and other refined oils has been found to contribute to increased intestinal permeability (leaky gut). Using these oils or consuming foods that contain them is thought to be a risk factor for developing ulcerative colitis, according to a study published in 2009 in the journal *Gut*. Other digestive disorders associated with a leaky gut may also be associated with these unhealthy fats, but more studies need to be done to determine if a connection exists. Nevertheless, if you have a condition like a past gastrointestinal infection, SIBO, ulcerative colitis, Crohn's disease, celiac disease, or an autoimmune condition, it might be safer to avoid omega-6-rich refined oils.

Refined oils can also skew your dietary ratio of omega-6 to omega-3 in the wrong direction. A high dietary ratio of omega-6 to omega-3 is associated with more inflammation. It is estimated that the standard American diet has 15 to 20 times more omega-6 than omega-3, while the ideal ratio should be close to one-to-one. A high ratio can contribute to accelerated aging and the development of associated chronic diseases, such as cardiovascular diseases, some cancers, arthritis, and other inflammatory and autoimmune conditions. Polyunsaturated fats include both omega-6 and omega-3 fats. Both are essential to health, but both have a very high oxidative potential. As a result, too much polyunsaturated fat can be deleterious for your health.

If you are struggling with digestive issues, you already have high inflammation levels in your body. Consuming refined oils can further worsen this inflammatory process. If you want to improve your digestive health, make your diet anti inflammatory by improving its omega-6 to omega-3 ratio. Unfortunately, you can't just take high doses of omega-3-rich fish oils to try to balance a high omega-6 intake. Too much oxidation-prone polyunsaturated fats, even the omega-3 kind, could also promote inflammation. If you want to improve your health and reduce inflammation, decrease your total polyunsaturated fat intake and improve your ratio simply by avoiding refined oils, which include the following:

Table 38: Refined Oils

Refined Oils
• Canola oil
• Soybean oil
• Peanut oil
• Cottonseed oil
• Corn oil
• Sunflower oil
• Safflower oil
• Vegetable oil
• Flaxseed oil
• Grapeseed oil
• Margarine
• Shortening (hydrogenated or partially hydrogenated oils)
• Trans fat

Sugar

Everybody "knows" sugar isn't healthy, but the food industry's aggressive marketing has managed to make us believe that sugar might just be more of a benign treat. Fat is now portrayed as the real devil, so much so that it can be difficult to eat bacon, red meat, or butter without having someone comment that fat is gross, is bad for you, and clogs your arteries. Most people don't feel guilty about adding a bit of sugar to their "healthy" whole grain oatmeal or drinking a big glass of fruit juice. But this conception is misguided.

CHRONIC DISEASES OF CIVILIZATION

Sugar has been associated with many of the chronic health problems attributed to the Western lifestyle. Fructose, which is found in table sugar, agave syrup, high-fructose corn syrup, honey, maple syrup, and most other types of sugar, seem to have a particularly deleterious effect on your health. Studies have associated sugar and fructose with weight gain, high levels of triglycerides and inflammation, fatty liver disease, insulin resistance (associated with prediabetes, type 2 diabetes, PCOS, and metabolic syndrome), gout, kidney disease, urticaria, accelerated aging, and even cancer.

NUTRIENT POOR

As for your digestive health, sugar can feed an imbalance in your gut flora. In addition to being devoid of nutrients, sugar also displaces more-nutrient-dense calories from your diet (instead of eating 200 calories of sugar per day, you could be eating 200 calories of nutritious vegetables). Despite the fact that sugars defined as more "natural" like honey and maple syrup do contain some *trace* minerals, don't count on them to get the nutrition your body needs.

FERMENTABLE CARBOHYDRATES

Many sugars also contain FODMAPs, which can be fermented in your gut. High-fructose corn syrup, agave syrup, and honey are especially high in fructose, while coconut sugar contains fructans and sugar alcohols are made of fermentable polyols. Sugars are also found commonly in processed foods that contain grains, starches, or other ingredients that are not compatible with digestive health for sensitive people. Sugars and processed foods can all contribute to feeding a bacterial overgrowth like SIBO, a candida overgrowth, or any other form of gut dysbiosis.

INFLAMMATION

Sugar can also promote inflammation, and you certainly don't need more of that. Eating inflammatory foods like refined oils and sugars is like pouring gasoline on a fire that's already blazing inside your digestive tract. In this case, sugar is contributing to the constant damage that prevents your intestines from healing.

COMPROMISED IMMUNITY

Sugar also lowers your body's ability to fight infections by decreasing your immunity. Every time you eat sugar, whether from regular sugar, honey, or orange juice, it suppresses your immune system by 50 percent within 10 minutes and for up to five hours. Try to imagine what would happen if you were to eat sugar at each meal: Your immune system would be functioning at half-capacity for most of the day!

REDUCED HEALING

Another good reason to avoid sugar and refined carbohydrates is that these foods can elevate your blood-sugar levels, which can be dangerous if they stay elevated for long periods of time, especially if you have diabetes, metabolic syndrome or PCOS. Even a slight increase in your blood-sugar can compromise your body's ability to heal. If you want your diet to be conducive to healing, stabilizing blood-sugar levels by avoiding foods that make them go on a roller coaster is a good place to start.

SUGAR ADDICTION

Giving up sugar can be scary. Many people already feel restricted by their diets and can be terrified of giving up sugar. Sugar can have a very calming effect, as well as be highly addictive. A 2007 study by a team of French researchers even showed that sugar can be *more* rewarding than cocaine! It can be even more difficult to give up sugar if you have a gastrointestinal infection or a gut dysbiosis. Parasites, yeasts, or the excess bacteria associated with SIBO can make you crave sugar even more intensely. The bugs in your intestines are begging you to feed them and they send sugar-craving signals directly to your brain. The good news is that, although your first days without sugar may be hard, your body will soon learn to function without it—and function better, too. If you can resist the first few weeks, you will notice that your cravings will decrease quickly and that you *can* live without sugar. You're sweet enough already. ☺

WHAT ABOUT ARTIFICIAL SWEETENERS?

It's probably best to avoid artificial sweeteners, too, at least in the beginning. For one, they certainly don't qualify as REAL food. There is also evidence that some of them may negatively alter your gut flora. They can also be addictive and perpetuate your sugar cravings. You're much better off without them.

Problematic Fruits and Vegetables

There is no doubt that vegetables, fruits, roots, and tubers are healthy, unprocessed, REAL foods. However, some of them contain compounds, including some types of carbohydrates, fiber, natural food chemicals, and alkaloid compounds that can interfere with the recovery of your digestive health. You won't have to avoid all of these foods forever, but it is best to remove them for a period of time during the elimination phase. Doing so will allow you to assess your personal tolerance to these foods when you start the reintroduction phase a few weeks later.

If you have a gut dysbiosis, which is very likely if you suffer from digestive problems, you don't want to be feeding bad microbes or an excess of bacteria in your small intestines. Avoid fruits and vegetables that are rich in FODMAPs, as well as higher-carbohydrate choices like starchy vegetables and fruits, at least at the beginning. Starchy vegetables include potatoes, sweet potatoes, yams, parsnips, plantains, yucca, cassava, and winter squashes. Some of the fiber in vegetables, fruits, and tubers, especially in peels, seeds, and membranes, can also be hard on your digestive system. This is why the first phase of the elimination diet only includes easy-to-digest and thoroughly cooked and peeled vegetables. Sometimes, de-seeding and puréeing your vegetables can make them gentler on your intestines to avoid interfering with the healing process.

NIGHTSHADES (*SOLANACEAE*)

It is also a good idea to avoid the family of vegetables, fruits, and spices called nightshades (or *Solanaceae*). Formerly used as ornamental and decorative plants, nightshades share a common compound called alkaloids. Members of the nightshade family include potatoes (but not sweet potatoes), eggplants, tomatoes, tomatillos, goji berries, ground cherries, paprika, bell peppers, and most kinds of peppers like chili peppers (including chili powder), jalapeños, cayenne peppers, and habaneros (but not black and white pepper), as listed in Table 39. Nicotine, and the herb ashwangandha, often used in Ayurvedic supplements, are also nightshades.

Table 39: Nightshades

Nightshades	
• Potatoes (but not sweet potatoes)	• Most kinds of hot peppers (chili powder, jalapeño, cayenne, chipotle, habanero; NOT black and white pepper)
• Eggplants	
• Tomatoes	• Curry (often contains pepper)
• Tomatillos	• Ashwangandha (Ayurvedic supplement)
• Goji berries	• Nicotine
• Ground cherries	
• Paprika	
• Bell peppers	

Avoiding nightshades isn't easy if you eat processed foods. The ingredient "starch" found in many foods and even prescription medications and supplements can hide potato, while the terms "flavors" and "spices" can hide paprika or peppers. Tomato is also omnipresent in sauces and condiments, including ketchup, salsas, and pasta sauces.

Some people feel addicted to many foods within the nightshade family, probably because all of them actually contain small amounts of nicotine. It is not uncommon for someone to eat nightshades at every meal, with goji berries in your morning yogurt or granola bar, a taco with salsa and jalapeño peppers at lunch, and a pizza with tomato sauce at dinner. You could very well be eating more alkaloid compounds than your body can handle.

The alkaloid compounds in nightshades act as natural pesticides to protect the plant against invaders. If you are sensitive to them, these alkaloids can promote inflammation if you eat enough of them. Most of the research on nightshades has been done in people with rheumatoid arthritis and joint pain, but anecdotal evidence shows that people with digestive disorders may also react to them. Some studies also indicate that many of the compounds found in nightshades, such as the alkaloid compounds (including saponins), lectins, and the capsaicin found in hot peppers are involved in increased intestinal permeability. It might be safer and more prudent to avoid them, at least at the beginning of your elimination diet, since you already have inflammation in your digestive system. In any case, most nightshades also have high levels of natural food chemicals (salicylates, glutamates, and amines) that can trigger an uncontrolled inflammation response, which is just another good reason to avoid them for the first month or two before determining how they impact you during the reintroduction phase.

Cruciferous Vegetables (Brassicaceae)

Vegetables in the *Brassicaceae* family, which includes broccoli, cauliflower, cabbage, and several others, can also contribute to bloating, gas, and bowel-movement problems if you are sensitive to them. Again, not everyone reacts to this food group, and the elimination diet will allow you to determine how your body responds to it. Some, but not all, of these cruciferous vegetables contain FODMAPs, but they may contain salicylates, glutamates, and amines that can trigger symptoms in people sensitive to them. You will find a list of all the vegetables in the cruciferous family in Table 40.

Table 40: Cruciferous Vegetables

Cruciferous Vegetables
• Horseradish (including wasabi)
• Kale
• Collard greens
• Broccoli (including Chinese broccoli, broccoflower, wild broccoli, broccoli romanesco, and rapini)
• Cabbage (including Chinese cabbage, Napa cabbage, red cabbage, and sauerkraut)
• Brussels sprouts
• Kohlrabi
• Cauliflower
• Bok choy, pak choy
• Turnip
• Rutabaga
• Canola/rapeseed
• Mustard seeds
• Arugula (rocket lettuce)
• Maca
• Watercress
• Radish
• Daikon

Yeast, Molds, and Mycotoxins

Yeast could be problematic for you, especially if you have an excessive amount of yeast (fungi) in your digestive system. Candida is probably the most well-known yeast that can overgrow in your intestines, but it is not the only one. As with SIBO, a yeast overgrowth can ferment some of the food you eat, especially starches and sugars, and induce bloating, abdominal pain, changes in your bowel movements, recurring vaginal infections, brain fog, joint pain, sinusitis, asthma, skin problems, and other systemic symptoms commonly associated with a leaky gut.

Although the topic of Candida overgrowth is controversial, it is one of the many possibilities you should consider when dealing with chronic GI symptoms. Some researchers from the Netherlands even hypothesize that Candida may be a trigger in the onset of celiac disease (and possibly non-celiac gluten sensitivity) since some of its proteins are very similar to gluten, as published in 2003 in the journal *Lancet.* You can determine whether you have a candida overgrowth with a stool test.

According to the theory, eating food that contains yeast or mold could contribute to worsening a Candida or yeast overgrowth. Whether or not you have a candida overgrowth, it's also possible to be sensitive to yeast, molds, and mycotoxins (toxins produced by yeasts and molds) in the same way you can be sensitive to gluten, dairy, or soy. The most common sources of yeasts and molds are found in Table 41. Many supplements, especially B vitamins, are also made from yeast. Mycotoxins are usually found in the same foods commonly contaminated with yeasts and molds. They are very resistant and can survive digestion, cooking, or freezing.

Table 41: Yeasts, Molds, and Mycotoxins

Yeasts, Molds, and Mycotoxins
• Grain products containing baker's yeast
• Nutritional yeast
• Alcoholic beverages
• Vinegars (with the exception of apple cider vinegar)
• Many condiments
• Fermented foods (sauerkraut, miso, soy sauce, tamari sauce, cheeses)
• Some fruits (berries, melons, grapes, dried fruits)
• Monosodium glutamate (MSG)
• Aged and cured meats (sausage, bacon, ham)
• Refined vegetable oils
• Some nuts (cashews, pistachios)
• Peanuts (including peanut butter)
• Citric acid
• Yeast extracts
• Overripe produce
• Yeast spreads (Vegemite or Marmite)
• B vitamins and other supplements made from yeasts

Alcohol

Not alcohol, too? Yes, I know. So many foods have been crossed off your list already, but if you really want to succeed and conquer your digestive problems, alcohol should stay out of your diet for a little while. It's a well-known fact that alcohol can irritate your intestines. A paper published in the journal *Alcohol* in 2008 even reported that alcohol can promote the growth of bad bacteria and contribute to increased intestinal permeability (leaky gut), as well as slow down your immune system.

You should avoid alcohol completely for at least the first three to six months, if not longer, to allow your gut to heal fully and prevent a breakdown of your digestive health. If you keep drinking alcohol, it can also prolong a leaky gut, making you sensitive to many foods and preventing you from increasing your food variety. Beer should already be out of the picture because of its gluten. Sugary alcoholic beverages (cocktails, port wines, and sweet wines) are also a big no-no because of their high sugar content that can feed a bacterial overgrowth. Although wine, liqueurs, and spirits are usually low in sugar and gluten free (if the liqueurs and spirits are distilled properly), the presence of alcohol alone could still be hindering your efforts. Give your digestive system a chance to recover and enjoy sparkling water with a twist of lime juice instead. You can have fun even without alcohol. ☺

Caffeine

Do you typically start your day with a cup of coffee, an energy drink, or a mug of black tea? Maybe it's time to let go of this habit for now. It's no secret that caffeine is irritating to the digestive system. It can also make your digestive system overactive; one study showed that coffee can induce a bowel movement within four minutes in some people. The same findings indicate that a cup of java has the same stimulatory effect on your colon as a *1,000-calorie meal*! Decaffeinated coffee induces a similar response, so it's not just the caffeine, sadly. The stimulatory effect of coffee is definitely not a good thing if you are prone to diarrhea. If you're prone to constipation, caffeine may help you have more regular bowel movements, but it's not a long-term solution.

Caffeine also keeps your intestines inflamed and irritated, preventing them from healing and recovering their normal function. One study showed that drinking only six ounces (200 milliliters) of coffee per day can increase the levels of multiple inflammatory markers in your blood (interleukin 6 or IL-6, C-reactive protein or CRP, tumor necrosis factor alpha or TNF-alpha, and white blood cells). With your current digestive problems, you certainly don't need more inflammation in your body.

One of the reasons people like caffeine so much is because it raises cortisol levels, making you more awake and alert. The problem is that your cortisol levels are probably already elevated, from the physical and emotional stress of living with digestive problems, in addition to all the other stresses of modern life. Forcing your body to produce more cortisol by drinking caffeine can exhaust your adrenal glands and put your body in a constant "fight-or-flight" mode. When your cortisol levels are high, your body switches to your sympathetic nervous system, in which digestion stops and stomach-acid production is inhibited, so you won't absorb as much of the nutrients you eat. It can also expose you to food-sensitivity reactions, put you at higher risk of all kinds of infections, and worsen your gut dysbiosis.

When in sympathetic ("fight or flight") mode, your body allocates all its resources and energy to address the emergency it thinks it is facing. Your body believes it is in a life-threatening situation and that it doesn't make sense to waste energy on digesting your food. Instead, your survival instinct prepares you to either fight the danger or flee from it.

If you want your digestive system to work properly, you need to feel calm, relaxed, and happy to activate your parasympathetic nervous system—the "rest-and-digest" mode that's the opposite of the "fight or flight" response. It's only when you're in a relaxed, calm state that your body can digest, heal, and repair itself—and you can help this by cutting out caffeine. Chapter 7 has more tips for managing your stress.

You may already be consuming more caffeine than you realize. Table 42 lists the caffeine content of different beverages and foods. Rooibos tea, green tea, and herbal teas can be safely consumed during the first phase of your elimination diet. Buy whole leaves if possible. If you buy tea bags, always read the ingredients to make sure your tea doesn't contain any added inulin, chicory root, or sweeteners that could compromise your digestive health.

Table 42: Caffeine Content of Various Foods

Food	Serving Size	Caffeine Content
Espresso	1 oz / 30 ml	40-75 mg
Brewed coffee	8 oz / 240 ml	95-200 mg
Decaffeinated coffee	8 oz / 240 ml	2-12 mg
Black tea	8 oz / 240 ml	14-61 mg
Green tea	8 oz / 240 ml	24-40 mg
Rooibos tea	8 oz / 240 ml	0 mg
Herbal teas (with the exception of yerba mate, guayusa, yaupon, and guarana)	8 oz / 240 ml	0 mg
Cola (regular, zero, diet)	12 oz / 355 ml	27-47 mg
Energy drinks	8 oz / 240 ml	70-80 mg
Dark-chocolate-coated coffee beans	10 pieces	120 mg
Dark chocolate (70-85% cacao)	3.5 oz / 100 g	70-90 mg

Also keep in mind that caffeine-rich foods like coffee and chocolate belong to the seed family, which means that they contain proteins that can trigger food sensitivity reactions. If you have digestive problems, you're very likely to have a leaky gut, which in turn puts you at risk for multiple food sensitivities. Gluten, eggs, dairy, nuts, and seeds like coffee and caffeine are common triggers and should be avoided during the elimination phase.

Processed Foods

Processed foods are everywhere, but you already know this is no reason to eat them. They often contain a combination of refined grains, gluten, soy, corn, sugars, FODMAPs, refined oils, and other mysterious, unpronounceable ingredients, all of which can be problematic for your intestinal *and* overall health.

Food manufacturers also seem to enjoy making it difficult to know what's in the food they engineer, turning food labeling into a complex word game and plumbing their thesaurus for new ways of describing ingredients. Plus, even if you read labels carefully, food manufacturers do not have to declare all the ingredients they use. The most frequent allergens must be identified, but other ingredients that can cause gastrointestinal problems in some people, such as paprika (nightshade), onion (FODMAP) and MSG (food chemical), can be hidden under the broad term "spices" and "flavorings." "Processing aids," such as the cornstarch used between slices of lunch meat to prevent them from sticking, also don't have to be listed. Mislabeling and cross contamination are also frequent problems with foods that come in a box, bag, or can. The bottom line is that it's impossible to be sure of what you're eating if your diet includes processed foods.

> ## "If it's a plant, eat it. If it was made in a plant, don't."
>
> – Michael Pollan

You best bet is to stick with REAL food! By now, you're probably realizing that a REAL food-based diet is not only a diet that you *need* to follow to improve your digestive health but one you also *want* to follow because it's simply the healthiest way to eat! REAL food will help you better manage and alleviate your digestive symptoms, as well as nourish your body.

> ## "Fake food—I mean those patented substances chemically flavored and mechanically bulked out to kill the appetite and deceive the gut—is unnatural, almost immoral, a bane to good eating and good cooking."
>
> – Julia Child (1912-2004)

Chapter 4: Nourishing Foods

What am I going to eat now? That's the question you're probably asking yourself. This next chapter will discuss what REAL foods are best for you to eat to help manage your gastrointestinal symptoms and nourish your body to facilitate the healing process.

> ## "Optimum nutrition is the medicine of tomorrow."
>
> – Linus Pauling

Keep in mind that no one really knows what *you* should eat. No dietitian, nutritionist, or doctor can give you a definitive list of what you can and can't eat. Don't trust anyone who says otherwise. You'll have a bit of work to do, as described in Chapter 5, to figure this out for yourself. But the good news is that most of the foods in this category should be well tolerated by all people with tummy troubles. Use the elimination diet protocol to introduce them one by one and assess your personal tolerance to each one. Your body will tell you what works for you—you just have to learn how to listen.

Animal Protein

Animal protein is underrated in this recent era of "Meatless Mondays." The truth is that vegetarian sources of protein, such as beans, lentils, soy, and nuts, can be very hard to digest, especially for an already-impaired digestive tract. The proteins in soy are highly allergenic, while beans and lentils are high in FODMAPs and starches that can feed a bacterial overgrowth. Animal protein is a safer, superior option, for reasons we'll discuss.

Protein from animal sources has the highest quality. Unlike vegetarian protein, animal protein is complete because it contains all the amino acids (protein building blocks) in balance. There are 21 different amino acids required for human health, and not having enough of only one of them is enough to prevent your body from accomplishing its daily tasks. The right balance of all amino acids is required to build and repair muscles and tissues as well as synthesize hormones, proteins for your immune system, and other proteins to transport vitamins, minerals, cholesterol, and fat inside your body.

Getting the right balance of all the amino acids is also important for the production of neurotransmitters like serotonin, dopamine, and GABA. These neurotransmitters are like messengers that communicate with your brain to help you feel happy and relaxed and calm anxiety and cravings. Serotonin, synthesized from the amino acid tryptophan found in animal protein, is thought to have an important role in promoting intestinal motility. Serotonin also influences the perception of pain and the amount of fluid secreted in your intestines, which can also play an important role in your IBS symptoms.

Healing, Repair, and Healthy Weight

Why is animal protein important for your digestive health? If your intestines are damaged, your body needs high-quality protein to repair them. Some people with digestive issues are underweight because the food they eat just seems to pass right through. If this is your case, eating animal protein at each meal is essential to prevent further wasting and help you put on weight.

Some people who struggle with their digestion actually have the opposite problem and can't seem to be able to lose weight. If you are overweight, it is most likely due to ongoing inflammation in your body, from food intolerances and constant damage to your intestines. Low-grade systemic inflammation levels lead to elevated cortisol, a stress hormone that decreases your body's ability to burn fat and promotes weight gain. Excess weight can also be attributed to uncontrollable cravings for sugars, starches, and other processed foods that result from a gut dysbiosis or gastrointestinal infection. Eating high-quality protein, the most satiating of all nutrients, at each meal can help you get your cravings under control and keep you feeling full longer to help you reach a healthier weight. A diet based on REAL food is the best place to start to normalize your weight, whether you are underweight or overweight.

Protein also has the advantage of not feeding a bacterial overgrowth (SIBO), a yeast infection, or any other source of gut dysbiosis. Little bugs like bacteria, yeast, and parasites *love* sugars, starches, and carbs, but fortunately don't seem to be really interested in protein.

If food moves through you too quickly or if your digestive system can't produce enough stomach acid or digestive enzymes, your body will unfortunately not be able to properly absorb the nutrients you eat. Even if you eat the most nourishing foods, you can end up malnourished and producing very expensive poop. And if you have SIBO, it's even possible that the excess bacteria in your small intestines are stealing nutrients from you.

Animal protein is also very nutrient dense and nourishing. You need your food to be rich in nutrients to recover from the nutritional deficiencies frequently associated with digestive issues, such as iron, vitamin B_{12}, and various fat-soluble nutrients. Animal protein sources such as beef, lamb, pork, poultry, bison, wild boar, and wild game are the richest in iron, vitamins A and B_{12}, zinc, magnesium, potassium, and selenium. Most of these nutrients are also more bioavailable (better absorbed and utilized) in animal sources than vegetarian ones. For example, the iron in animal protein is in the heme form, which is easier to absorb than the non-heme form found in vegetarian sources. Fish and seafood are rich in anti-inflammatory omega-3 fats, and eggs are rich in choline. Organ meat (liver, kidney, heart, sweet breads, tongue, and testicles) truly is a super food because it's an even more concentrated source of these nutrients, with the added bonus of being a good source of vitamin D, CoQ10 and, choline.

Animal protein and eggs are also great sources of cholesterol. Although cholesterol has gotten a bad rap, it's essential to life. Cholesterol is part of each and every cell of your body. It's required to synthesize hormones, produce vitamin D from sun exposure, help your brain work optimally, and act as an antioxidant to protect your body from age-related damage. You also need cholesterol to produce bile and digest the food you eat. It has been established for over a decade that dietary cholesterol does *not* contribute to cardiovascular disease or any other diseases (unless you have a rare genetic defect).

Bottom line: Animal protein is vital.

Common Anti-Animal-Protein Arguments

Are you afraid of eating meat? Animal protein has been vilified in the media and accused of causing just about every common ailment. Here are the three most common health arguments against the eating of animal flesh:

1. Animal protein is hard to digest!
2. Animal protein causes kidney damage!
3. Red meat is unhealthy!

Fortunately (or unfortunately, depending on which side you're on), all these claims about the dangers of meat are false. Let's tackle them one by one.

HARD TO DIGEST

Red meat *can* be hard to digest, but only if you have low stomach acid. You can stick to poultry, eggs, fish, and seafood if you find that red meat sits too long in your stomach. If you want to be able to enjoy a tasty, juicy steak, try supplementing with digestive enzymes and betaine HCl to assist your digestion (see Chapter 6 for more on supplementation), or make your stomach more acidic by taking a tablespoon or two of apple cider vinegar mixed in warm water five to ten minutes before you eat. Discontinue the use of any of these protocols if you experience a burning sensation or take anti-inflammatory medications, as explained in the supplement chapter.

You can also try slow-cooked meat since the slow cooking makes it easier to digest. Make good use of the Crock-Pot collecting dust in your cupboard, or invest in a new one. This is a great way to prepare wholesome meals without spending hours in the kitchen. Even if you don't have a slow cooker, you can use a large stock pot to make convenient, easy-to-digest, all-in-one slow-cooked meals.

THINK OF THE KIDNEYS!

But won't protein damage your kidneys? First, eating animal protein at every meal doesn't necessarily mean you're on a high-protein diet. Yes, meat is a good source of protein, but you probably won't be eating a 16-ounce steak at each meal. Eating four to six ounces of protein three times per day only adds up to between 96 and 144 grams of protein. This is probably higher than what some people on the standard American diet or on a vegetarian diet eat, but it is well within the recommended range.

You may know that people with kidney disease need to restrict their protein intake, but this doesn't mean that dietary protein *causes* kidney damage. What does, then? Inflammation, high blood pressure, and elevated blood sugar are actually the most common culprits. It is only *once* the kidneys are damaged that too much protein can worsen their condition. You can ask your doctor to check your kidney health with a simple urine test if you're worried.

THE RED (MEAT) SCARE

The media has done a great job of vilifying animal protein—especially red meat. Every few months, a new study seems to come out proclaiming that "red meat will kill you." However, almost all such studies are *epidemiological* studies, ones that look at large numbers of people to see if there are associations between what they eat and their risk of dying after a certain number of years.

The problem with epidemiological studies is that they are meant to formulate *hypotheses*, but they are unsuitable to establish *causation*. The associations found in epidemiological studies need to be further evaluated because they can be confounded by so many other variables. In these studies, participants usually report what they eat by filling out a food-frequency questionnaire every four years or so. Can you remember how often you ate red meat in the last year? That's the kind of question participants have to answer.

Besides obvious recall issues, bias is also frequent in epidemiological studies. Health-conscious people may select answers that are considered more socially acceptable by indicating that they eat more fruits and veggies and less meat than they actually do. On the other hand, people diagnosed with a medical condition like diabetes or heart disease may feel guilty and put the blame on foods that are considered unhealthy (such as meat and fat) by over-reporting the quantities they actually consume.

In addition, these studies often don't account for the types of food commonly eaten with red meat. Only a minority of people eat their steak with a healthy serving of vegetables and olive oil, while most red-meat eaters have their meat with a bun made with refined flour along with French fries and a soft drink. If the data is not carefully analyzed (and it rarely seems to be), the blame is often placed regrettably on red meat instead of the processed foods that usually accompany it. Moreover, these studies almost never differentiate between conventional grain-fed meat and grass-fed and pastured meat.

One such recent study, published in 2012 in *Archives of Internal Medicine*, observed an association between red meat and increased mortality many factors could be responsible for this association. In the study, the group that consumed the most meat also happened to smoke more, exercise less, consume more alcohol, have a higher body weight, and eat more calories. You think that might have skewed the results a bit?

The best study to determine the real health effects of meat would be a randomized, controlled trial, considered the gold standard of research, in which participants with the *same* baseline characteristics either consume red meat or non-animal protein for years (decades, ideally) until we can observe differences in their health status. This would be the *only* way to determine once and for all if red meat really is problematic for human health. However, don't expect to see any such studies anytime soon. Recruiting people to commit to eat only the food provided by the researchers, for years on end, is practically unthinkable. Just the cost alone would be a hindrance, bolstered by the fact that most of the funding for these kinds of studies usually comes from pharmaceutical companies.

Since studies will likely never be able to offer a definitive answer about red meat, your best bet is to do your own personal experiment. If you're still worried about red meat, try eating animal protein regularly while you keep track of some key health markers. You can measure your weight (especially your waist circumference) yourself and ask your doctor to track your blood sugar (fasting, post-meal levels, and hemoglobin A1c), blood cholesterol levels (especially triglycerides and HDL cholesterol), inflammatory makers (such as CRP), and kidney function (creatinine and glomerular filtration rate or GFR). Use the chart in Appendix 18 to keep track of your numbers. If everything is in check even after three to six months of eating red meat, you shouldn't have anything to worry about. You can have your steak and eat it, too!

HOW MUCH PROTEIN?

Popular dietary recommendations advise people to eat a *minimum* of 0.4 grams of protein per pound of body weight (about 0.8 grams of protein per kilogram of body weight). Most people do better with between 0.7 and 0.9 grams per pound (between 1.5 and 2.0 grams per kilogram). You can calculate the amount of protein you need with this simple formula:

Units	Your Body Weight	Formula	Your daily protein range	
US	_____ lbs	Multiply by 0.7	= _____ g	Minimum
		Multiply by 0.9	= _____ g	Maximum
Int'l	_____ kg	Multiply by 1.5	= _____ g	Minimum
		Multiply by 2.0	= _____ g	Maximum

*One pound corresponds to approximately 2.2 kilogram, and one kilogram corresponds to approximately 0.45 pounds.

For example, if you weigh 150 pounds (68 kilograms), you probably need somewhere between 105 and 135 grams of protein per day. Your daily protein range will be a bit lower if you weigh less and a bit higher if you weigh more. This corresponds to a moderate, not high, protein intake.

What does this mean in concrete terms? Generally, one ounce (30 grams) of protein-rich foods like meat, poultry, fish, or seafood provides six to nine grams of protein (see Table 43). Make sure you don't confuse the grams of protein with the weight of the food itself.

Table 43: Protein Content of Protein-Rich Foods

Protein-Rich foods	Reference Serving (weight of the food)	Protein Content
Meat, poultry, fish, and seafood	1 oz (30 g)	6-9 g
Eggs	1 large to jumbo egg	6-8 g
Nuts	1 oz (30 g)	2-6 g
Nut butters	2 tbsp. nut butter	

Most people can get their daily protein requirements by consuming a total of about 12 to 24 ounces (360 to 720 grams) of protein-rich food per day, which corresponds to somewhere between four and eight ounces (120 to 240 grams) at each of your three daily meals.

Animal Welfare

You don't have to be a vegetarian to care about animals. If you are concerned about animal welfare—and want to get even more nutrition from the animal protein in your diet—go for pastured and free-range animals or wild-caught seafood. Like us, animals were not meant to eat grains. Cows, pigs, chicken, and fish are healthier without wheat, corn, soy, and other non-species-appropriate foods. Ruminants, like cows and bison, should only eat grass from the moment they are weaned until the ends of their lives. Chickens are omnivorous, and they need and enjoy worms and insects; they even love to nibble on dead carcasses.

What's more, pastured and free-range animals constitute a more ethical choice for both the animals and the environment. There is no doubt that conventionally raised animals, which spend their lives confined in small, closed spaces or cages, are treated cruelly. These poor creatures can't even stretch their legs or gain exposure to real sunlight. They are often given regular doses of antibiotics because their poor diet and lifestyle make them more prone to getting sick. They may also receive hormones to make them grow faster.

Many people switch to vegetarianism as a way of protesting animal cruelty, but you don't need to choose a vegetarian lifestyle to ease your worries about animal welfare. Choose pastured meat instead. Get to know your farmers at the local farmers' market, and buy from the ones who treat their animals with care. Show respect to the animal your meat came from by trying to use every part of it. Eat the organ meat and use the bones to make homemade bone broth. Remember that a single cow can feed a family for almost a year!

Also remember that eating meat is part of the natural cycle of life. Plus, vegetarians can't really claim that their way of eating results in the death of fewer animals. How many animal lives are lost when their natural habitat is destroyed to make way for fields of wheat, corn, and soy? How many small animals like rodents, birds and snakes die during the harvesting of these crops? One could argue that eating animal protein and avoiding grains and processed foods actually results in a lower death toll.

NUTRITIONAL BONUS

Happy, healthy animals make more nutritious meat, too. Grass-fed beef has two to four times more omega-3 fats, four times more vitamin E, three to five times more CLAs, and more iron, zinc, B vitamins, beta-carotene, magnesium, potassium, and selenium. Eggs from hens that can forage outside for worms and insects have two to 10 times more omega-3 fats, twice as much vitamin E, and more A, D, and B vitamins (especially folate and B_{12}) and eye-protecting antioxidants (lutein and zeaxanthin). You'll notice that the yolks from these eggs are a lot darker too, a good sign of their greater nutritional value. Since pastured animals are less likely to be infected with dangerous bacteria, they are naturally free of antibiotics and hormones. Visit your farmers' market, eatwild.com, localharvest.org, U.S. Wellness Meats or your local chapter of the Weston A. Price Foundation to find good sources of quality meats and eggs.

If Money is Lean, Go Lean

If you can't always afford the best-quality meat or you don't have control over where your meat comes from, choose leaner cuts. It's not that fat is necessarily bad (as you'll discover in the next section). The problem is that toxins and harmful compounds tend to accumulate in the animals' fat deposits. There's nothing wrong with eating fatty cuts of meats from pastured animals since these animals have had minimal exposure to pesticides, chemicals, and other toxins. With conventionally raised meat, however, choosing leaner cuts, trimming the fat, or using cooking methods that allow excess fat to drip off will help you minimize your exposure to potentially harmful compounds.

Sensitive to Eggs, Chicken, or Meat?

Some people are sensitive to different types of meat or fish, not because of their protein, but because of the toxic compounds and protein residues (from a species-inappropriate diet) they often contain. For example, it is possible for someone sensitive to soy or corn to react to a serving of fish, steak, or chicken if those foods were part of the animal's feed during its life. Unless you have a true food allergy to chicken, beef, or eggs, it might be worth experimenting with higher-quality wild-caught, grass-fed, or pastured versions of these animal proteins. Properly raised animals and fish should *never* be fed soy, corn, or gluten and are usually better tolerated by most people.

"You are what what you eat eats." – Michael Pollan

Protein Exceptions

The only animal protein options you should avoid during the first weeks of your elimination diet are shrimp, smoked fish, and aged and cured meats like bacon, ham, and sausages. In general, these foods fall in the category of REAL food *if* properly prepared and not cooked or mixed with gluten, sugar, or MSG. The problem with shrimp is that it is soaked in a sulphite-containing mixture on the ship right after it's caught, making it high in food chemicals. Fish and meats that are smoked, aged, or cured develop natural food chemicals (glutamate and amines) as a result of their protein breaking down. You will be able to reintroduce these foods during the reintroduction phase of the elimination diet to determine if you can add them safely back to your diet.

A SPECIAL NOTE ABOUT EGGS

Eggs are highly nutritious and are one of the only dietary sources of choline (besides liver). The protein in eggs is divided equally between the white and the yolks, but almost all the other nutrients, including cholesterol, omega-3 fats, vitamins A and E, and other vitamins, minerals, and antioxidants, are found exclusively in the yolk. Although the concerns about its high cholesterol content have been invalidated, too many people unfortunately still eat egg-white omelets and discard one of the most nutrient-dense foods out there.

Despite being highly nutritious, eggs are still a common allergen that can be responsible for food-sensitivity issues in some people. For this reason, it is a good precaution to avoid them during the first phase of your elimination diet. As soon as your symptoms subside, you can try reintroducing egg yolks. If you tolerate egg yolks, you should then be able to experiment with whole eggs. The reason to start with egg yolks is simple: They're less likely than egg whites to cause a reaction (and they're more nutritious!). Some people may not tolerate eggs at all, some can do yolks only, and some tolerate whole eggs without any problems. Following the steps outlined in Chapter 5 will help you find your place on that spectrum. It goes without saying that you should *never* reintroduce any foods to which you find you are allergic.

Traditional Fats

The energy you get from food has to come from one of the three macronutrients: carbs, protein, or fat. The first step to try to control your gastrointestinal symptoms is to eliminate most carbohydrates from sugars, grains, and starchy foods to prevent excessive fermentation from occurring in your digestive system. You will then get some of the calories you need from animal protein, but there is a limit to the amount you can eat (because it's highly satiating). The bulk of your energy will therefore come from (drum roll…) fat!

Not just any type of fat, though. You don't want trans fats, shortening, or hydrogenated oils, as well as those from refined and potentially rancid vegetable oils high in omega-6 fats (canola oil, corn oil, soybean oil, and other vegetable oils), and no margarine or commercial mayonnaises or salad dressings, either.

What you need is fat from REAL food. Traditional fats that have been a safe part of human diets for centuries. These fats are more stable, less susceptible to oxidation and rancidity, and naturally packaged with valuable nutrients.

What About My Heart Health?

After being told for years that the saturated fats in meat, butter, and tropical oils are bad for you and cause heart disease, this belief may be ingrained in your mind. Unfortunately, the evidence for this stance was never based on sound science. The main driver behind the campaign against fats and saturated fats is political more than scientific, as explained in detail by Gary Taubes in "Good Calories, Bad Calories." Regrettably, this information seems to be taking a long time to reach doctors, dietitians, and health authorities.

The good news is that many recent studies have exonerated saturated fats, including a large meta-analysis of almost 350,000 subjects followed for between five and 23 years and published in 2010 in the *American Journal of Clinical Nutrition*.

Just so we're clear: There is *no* association between saturated fats and the risk of dying of a heart attack. *Saturated fats do not cause heart disease.*

In fact, eating a high-fat diet, which is consequently lower in carbohydrates, can increase your heart-protecting HDL cholesterol, decrease your (bad) triglycerides (TG), and reduce your blood sugar levels and your blood pressure. This way of eating can even make your "bad" LDL cholesterol less atherogenic (less likely to clog your arteries) by making your LDL particles larger and fluffier (as opposed to small and dense).

If you are still concerned or reluctant to increase your fat intake, have your doctor run a complete blood panel that includes your total cholesterol, LDL cholesterol, HDL cholesterol, TG, blood sugar, hemoglobin A1C, and CRP, in addition to your waist circumference and blood pressure, as shown in Table 44, then repeat these measurements in three to six months to see the effects of your high-fat diet (see Appendix 18 for a convenient table to track your heart-health and other markers). You can also have a heart scan to track the amount of plaque in your arteries, which is the best way to determine your risk for heart disease. Most people actually see improvements in many of these heart-health markers when they eat REAL food, even if they consume a lot more fat. You'll see for yourself.

Table 44: Measures to Monitor Your Health

Monitor Your Health		Target US values	Your Values Int'l values	Date: _____	Date: _____
Total Cholesterol		Below 200 mg/dL	Below 5.2 mmol/L		
LDL Cholesterol		Below 100 mg/dL	Below 2.6 mmol/L		
HDL Cholesterol		Above 60 mg/dL	Above 1.5 mmol/L		
Triglycerides (TG)		Below 150 mg/dL	Below 1.7 mmol/L		
Fasting Blood Sugar		Below 100 mg/dL	Below 6.1 mmol/L		
Post-Meal Blood Sugar (1-2 hours post meal)		Below 140 mg/dL	Below 7.8 mmol/L		
Hemoglobin A1C		Below 5.7%	Below 5.7%		
CRP (C-reactive protein)		Below 1.0 mg/dL	Below 10 nmol/L		
Waist	Women	Below 35 in	Below 88 cm		
Girth	Men	Below 40 in	Below 102 cm		
Blood Pressure		Below 130/90 mm Hg	Below 130/90 mm Hg		
GFR (glomerular filtration rate)		90 or above	90 or above		
Creatinine		0.5-1.2 mg/dL	44-106 umol/L		

What About My Weight?

But doesn't fat make you fat? The short answer is no! The human body is complex and the simple fact of eating fat does not make you fat. Many hormones are involved in body-weight regulation, and trading carbohydrates for fat can actually help these hormones work better and help you achieve a healthier weight.

Studies show that diets with more fat and fewer carbs are more satiating and can actually help you lose weight by better controlling your hunger and cravings. Plenty of studies have shown that low-carb, high-fat diets are actually as effective as, if not more effective than low-fat, low-glycemic, low-calorie, and even "Mediterranean" diets.

Yes, "fatty" foods like donuts, French fries, pizzas, burgers, and cookies can make you fat. But these are not REAL foods; they are processed foods that contain refined carbohydrates from flours and sugars. Exactly what makes you fat is beyond the topic of this book, but rest assured that processed foods are more likely to make you fat than REAL food ever will. If you want to learn more about this aspect of health, read "The Art and Science of Low Carbohydrate Living" by Stephen D. Phinney, M.D., Ph.D., and Jeff S. Volek, Ph.D., R.D.

If you're underweight, eating more fat can also help you reach a healthier weight by helping you get more calories. The meal plan in Chapter 11 will help you ensure you eat enough to prevent further weight loss and even put on a few much-needed pounds.

Fat Advantages

Now that you understand fat is hardly the devil, it's time to learn about the benefits of eating a higher-fat diet, especially if you have digestive problems. Here are seven reasons to eat more fat:

1. Fat is satisfying and satiating.
2. Fat provides long-lasting energy.
3. Fat can help you starve a bacterial overgrowth or gut dysbiosis.
4. Fat can offer a variety of precious and hard-to-obtain nutrients.
5. Fat enhances the absorption of fat-soluble nutrients.
6. Fat supports many important functions in your body.
7. Last but not least, fat is tasty!

SATIETY

Protein is the most satiating nutrient, but it is followed closely by fat. Carbs are far behind. Fats combined with grains or sugars seem to lose their satiating power, though. Is it easy to eat only one potato chip or cookie? Not really! But have you ever overeaten coconut oil, butter, or avocado? Your body enjoys fat because it is a concentrated source of long-lasting energy, making it both satiating *and* satisfying.

LONG-LASTING ENERGY

You can of course get energy from starches and sugars, but it won't last long. And you can only store a very limited amount (about 2,500 calories' worth) of carbohydrates in your muscles and liver for later use. On the other hand, even lean individuals have thousands of calories stored as body fat (over 110,000 calories in a very lean adult). Eating a higher-fat diet can actually help your body better tap into this vast energy supply by making it more efficient at burning fat instead of sugar! While carbohydrates are like kindling that gives you a quick burst of energy, fats are slow-burning logs that will help you keep your energy levels more stable all day long.

DIGESTIVE HEALTH

Another advantage of eating a high-fat diet is that it can help you control your digestive symptoms. Since bacteria don't eat fat, eating this way helps ensure that you're not feeding a gut dysbiosis or giving it substrates that can be fermented excessively inside your digestive tract.

NUTRIENT DENSITY

Although fat won't feed a bacterial overgrowth, it can certainly feed *you*. Many people think of fat as an icky substance that only provides empty calories, but this couldn't be further from the truth, as long as you stick to natural and traditional fats from REAL food:

- Olive oil and avocado are rich in vitamin E and antioxidants called polyphenols that protect your health against inflammation and free radicals.
- Unrefined red palm oil is rich in the health-protective antioxidants beta-carotene, lycopene, vitamin E, and CoQ10.
- Butter and ghee, especially if made from the milk of grass-fed cows, are rich in vitamin A, vitamin K_2, and CLAs.
- Meat from grass-fed animals, eggs from pastured fowl, and wild-caught fish are also great sources of omega-3 fats, which can help reduce inflammation.

We have already seen how nutrient dense these sources of animal protein can be, especially if they come from animals that lived a healthy life and were fed their natural diet. Best of all is that many of these nutrients are prepackaged with the fat they require to be absorbed properly.

Many different antioxidants found in vegetables also need fat to allow you to absorb them. One study showed that eating a salad with a full-fat dressing is better than eating it with a fat-reduced dressing in helping the body utilize the carotenoids and other protective compounds found in the vegetables. Not only do traditional fats provide important nutrients, they come in a perfect package that helps make sure your body can utilize those nutrients. And doesn't broccoli taste better sautéed in coconut oil or drizzled with butter, anyway?

Antioxidants also seem to be better absorbed when consumed with fats that are low in polyunsaturated fats (PUFAs). Refined oils like soybean oil, corn oil, or canola oil are rich in PUFAs, but traditional fats are all low in PUFAs. Skip these oils in favor of adequate amounts of traditional fats at each meal to allow your body to make use of the nutrient-dense food you're eating.

OTHER ROLES OF FAT

Fat is part of the membrane of each and every one of the ten trillion cells in your body, in addition to being a major constituent of your brain and nerves. Your body also needs fat to synthesize hormones and molecules that aid in the transport of nutrients in your blood. Some fats even have anti-inflammatory properties (omega-3 fats in fish oils and butyric acid in ghee and butter), anti-cancer properties (CLAs in butter and ghee), and anti-microbial properties (MCTs in coconut oil).

> "As for butter versus margarine, I trust cows more than chemists."
>
> – Joan Gussow

Choosing the Right Fats

Hopefully, you now understand the importance of including natural fats in your diet, especially to help control your digestive problems. The next table shows you different REAL-food sources of fat that to include at each meal. Depending on their stability, some of these fats should be reserved for cold use only, while others are appropriate for cooking. Fats in the "for cold use" category can lose some of their antioxidants or risk being damaged by high heat. Traditional fats in the "for cooking" category can tolerate higher temperatures without being altered or losing nutrients.

Table 45: Uses of Various Healthy Fats

For Cooking	For Cold Use	Other Good Sources of "Hidden" Fat
• Coconut oil (extra-virgin)	• Olive oil (cold-pressed**)	• Egg yolks*
• Palm oil*** (red and unrefined)	• Macadamia oil (cold-pressed**)	• Fatty cuts of meat
• Ghee (clarified butter)	• Avocado oil (cold-pressed**)	• Fatty fish
• Butter*	• Avocado*	• Bone marrow
• Duck fat	• Olives*	• Coconut milk*
• Tallow	• Homemade mayonnaise*	• Coconut cream*
• Lard	• Homemade salad dressings	• Coconut butter*
• Cacao fat***		• Unsweetened dried coconut*

* Shouldn't be used in the first phase of your elimination diet; ** Synonymous with extra-virgin; *** Very strong taste

Fat will be your main source of calories during the first phase of your elimination diet. Fortunately, the fats above provide more than just calories, unlike refined oils (canola oil, corn oil, and shortening), and you can of course further boost your nutritional intake by choosing fats that come from healthy, pastured animals.

AREN'T OLIVE OIL AND COCONUT OIL REFINED OILS?

Eating REAL food is what this book is all about. Chapter 3 explained that refined oils are not REAL foods. You now know that extracting oils from seeds or legumes can be a messy business that involves many chemicals and can damage the oils' fragile polyunsaturated fats. But how are they different from the oils listed in Table 36, which also require processing to be extracted?

Of course, not all olive oils and coconut oils on the market are created equal. Regular olive and coconut oil are treated with many chemical products and heat, making them processed and refined oils. But extra-virgin coconut oil and cold-pressed olive oil are extracted without chemicals or heat, using a simple cold-press system that preserves the integrity of their fatty acids as well as their natural vitamins and antioxidants.

It's important to keep in mind that extracting oils from olives has been done for thousands of years simply by pressing these oily fruits. Cold pressing only requires rudimentary installations—you could do it yourself in your kitchen if you wanted! Cold-pressed, extra-virgin coconut oil, olive oil, macadamia oil, avocado oil, and red palm oil are all unrefined and free of chemicals. Unlike unrefined oils that are loaded with rancid and oxidized polyunsaturated fats, these more natural fats are composed primarily of stable saturated and monounsaturated fats, which are left intact during the gentle heat-free, chemical-free extraction process.

You can use these fats as part of your REAL-food diet to improve both your digestion and overall health, but keep in mind the vitamins and antioxidants in extra-virgin olive oil, avocado oil, and macadamia oil (though not those in coconut oil) are sensitive. Avoid buying oils in clear glass bottles because light can damage their fragile nutrients. Store your oils away from light, heat, and air to preserve and protect their beneficial compounds.

SPECIAL CASE 1: MEDIUM CHAIN TRIGLYCERIDES (MCTS)

The majority (over 98 percent) of the fats you eat from animal products, oils, and avocado are long-chain fatty acids. Medium-chain triglycerides (MCTs) have a shorter chain than long-chain fatty acids and are found only in very specific foods like coconut oil and human milk. Unlike the regular long-chain fatty acids found in most foods, MCTs do not require bile to be digested. They are thus absorbed easily and provide an efficient source of energy. If you're worried about gaining weight on a higher-fat diet, go for MCTs such as coconut oil because your body uses them immediately to produce energy and can't store them as fat. And because MCTs don't require bile to be digested and absorbed, coconut oil is also an excellent choice for people with gallbladder issues or no gallbladder.

The energy-producing effect of MCTs can be similar to the energy boost from caffeine. Some people even feel warmer in the hours after eating coconut oil because of how it can increase your metabolism. The advantage of coconut oil over caffeine, though, is that the energy increase from coconut oil is steadier and won't lead to a sudden energy crash a few hours later. While MCTs have been shown to be helpful for people trying to lose weight because your body prefers not storing them, they can also help people who are underweight and malnourished get the energy they need.

MCTs can also help your digestive health. Using coconut oil as a way to get your daily fat can provide your body with the energy it needs to function better and heal without putting more strain on your digestive system. MCTs can also boost your immune system to help you fight infections and protect you from illness. On top of that, one type of MCT, lauric acid, has strong antimicrobial properties, which is why Mother Nature put it in human breast milk to protect infants' immature immune systems from disease.

Making coconut oil one of your regular sources of dietary fat could help you fight harmful bacteria, fungi/yeasts, viruses, and even parasites more effectively to prevent getting sick. Any type of infection can compromise the recovery of your digestive system and unravel all the good work you've been doing to improve your digestive health. Coconut oil truly is a superfood to include in your diet to optimize your digestive and overall health.

There are no health risks associated with taking coconut oil, but it can cause some nausea or gastric discomfort in some people at first, especially if you start by taking large amounts. Start gradually with one quarter to one half teaspoon (one to two milliliters) at each meal or snack and build up gradually to allow your body to adapt and prevent any possible side effects.

Although coconut oil is the best source of MCTs, other coconut-based products such as coconut cream, coconut butter, and dried, unsweetened coconut also contain these unique fats. Table 46 will help you understand the differences between the panoply of coconut products available to you.

Table 46: Characteristics of Various Coconut Products

Coconut-Based Products	Characteristics
Coconut Oil	• 100% fat • Oil extracted from coconut meat • Allowed in the elimination phase
Fresh Coconut meat	• Mostly fats with a bit of protein, carbs, and fiber • Not recommended in the elimination phase, but can be trialed in the reintroduction phase (if desired)
Coconut Water	• Mostly carbs and electrolytes • Not recommended in the elimination phase, but can be trialed in the reintroduction phase (if desired)
Coconut Butter (also called coconut cream concentrate or coconut manna)	• Mostly fats with a bit of protein, carbs, and fiber • Ground up coconut meat (similar to nut butter, but with coconut) • Not recommended in the elimination phase, but can be trialed in the reintroduction phase (if desired)
Coconut Chips	• Mostly fats with a bit of protein, carbs, and fiber • Dried unsweetened coconut flakes • Not recommended in the elimination phase, but can be trialed in the reintroduction phase (if desired)
Unsweetened Dried Coconut	• Mostly fats with a bit of protein, carbs, and fiber • Dried unsweetened coconut flakes, grounded more or less finely • Not recommended in the elimination phase, but can be trialed in the reintroduction phase (if desired)
Coconut Milk	• Mostly fats with a bit of protein, carbs, and fiber • Liquid extracted comes from grated coconut meat • Not recommended in the elimination phase, but can be trialed in the reintroduction phase (if desired) • Commercial coconut milks often contain added sugars, gums, or other thickeners that can cause digestive problems in some people
Coconut Cream	• Mostly fats with a bit of protein, carbs, and fiber • Same as coconut milk, but with less water (and therefore more fat) per serving • Not recommended in the elimination phase, but can be trialed in the reintroduction phase (if desired) • Commercial coconut milk often contain added sugars, gums or other thickeners that can cause digestive problems in some people
Coconut Flour	• Mix of carbs and fiber with some protein and a little fat • Ground coconut meat from which the oil has been extracted (to make coconut oil) • Not recommended in the elimination phase, but can be trialed in the reintroduction phase (if desired)

SPECIAL CASE 2: BUTYRIC ACID

Butyric acid is another special fat found in some traditional fats that deserves special attention. How is it special? The cells lining your colon love butyric acid as a source of energy. Butyric acid also has anti-inflammatory properties. It belongs to the small family of short-chain fatty acids and is also involved in improving intestinal permeability to seal your leaky gut.

Lower levels of butyric acid have been found in people with digestive disorders. The major source of butyric acid in food is the milk fat of pastured animals like cows and goats. Butyrate, which is very similar to butyric acid, can also be produced as a result of the fermentation of indigestible fiber by bacteria in your intestines, *if* you have a healthy gut flora.

The best way to tap into this fatty wealth is to incorporate ghee (and butter, once tolerated) into your diet. You can learn how to make your own ghee in the recipe chapter. Ideally, these fats should come from the milk of healthy, grazing animals to make them even more nutritious for you. Down the road, as your digestive health improves and as you reestablish a healthy gut flora, you should be able to incorporate more fiber and carbohydrates from tubers that can serve as a substrate to make your own internal supply of butyrate and keep your intestines happy.

How Much Fat?

Fat will become your principal energy source once you start the elimination diet. Protein will provide a moderate amount, and carbs a very small amount. In addition to the fat present in some animal protein, it will be very important to eat extra fat at each meal.

macronutrient balance for digestive health

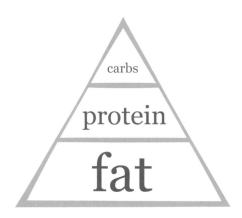

Most people require *at least* one to three tablespoons (15 to 45 milliliters) of fat *at each of their three meals* and possibly at snack time, too. Some will need more, but definitely won't need less. These fats can be used either to cook or accompany your meals. It's as simple as cooking your eggs and spinach in ghee and drizzling them with olive oil for breakfast, accompanying a serving of salmon with half or a whole avocado for lunch, or adding a generous amount of butter to your broccoli and steak at dinner. Homemade mayonnaise and salad dressings are also good ways to add healthy traditional fats to your diet.

WHY DO TYPICAL IBS DIETS SAY TO AVOID FATS?

Does fat worsen IBS and similar digestive problems? Most nutritional recommendations given to patients with IBS, inflammatory bowel diseases or other gastrointestinal conditions promote a low-fat diet. Processed foods like chocolate bars, French fries, and pizza can be problematic for people with IBS, but is this due to the fat or is it the refined-carbohydrate content? Or maybe the FODMAPs in the wheat flour or sugar? Or the types of fat, which are usually refined oils high in inflammatory omega-6 fats?

It's almost impossible to know for sure, but one thing is certain: these high-fat foods are *not* REAL food. Everyone is different, but most people, even with digestive issues, can tolerate traditional fats from REAL food. Just make sure to introduce them gradually, especially if you're accustomed to a low-fat diet. Start with small amounts at each meal and increase slowly to give your body a chance to adjust and produce more bile and digestive enzymes to break down the additional fat.

WHAT IF YOU HAVE GALLBLADDER ISSUES (OR DON'T HAVE ONE)?

If your gallbladder has been removed (via a cholecystectomy), you no longer have the ability to accumulate bile and release it in bulk whenever you eat fat. Instead, bile drips slowly from your liver into your intestines. If you eat more fat, it's likely the small amount of bile in your intestines won't be sufficient to digest it. An inability to digest and absorb the fat you eat can lead to a race to the bathroom and steatorrhea.

If you still have your gallbladder but find that your ability to digest fat is limited, try some of the following strategies to prevent bathroom drama:

- **Increase your fat intake gradually** to allow your liver time to increase bile production. Some people without a gallbladder are able to train their liver to produce more bile, permitting them to digest fat effectively without problems.
- **Eat fats rich in MCTs**. Unlike other fats, they do *not* require bile to be digested and absorbed. A little more than half the fat in coconut oil is in the form of MCTs. Replacing most of your fats with coconut oil should help you tolerate a higher-fat diet without unwanted side effects. If this doesn't seem to be enough, you can also experiment with MCT oil, which is 100-percent pure MCTs extracted from coconut oil. MCT oil has a neutral taste and can be used for cooking at low temperatures or to make mayonnaise and salad dressings.
- **Try using digestive aids** like ox bile, digestive enzymes, and/or betaine HCl. There are no recognized side effects or contraindications from taking ox bile. All it does is supplement your body with the bile it can't produce so you can digest and absorb the fat and fat-soluble nutrients. Consult the supplement chapter for more details. This option can be used in combination with the two previous strategies.

Now that you know about the importance and healthiness of fats in your diet, you have no excuse not to eat more of them. Let's move on to the other components of your REAL-food-based diet for optimal digestive health.

Bone Broth: A Gut-Healing Whole-Food Supplement

Bone broth? This isn't a French cookbook, is it? What does bone broth have to do with digestive health? A lot, actually! Bone broths are a culinary tradition in many cultures and the foundation of many cuisines, but they've been largely replaced by packaged broths, bouillon cubes, liquid meat extracts (such as Bovril), and artificial broth powders. Artificial broths have no nutritional value and can contain ingredients that could contribute to IBS symptoms, such as onions (FODMAPs), MSG, and other questionable ingredients. They also lack the nourishing minerals and gelatin of homemade bone broths. This may be why commercial chicken soup is not as soothing as the home-cooked kind when you have a cold. Unlike their pale imitation, authentic bone broths are an invaluable source of nutrition you can't get anywhere else.

Doctors used to prescribe bone broths for many ailments until around 1930, when drugs began to take over. Bone broth was even added to infant formulas to treat colic. "Gelatin [a component of bone broth] may be used in conjunction with almost any diet that the clinician feels is indicated," said Dr. Francis Pottenger in 1937 at the Annual Meeting of the American Therapeutic Society in Atlantic City. "Its colloidal properties aid the digestion of any foods which cause the patient to suffer from 'sour stomach.' Even foods to which individuals may be definitely sensitive, as proven by the leucopenic index and elimination diets, frequently may be tolerated with slight discomfort or none at all if gelatin is made part of the diet."

Bone broth is the best source of gelatin, a protein rich in the amino acids proline, hydroxyproline, and glycine. Gelatin can assist digestion by normalizing stomach-acid levels and promoting the flow of gastric juices. This explains why many people find meat on the bone cooked in soups or stews easier to digest. In addition to aiding digestion, gelatin is also soothing for the GI tract. Back in 1905, Erich Cohn of the Medical Polyclinic of the University of Bonn noted how "[g]elatin lines the mucous membrane of the intestinal tract and guards against further injurious action on the part of the ingesta." Cohn recommended gelatin routinely to treat "intestinal catarrh," an inflammation of the digestive system now known as IBS.

Bone broth is known to facilitate digestion and promote intestinal healing. In addition, bone broth may be helpful for your cartilage and joints, immune system, liver detoxification, bones, and skin health. Besides its gelatin and amino acids, bone broth also contains many minerals. As you would expect, bone broth contains exactly the same minerals found in your bones (and in the same proportion): calcium, phosphorus, magnesium, sulfur, and potassium. These minerals can help you develop and maintain strong bones and teeth even without consuming dairy.

Making Bone Broth

Don't fall for the convenience of commercial bone broth. It contains artificial flavors and added MSG, in addition to lacking gut-healing gelatin and bone-building minerals. Homemade is the only way to go, and daily is best. Think of it as a supplement. You can drink it instead of coffee in the morning, add it to soups and stews, or use it to make sauces to accompany your meals. Homemade bone broth is a great tool to speed up your recovery.

The recipe chapter explains how to make this valuable gut-healing potion. Even better, it's simple and inexpensive. If time is a constraint, you can simply make a large batch every weekend or even once a month. Freeze extras and thaw as you need. Investing in a slow cooker can make this process even easier.

All you need to make bone broth is bones or a chicken carcass, water, and some seasonings. Simmer for six to 24 hours with a little vinegar to help leach more minerals from the bones. You'll know that your bone broth is rich in gelatin if it gels when you chill it. Bone broth is good for about five to six days in the fridge and keeps for months in the freezer. Just make sure you never use the microwave to thaw it or heat it, as a study showed microwaves could alter the broth's beneficial amino-acid profile.

Avoid adding onions and garlic to your broth at first because the fructans (FODMAPs) they contain are water soluble and stay in the broth even if you remove the garlic and onion pieces. If you still seem to have problems tolerating your bone broth, start with meat broth for a few weeks before trying bone broth again.

IF YOU REACT TO BONE BROTH:

Natural glutamates (similar to MSG) can form naturally in your bone broth if it's heated at too high a temperature. These glutamates can cause a reaction if you're sensitive. Make sure the water is *barely* simmering next time. Some slow cookers unfortunately do not have a low enough setting. Use a large pot on the stove or find another slow cooker that allows you to better control the temperature.

Did you use onions, garlic, or celery? Most FODMAPs are water soluble. Even if you discard the vegetables, the FODMAPs they contain stay in the liquid broth and can be responsible for your symptoms. Instead, add a pinch of asafoetida powder or garlic-infused oil to season your bone broth.

If you really can't tolerate bone broth, try meat broth instead for a few weeks. You should be able to reintroduce real bone broth in a few weeks.

"A big stock pot is the most important gift a bride could receive."

– Dr. Francis Pottenger

Plant Matters

Vegetables, fruits, and tubers are all healthy REAL foods, but some of them can worsen your symptoms or set back your healing if you are dealing with digestive issues. Plant matter tends to be harder to digest because of their fiber, seeds, and membranes. Many plant foods also contain fermentable carbohydrates such as sugars, starches, and FODMAPs, as well as irritating compounds like food chemicals (salicylates, glutamates, and amines) you may have trouble tolerating. Some people also react to nightshades or cruciferous vegetables.

The first goal of using REAL food is to improve your digestive health to get your symptoms under control as quickly as possible, and you'll get better results by playing it safe. The first few days or weeks, depending on how quickly your symptoms subside, may be a bit more restrictive in terms of food variety, but this will allow you to reset your digestive system more quickly. You can then start experimenting slowly with new vegetables to see how your body tolerates them. Be patient. The elimination diet is a rigorous process in the beginning, but it is the best way to create a diet that is customized for you and only you.

Safe Vegetables

At first, a limited selection of safe vegetables is best. The fewer factors in the equation, the easier to figure things out. But what vegetables in the world are non-starchy, non-nightshade, non-cruciferous, low in FODMAPs, low in food chemicals, and low in fiber? The truth is, not many. But don't worry—limited food variety is okay for a little while, especially if it helps you recover your digestive health more quickly. Digestive issues prevent you from properly absorbing the nutrients you eat, so until you correct your digestion, you remain at risk for nutrient deficiencies, even on a varied diet.

So what are the *safest* vegetables with which to start? Zucchini, carrots, green beans, and spinach. Zucchini are very safe, especially if peeled and de-seeded. Carrots and spinach are a bit higher in food chemicals, but since the serving size will be limited at first and since almost no other foods in your diet contain food chemicals, you shouldn't be exceeding your tolerance threshold by eating them. Green beans contain some polyols but should be fine in small amounts. Since you won't have any other sources of FODMAPs in your diet, you should be well below your personal tolerance.

Table 47: Safe Vegetables and Ones to Trial Later

Categories	Vegetables	
Safest Vegetables*	• Zucchini • Carrots • Green beans** • Spinach	Thoroughly cooked, peeled, de-seeded, and even puréed
Vegetables to Trial Later	• Cruciferous vegetables (cauliflower, broccoli, cabbage) • Nightshades (tomatoes, bell pepper, eggplant, potatoes) • FODMAPs (onions, garlic, cabbage, avocados, mushrooms) • Fermented vegetables (sauerkraut, kimchi, fermented pickles) • Raw vegetables (salads, tomatoes, cucumbers, avocados) • Winter squashes (butternut squash, pumpkins, spaghetti squash) • Tubers, roots, and starchy vegetables*** (potatoes, sweet potatoes, plantains, cassava, yucca, etc.)	

*These choices are usually safe for most people but it's not impossible to react to them; avoid any items to which you know you are sensitive;
**Although green beans are technically legumes, they don't contain the same problematic galactans (FODMAPs) and anti-nutrients in beans and lentils;
***Best avoided if you have SIBO, a yeast infection, or a similar gut-dysbiosis problem.

To minimize reactions like bloating, abdominal pain, gas, diarrhea, or constipation, it is important to cook your vegetables thoroughly, and to even peel, de-seed, and purée them if applicable. You want to make them easier to digest to ensure your body can make good use of them, instead of allowing them to end up as food for the bacteria and other microorganisms in your intestines.

As Dr. Campbell-McBride (author of the GAPS diet) says, "When the gut wall is inflamed, no amount of fiber can be tolerated. That's why you do not rush to introduce vegetables (even very well-cooked)." The same is true if you experience other digestive symptoms like bloating and constipation. Of course, the severity of your symptoms is an important factor to consider. If you're feeling very poorly, eliminate all vegetables for a few days and rely on bone broths, animal protein, and fats to nourish your body.

The amount of vegetables you eat can also make a BIG difference. Even though these vegetables are usually safer for most people, eating two cups at a time may be too much for your intestines. See how the cumulative effect can work in Figure 13. Start with small amounts, like one quarter to one half cup (60 to 125 milliliters) per meal or snack. If you are a vegetable lover, it can be hard to eat so little of them, but remember that it's only for a short while. This is a necessary step to give your digestive system a break and a chance to heal. Think long-term. If you do this, your digestive health is likely to improve more quickly so you can start enjoying a larger variety and larger quantities of REAL food again.

Figure 13

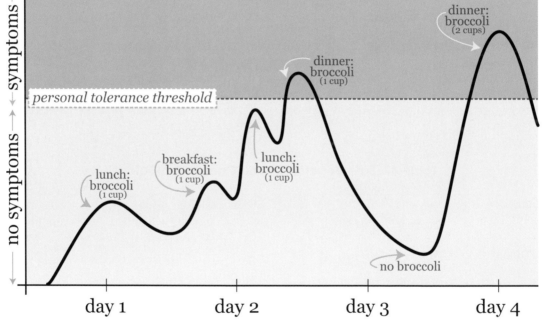

Identifying problematic foods can be confusing if you seem to react to a food one day but not another. In this example, it may seem like you are having random reactions to broccoli when it's actually due to a cumulative effect. You will experience symptoms only when you have an amount of broccoli, or any other food to which you are sensitive, exceeding your personal tolerance threshold. This doesn't mean you shouldn't eat that food, but that you should space out your consumption and moderate your serving sizes.

ONIONS AND GARLIC: BE WARY

Onions and garlic are common ingredients in stews and bone broths, but they should be avoided in the beginning because of their high FODMAP content. Even if you strain your broth or remove the onions and garlic from your stew, the fructans they contain are water soluble, which means they could still be causing symptoms if you are sensitive to them. You can use carrots and all the seasonings you like in your stews, broths, and soups at first. Once you're ready for the reintroduction phase, you can trial onions and garlic to determine whether you can incorporate them back into your diet.

To add flavor to your meals, try using asafoetida powder to give an onion-like flavor to stews, broths, and other recipes. Asafoetida is a pungent Indian spice with a long history of use that works surprisingly well to enhance the flavor of onion-less dishes. Rest assured, its flavor and taste become more pleasant and milder once you heat it up. Just remember that you don't need a lot of it. As an added benefit, this spice is said to have anti-flatulent and antimicrobial properties by helping you keep your gut flora under control.

If you love the taste of garlic, you can prepare garlic-infused ghee or oil to keep this flavor in your diet without its potentially problematic fructans. Since garlic is water soluble, using it in fat will allow you to extract its flavor sans the FODMAPs. All you need to do is heat ghee or oil with pieces of garlic in a skillet for a few minutes until fragrant. Let your oil cool and filter it to discard the garlic pieces. Use this oil to cook your vegetables or meat or to prepare a soup or stew, or simply drizzle it over your food before serving.

PROGRESSION: ADDING VEGETABLES

You won't have to limit yourself to these four vegetables for more than a few weeks. Soon after your symptoms settle, you should be able to experiment with new vegetables to add variety to your diet. The next chapter will explain how to proceed to help you determine which vegetables you can keep in your diet and which you should continue to avoid. You'll soon be able to experiment with cruciferous vegetables, nightshades, and high-FODMAP and high-food-chemical vegetables, and construct a diet that agrees with your digestive system.

All vegetables should be thoroughly cooked at the beginning, but you can experiment with different cooking methods once your symptoms are more under control. Don't feel discouraged if you don't seem to tolerate FODMAPs and cruciferous vegetables right after the elimination phase. Be patient and your intestines may feel ready to accept these foods again after a few more weeks or months of healing. After a while, you should even be able to experiment with raw vegetables if you like. At any point, if you notice a worsening in your digestive health, back up a few steps and go back to your safe foundation diet.

Winter squashes are a good source of nutrient-dense carbohydrates in your REAL-food-based diet. Winter squashes include pumpkin, butternut squash, acorn squash, spaghetti squash, and other similar varieties. They can be added to soups and stews or cooked and puréed to accompany your meals. You can even use puréed winter squash mixed with cinnamon and butter or coconut oil for a delicious, sugar-free treat.

Unfortunately, not everyone reacts well to carbohydrates, especially if you have SIBO, a yeast infection, or another form of gut dysbiosis. Trial winter squashes as you would any other foods you want to add to your diet.

Potatoes, sweet potatoes, yucca/cassava, plantains, beets, and parsnips are also great sources of nutrient-dense carbohydrates on a grain-free, sugar-free diet. Like fruits and winter squashes, however, not everyone tolerates them. These foods should actually be avoided for a few months to up to a few years for people diagnosed with or who suspect SIBO or a Candida overgrowth. The GAPS diet and the SCD both recommend avoiding these starchy foods for one or two years if you have gut dysbiosis.

If you find you can tolerate them during the reintroduction phase with no bloating or altered bowel habits, though, there's no reason to keep them out of your diet. Some people actually feel better with more starches in their diet since starches can help feed the good bacteria in the digestive system. But this is highly dependent on your individual situation and gut flora. The amounts and types of plant matter tolerated can vary a lot between people and over time. Be patient and follow the tips in the next chapter for help designing your own optimal diet.

Fruit

It's best to avoid fruit during the first few weeks of your elimination diet in case you have SIBO or another similar form of gut dysbiosis. Even though the sugars in fruits are natural, they can still feed an overgrowth and trigger digestive symptoms. To make things even more complicated, the fruits that are low in food chemicals are high in FODMAPs and vice versa. This doesn't mean you won't be able to eat fruits at all, but that you need to get your symptoms under control before experimenting with them. As with everything else, tolerance is highly individual.

Cooked fruits, such as baked apples, unsweetened applesauce, baked pears, or fruit purées can be easier to digest for some. Others may do fine with berries or ripe banana. The key is to follow the elimination diet protocol to determine what fruits *your* digestive system tolerates. *How much* you eat can also make a big difference. You may be fine with half a banana, but eating a whole one could put you over your personal tolerance threshold. Some people can't tolerate fruits at all or only very occasionally. If this is the case, don't worry. You can still get all the nutrients you need from vegetables and other REAL foods. Vegetables are actually much more nutrient dense than fruits, anyway. You don't need fruits at all to get all the vitamins, minerals, fiber, and antioxidants you need.

Is Organic Worth It?

If you can afford it, choose organic produce whenever possible to maximize your nutrient intake while minimizing your exposure to chemical residues that could compromise your health. But it's still better to eat conventional produce than no produce, provided you wash it thoroughly.

According to the Environmental Working Group's *Shoppers Guide to Pesticides in Produce,* the vegetables that harbor the least pesticide residues and are therefore safest to eat non-organic are asparagus, avocado, cabbage, eggplant, mushrooms, and onions. On the other hand, bell pepper, celery, cucumber, lettuce, spinach, green beans, kale, and other greens often contain significant amounts of chemical residues. To minimize your exposure to these toxic compounds, you can either choose to avoid these more contaminated varieties or buy their organic versions, as detailed in Table 47.

Table 47: Prioritizing the Foods to Buy Organic

Most Contaminated [avoid or buy organic]	Least Contaminated [safer to buy non-organic]
• Apple	• Onions
• Celery	• Pineapples
• Sweet bell peppers	• Avocado
• Peaches	• Cabbage
• Strawberries	• Sweet peas (frozen)
• Nectarines	• Asparagus
• Grapes	• Mangoes
• Spinach	• Eggplant
• Lettuce	• Kiwi
• Cucumbers	• Cantaloupe
• Blueberries (domestic)	• Sweet potatoes
• Potatoes	• Grapefruit
• Kale/collard greens	• Watermelon
• Cherries	• Mushrooms
• Hot peppers	• Winter squash
• Pears	• Plums (domestic)
• Green beans	• Cauliflower

*Adapted from the Environmental Working Group's 2012 Shoppers Guide to Pesticides in Produce.

Fermented Foods

Probiotics are an important component of your nutritional protocol to help rebalance your gut flora. The gut-friendly bacteria and yeast that constitute probiotics can help you better digest the foods you eat, protect you from harmful microorganisms, detoxify your body, produce important nutrients, and even boost your immune system—all crucial elements of support, especially if you're dealing with digestive issues. Unfortunately, most people think of supplements when they hear probiotics. But fermented foods are actually the best and most affordable source of probiotics you can find.

What are fermented foods? If you're unfamiliar with them, the term may be a bit off-putting. But don't worry, fermented doesn't mean spoiled. It's more like a good wine that gets better with time (although wine is fermented, it doesn't contain probiotics, unfortunately).

The fermentation process actually enhances the nutritional value of fermented foods. An example of a well-known fermented food is yogurt. Each culture around the world seems to have developed its own probiotic foods: kefir in Russia, sauerkraut in Germany, and kimchi in Korea. Table 48 lists more fermented-food examples based on the type of probiotics they contain and the medium in which they are delivered.

Table 48: Ferments and their Probiotic Content

Type of Ferment	Bacteria Only	Bacteria + Fungi
Dairy Based	• Yogurt • Sour cream • Crème fraîche	• Kefir
Non-Dairy Based	• Sauerkraut (fermented cabbage) • Kimchi (spiced fermented cabbage) • Lacto-fermented vegetables (pickles, carrots, beet kvass and other vegetables) • Coconut milk yogurt	• Coconut milk kefir • Water kefir • Coconut water kefir • Kombucha (fermented tea)

These foods have to be prepared traditionally to deserve to be called probiotic foods. Most *commercial* yogurts, sour creams, crème fraîches, and sauerkraut are pasteurized, which kills all their beneficial bacteria. Pickles and sauerkraut, which have been prepared traditionally for hundreds of years using a natural fermentation process, are now prepared *commercially* without any fermentation, by simply marinating them in vinegar.

If you decide to buy fermented foods instead of making them yourself, you should ensure they've been prepared properly and are in their raw, unpasteurized state. A good tip is to look for fermented foods that are refrigerated. Sauerkraut and pickles sitting on the shelf are less likely to contain any probiotics.

Your best bet is to make your own ferments. It is not as complicated as it sounds. It is probably best to start with vegetables in case you are sensitive to dairy products. If you choose to start making your own sauerkraut, all you need to do is to shred your cabbage, put it in a glass container, and pound it until it releases its juice. Add salt to inhibit the growth of harmful bacteria. You can also add seasonings to taste. Put a lid on the glass container, but not too tightly since gas produced by the fermentation process will need to escape. Wait two to three weeks, depending on the ambient temperature, and your sauerkraut should be ready.

The bacteria naturally present on the cabbage will grow and start fermenting (eating) the cabbage. Even though cabbage contains FODMAPs, the fermentation process gets rid of most of them. Remember that bacteria eat by fermenting, so by producing your own ferments, you're allowing the bacteria to carry out their fermentation inside a glass container instead of your intestines.

Once your sauerkraut is ready, it will keep in the fridge for months. Use a little bit every day to top your meat, vegetables or stews. Just make sure you don't heat your sauerkraut as this will kill its precious probiotic bacteria. The recipe chapter provides more details and shows you how to make fermented carrots and 24-hour fermented yogurt.

You might also be able to tolerate fermented dairy, such as yogurt and kefir, especially if you prepare it yourself. By allowing your yogurt and kefir probiotic strains to ferment the milk for 24 hours (as opposed to only four to 10 hours with commercial yogurt), you can ferment all the lactose. Even severely lactose-intolerant people can tolerate homemade 24-hour-fermented yogurt.

If you react to 24-hour fermented yogurt, this is likely due to an intolerance to casein, the main protein found in milk. If this is your case, avoid fermented dairy and stick to non-dairy-based fermented foods, such as lacto-fermented vegetables and coconut-milk yogurt.

If you choose to introduce fermented foods, it is important to remember probiotics are live microorganisms and too much heat can kill them, so *never* cook or heat them. You don't necessarily have to eat raw sauerkraut and other fermented foods cold, though. Add them to the top of warm (not hot) foods. If you can touch your food without burning yourself, it's probably a safe temperature for your friendly bacteria.

Fermented Foods vs. Probiotic Supplements

The advantage of getting your probiotics from fermented foods instead of supplements that fermented foods *always* comprise a combination of probiotic strains. The proportion of each strain can also vary from batch to batch. Since everyone's gut flora differs, it is difficult to know what types of probiotics will work best for you. If you eat fermented foods on a regular basis, you'll always be getting a different mix of probiotics, making it more likely to provide your gut flora with what it really needs.

In addition to offering various strains, using fermented foods as a delivery method for your probiotics guarantees that you'll be consuming the greatest number of live beneficial microorganisms. Unfortunately, many of the probiotic supplements on the market don't contain enough live bacteria to contribute to your digestive health. A large proportion of the probiotics are often already dead inside the capsule.

These supplements might be sufficient to *maintain* a good digestion if you are already healthy, but they might not be sufficient to *restore* a compromised digestion. Some brands of probiotic supplements test each batch to ensure they contain the right amount of live bacteria, and some companies even conduct scientific studies to assess the efficacy of their products. These high-quality probiotic supplements are a good alternative to fermented foods, but they don't come cheap, unfortunately. With probiotics more than with any other supplements, you really get what you pay for.

Fermented foods, though, are by far more affordable. You can get your daily dose of probiotics from sauerkraut or homemade yogurt for less than one dollar per day, while it could cost you at least three times as much to get a similar dose from reliable supplements. This may not sound like a big difference, but it can add up to hundreds of dollars at the end of the year. Wouldn't you rather spend this hard-earned money on something other than pills? The supplement chapter (Chapter 6) discusses probiotics in more details.

The Controversy over Probiotics

"Gut health and gut flora are a very chicken-and-egg type of thing," says naturopathic doctor Tim Gerstmar. Will improving your digestive health by eating REAL food and following an elimination diet protocol correct your gut dysbiosis? Or will correcting your gut dysbiosis improve your digestive problems? There's still so much not known about probiotics and human gut flora that it's impossible to answer these questions. Fortunately, there is one thing that seems clear: digestive health and a balanced gut flora seem to work together in a synergistic way. If you don't have one of these two things, you can't have the other, and vice versa.

Probiotics have mixed reviews in the scientific literature, probably because there is such tremendous variety in the strains and quantities of live bacteria in different supplements. Many studies have shown promising results for probiotics, while others show limited benefits. The good news is that none of them showed that they could cause any harm (unless you are severely immunocompromised or have short-gut syndrome).

Current technology only allows us to grow about 20 percent of the bacteria found in the human gut, so the remaining 80 percent can't yet be used in supplements. The importance of these little-known strains on digestive health is still unknown and more studies are needed in order to better understand their potential for health. It's also worth noting that very few studies have looked at the benefits of fermented foods as a delivery method for probiotics and it would be interesting to know how their beneficial effects compare to supplements.

If you have SIBO, taking probiotics may do more harm than good in some cases—but this depends on the cause of your SIBO, which is not always easy to identify. If the excessive accumulation of bacteria in your small intestines is due to ineffective cleansing waves in your intestines, taking in more bacteria may exacerbate the problem by worsening the chronic bacterial overgrowth. Remember that the bacteria that overgrow are not necessarily bad, so even the "good" bacteria you get from probiotics could join the party already raging in your small intestines. On the other hand, one study showed that probiotics may help stimulate these cleansing waves, which could be beneficial for people with SIBO. So should you take probiotics? It depends. No one can say how probiotics will affect *you*, so self-experimentation is your best bet to find the right answer for you.

Many digestive-health experts promote the use of probiotics. Elaine Gottschall, creator of the SCD, and Dr. Natasha Campbell-McBride, author of the GAPS nutritional protocol, both advocate the use of probiotics for all kinds of digestive disorders and recommend the use of a therapeutic-strength probiotic supplement in addition to the regular consumption of fermented foods. Dr. Campbell-McBride prescribes a minimum of 15 to 20 billion colony-forming units (CFU) per day for adults. Children require special formulations with smaller amounts.

If your gut flora is compromised, as is almost always the case in people with digestive issues, you definitely need to take action. Your gut flora is unlikely to change on its own. Remember that the bacteria in your gut outnumber the number of cells in your body tenfold and play a vital role in your digestive health. But also keep in mind that everyone is different and has a unique gut flora. Until more studies are conducted, there is no definitive probiotic prescription that works for everyone. Finding the types of probiotic supplements, fermented foods, or both that work *for you* will take some trial and error but is worth the effort.

Take It Slowly

Although fermented foods can be helpful for recovering your digestive health, it may be best to introduce them only once you start getting your symptoms under control. Probiotics from fermented foods offer many benefits, but they can be hard to tolerate at first, especially if you have SIBO or another severe type of gut dysbiosis. By causing shifts in your gut flora, a sudden overdose of probiotics could cause or worsen diarrhea, constipation, bloating, fatigue, and other similarly unpleasant symptoms.

Once you're able to better manage your digestive problems on the elimination diet, you should be able to start introducing tiny amounts of fermented foods or probiotic supplements: one quarter teaspoon (one milliliter) of sauerkraut juice or yogurt per day, for example. Then, gradually increase, to one half teaspoon (two milliliters) per day for the next few days and a little more every few days until you can tolerate at least one quarter to one half cup (60 to 125 milliliters) or even one cup (250 milliliters) of sauerkraut and its juice, yogurt, or other fermented foods on a daily basis.

Avoid *Prebiotics*

The term *probiotics* refers to healthy gut-friendly bacteria, while *prebiotics* means food for the bacteria. People with a *healthy* digestion benefit from taking prebiotics, especially those foods in vegetables and fruits, to nourish and maintain their balanced gut flora. If you have digestive issues, though, giving too much prebiotics to the bacteria in your gut could be counterproductive. In the context of gut dysbiosis, almost any carbohydrate, including lactose, FODMAPs, sugars, and starches, can have a prebiotic effect, contributing to a bacterial overgrowth and resulting in excessive intestinal fermentation with the accompanying digestive problems.

The elimination diet removes most natural prebiotics for a few weeks to give your digestive system a break and prevent excessive fermentation. Keep in mind, however, that many probiotic supplements contain added prebiotics. Before buying a probiotic, check the ingredient list and avoid any with inulin, chicory root, or fructooligosaccharides (FOS), or with the word "prebiotic" on the label.

Cautionary Notes: Thyroid Disorders and Candida

If you have a thyroid disorder, be aware that fermenting goitrogenic foods (like cabbage) increases their goitrogenic potential. Goitrogens include all cruciferous vegetables (bok choy, broccoli, Brussels sprouts, cabbage, cauliflower, collard greens, kale, kohlrabi, radishes, rapini, rutabaga, and turnips), spinach, sweet potatoes, and some fruits (strawberries, pears, peaches). The goitrogenic potential of cruciferous vegetables is higher in their raw state and is increased further by fermentation. Table 49 lists all the goitrogenic foods.

Table 49: Goitrogenic Foods

Food Categories	Goitrogenic Foods

REAL Foods	• Cruciferous vegetables (especially raw and fermented)
	   ○ Bok choy
	   ○ Broccoli
	   ○ Brussels sprouts
	   ○ Cabbage
	   ○ Cauliflower
	   ○ Collard greens
	   ○ Kale
	   ○ Kohlrabi
	   ○ Radishes
	   ○ Rapini
	   ○ Rutabaga
	   ○ Turnips
	 • Spinach
	 • Sweet potatoes
	 • Some fruits (strawberries, pears, peaches)

Foods Already Eliminated	• Canola • Soybeans • Peanuts • Millet

Keep an eye on your thyroid if you start eating sauerkraut or kimchi regularly because goitrogenic foods can interfere with its functioning. Taking iodine can help you better tolerate goitrogens, but you should work with a qualified health professional to decide if this is an option for you and determine an appropriate dose. If you don't want to take any chances, try getting your probiotics from fermented carrots, pickles, or coconut-milk yogurt instead.

Also, if you have a yeast or Candida overgrowth, avoid fermented foods and probiotics that contain yeast, such as kefir and kombucha. Stick to those that provide only bacteria to help you correct your gut dysbiosis.

Natural Seasonings

Processed foods are loaded with artificial ingredients that transform them into super-stimulating foods. The over-the-top flavors in packaged foods can numb your ability to enjoy the taste of REAL food. The good news is that, as you wean your taste buds from flavor-enhanced processed foods, they can and will adapt, and you'll rediscover the original delicious taste of REAL food.

Of course, you can also enhance the flavor of your meals with natural seasonings. Avoid commercial sauces, salad dressings and gravies that contain sugars, MSG, or gluten. Use fresh, unprocessed ingredients such as fresh herbs, lemon or lime juice, and vinegars. Table 50 lists the seasonings that are safe to use in the first phase of your elimination diet as well as those you'll be able to experiment with once you move on to the reintroduction phase.

If you find your meals become a bit repetitive during the elimination phase, make your food more varied and interesting by creating new combinations of protein, fat, plant matter, and seasonings. Once you learn to enjoy the simple satisfaction of REAL food, you may not even feel the need for much seasoning!

Table 50: Safe Seasonings and Ones to Trial

The Seasoning Safe List*	Seasonings to Trial Later
• Unrefined salt • Chives • Asafoetida powder • Cinnamon • Lemon or lime juice • Apple cider vinegar • Ginger • Fresh herbs (basil, rosemary, thyme, parsley, peppermint, sage, tarragon, oregano, dill, cilantro, bay leaves) • Green part of green onions (small amounts, FODMAP free) • Garlic-infused ghee or oil (FODMAP free) • Herb-infused oil	• Balsamic vinegar (aged and sugar free) • Red wine vinegar • Pepper (black and other kinds) • Hot peppers, chili powder, Tabasco sauce, curry powder, paprika (nightshades) • Coconut aminos • Tamari sauce (wheat- and gluten-free) • Sun-dried tomatoes (nightshade) • Onions and garlic (FODMAPs; in salad dressings and mayonnaise) • Sea vegetables (kelp, nori) • Nutmeg, anise seeds, black caraway seeds, celery seeds, cumin seeds, dill seeds, fennel seeds, fenugreek, mustard and poppy seeds

*These choices are usually safe for most people but it is not impossible to react to them; avoid any items you know you are sensitive to.

Keep in mind that many seasonings belong to the nightshade or seed family. Pay close attention to how you react to these groups of plants.

Salt Is Mandatory

The one and only seasoning that you *must* include in your diet is unrefined salt. As with saturated fat, most people have been brainwashed into thinking salt is bad and that it leads to high blood pressure and heart disease. One of the main problems with this claim is that it is based on epidemiological studies that observed the salt intake of different people in relation to their risk of suffering a heart attack (epidemiological studies). And where did most of the people in these studies get their salt? Processed foods. So can we really blame the salt and sodium, or could the health problems attributed to salt actually be due to the sugar, refined carbs, refined oils, trans fats, and other artificial ingredients found in the processed foods consumed by people with a higher sodium intake? It could also be due to the fact that people eating a standard American diet are not getting a balance of minerals? Potassium and magnesium are examples of minerals present mainly in plant-based foods that can help prevent high blood pressure and contribute to heart health if consumed in balance with sodium.

Several recent studies have even showed that a low salt intake is associated with a *higher* risk of dying from cardiovascular disease and type 2 diabetes. Clearly, we can't just single out nutrients without looking at the whole picture. Salt is not evil, especially if you choose unrefined, mineral-rich varieties and use it to season REAL, nutrient-rich food.

Why do you need sodium? First, unprocessed REAL food contains very little sodium. You require an estimated minimum of 500 mg of sodium per day (one fifth of a teaspoon or one milliliter) to allow your body to perform its basic functions, such as maintaining fluid balance and helping with nerve transmission and muscular functions.

Salt is also critical for proper hydration. A lower-carb diet, such as the grain-free, sugar-free one you're starting, can have a slight diuretic (dehydrating) effect. Replenishing your electrolytes, especially sodium, is necessary to help you stay hydrated. This is even more important if you experience regular diarrhea or vomiting.

Getting enough sodium in your diet also supports the function of your adrenal glands. The adrenals sit on top of your kidneys and help orchestrate many of the body's regulatory functions. If you have been suffering from chronic stress, inflammation, gastrointestinal infections, or intestinal problems, or have been simply eating the wrong foods, your adrenal glands are likely to be fatigued. Getting enough sodium in your diet can help them recover and do their job.

WHAT KIND OF SALT?

Avoid processed table salt. It's highly refined, bleached and stripped of the other minerals with which it is naturally found. It's much better to stick with unrefined, more natural alternatives that fit in the REAL food category. The mineral content of unrefined salt can vary depending on where it is from, but these salts always provide small amounts of calcium, potassium, magnesium, sulfur, zinc, and iron. The variety of minerals found in unrefined salt enhances its taste and make it more enjoyable to eat.

Sea salt and Celtic sea salt are good unrefined-salt choices. Avoid Dead Sea salt because it's high in bromide and can be toxic over time. And if you're concerned with the high levels of ocean pollution that could contaminate sea salts, go for Murray River salt from Australia, Utah beds salt, or Himalayan pink salt.

HOW MUCH SALT?

The lowest risk for diseases is associated with a salt intake of between 1.5 and three teaspoons (7.5 to 15 milliliters) per day. You always get a little bit of sodium from food, even REAL unprocessed food, so aim to add at least one half to one full teaspoon of unrefined salt to your food every day. Measure it at the beginning of the day in an empty salt shaker and make sure you use it up over the day. You can add unrefined salt during the cooking process or directly to your food.

> Aim for ½ to 1 teaspoon (2 to 5 ml) of salt a day.

If your kidneys are healthy, don't worry too much about restricting your salt intake. Use as much as you need to make your food tasty to *your* taste buds. If you take a little too much, rest assured that your kidneys regulate the amount of sodium in your body closely and will excrete any excess.

SALT PRECAUTIONS

If you have kidney problems or if your doctor has told you to restrict your sodium intake, be a bit more careful with your sodium intake, and consult a health professional before making any changes.

If you're worried about your blood pressure and heart health despite the lack of evidence that salt is the culprit, just keep track of your blood pressure and other health markers, with the help of your doctor, to reassure you (see Appendix 18).

Be aware that unlike refined table salt, unrefined salts do not contain added iodine. Iodine deficiency is common and supplementation is sometimes necessary. Consult a qualified health professional to know if you need iodine supplements, or introduce iodine-rich REAL food like seaweed into your diet (once you are ready for the reintroduction phase). Kelp is a good sea vegetable to include in your diet because of its high iodine content; a little every day is enough to cover your dietary iodine requirement. Sprinkle dried kelp over your food as a seasoning, or try kelp noodles once or twice a week, if tolerated, once in the reintroduction phase. These noodles are gluten free and go well with a stir-fry of meat, chicken, or shrimp with vegetables, coconut aminos (or gluten-free tamari sauce), and grated ginger.

Fluids

Staying hydrated is important to keep things moving smoothly through your gastrointestinal tract and prevent constipation. It's also helpful to replenish the fluids you lose if you suffer from diarrhea or vomiting. Getting enough fluids can also help you adapt to a lower carb intake when switching to a grain-free, sugar-free, REAL-food-based diet. Carbohydrates from flours and sugars can make your body retain water. Eliminating these foods can have a diuretic effect and allow your body to rid itself of the extra water it's retaining. The only problem is that if you don't replenish your body with enough water and electrolytes to maintain the right hydration level, you may become mildly dehydrated and suffer from headaches, constipation, dizziness, or irritability.

HOW MUCH FLUID?

The traditional recommendation to drink eight glasses of water a day is a good place to start, but you might need more. The color of your urine is a good marker of proper hydration. It should be very light yellow; dark-colored urine means you need to drink more fluids. Keep in mind some supplements like C and B vitamins can make your urine bright yellow even if you're hydrated.

Table 51: Safe Fluids and Ones to Avoid

Safe List*	Avoid for a While
• Water	• Black tea
• Sparkling water	• Coffee (regular and decaf)
• Water with lemon/lime juice	• Hot cocoa
• Water with fresh rosemary, mint, or other herbs	• Soft drinks (even diet)
• Rooibos tea	• Alcohol
• Green tea	
• Ginger tea (made with fresh ginger root)	
• Chamomile tea (no added ingredients)	
• Herbal tea (no sweeteners or added ingredients)	
• Homemade bone broth	

*These choices are usually safe for most people but it's not impossible to react to them; avoid any items you know you are sensitive to.

WHEN SHOULD YOU DRINK?

While it's important to stay hydrated, try to take your fluids *between* meals as much as possible since drinking too much with meals can dilute your gastric juices. This can make your stomach acid and digestive enzymes less effective, potentially compromising your digestion.

Start your day by drinking at least one to two cups (250-500 milliliters) of water upon waking to rehydrate yourself and "wake up" your organs. Water is absorbed within minutes, especially when your stomach is empty, so you can drink as much as you like up to 10 to 15 minutes *before* your meals. Drink a little during and after meals if you need to, but try to keep the amounts to a minimum. Then, try to wait at least one to two hours *after* your meals before drinking more generous amounts of liquids.

Elimination Diet: Common Concerns

Now that you're starting to get a better idea of what your elimination diet should look like, you still be worried about the fact that this way of eating is so different from the conventional nutritional recommendations you've been given by doctors, dietitians, and the media. But try to remember how well your low-fat diet, replete with whole grains, fruits, and vegetables, has been working for you so far. Not too well, or you probably wouldn't be reading this book. Don't be scared of changing your diet to find one that fits your individual needs and tolerances. Trust that your body will let you know what makes it feel at its best.

IS THIS JUST ANOTHER VERSION OF THE ATKINS DIET?

Your carb intake on this diet will be lower as a result of avoiding grains, starchy foods, and sugars. The REAL foods you will use to build your diet are also lower in carbohydrates and higher in fat than the foods most Americans eat on a daily basis. So is this diet like the Atkins diet? Not exactly. While it is true that the Atkins diet is low in carbs, it's not necessarily based on REAL food and does not focus as much on food quality.

Dr. Robert Atkins actually did a great job helping people lose weight and better control their diabetes and heart disease by going against the low-fat paradigm and advocating carbohydrate restriction. However, the focus of Atkins' plan is on keeping one's carb intake below 20 to 50 grams per day, according to your personal carb tolerance threshold, which doesn't prevent the bulk of your diet coming from nutrient-poor, inflammatory, and hard-to-digest foods made with refined oils, artificial sugars, nuts, glutenous food products, and chemical ingredients.

Although the macronutrient ratio of carbohydrates, fat, and protein of the REAL-food-based diet for optimal digestive health may be similar to that of the Atkins diet, the foods you will eat may be very different, based as it is on anti-inflammatory, easy-to-digest, and nutrient-rich REAL foods.

Carbohydrate-restricted diets are not dangerous for your health, on the contrary. Our ancestor hunter-gatherers, which are not that different from us genetically, have not only survived but also thrived on these types of diets for thousands of years. Some of these traditional tribes still exist today, such as the Greenland Natives, Inuit, and Pampas indigenous people, and still benefit from excellent health without the chronic diseases of civilization despite eating very few carbohydrates.

The Institute of Medicine, the scientific institution in charge of setting dietary requirements, even states that, "the lower limit of dietary carbohydrate compatible with life apparently is zero, provided that adequate amounts of protein and fat are consumed." While they acknowledge this fact, they later go on to recommend getting between 45 and 60 percent of your calories from carbohydrates, a confusing conclusion considering their earlier acknowledgement. Carbohydrates are not essential, unlike protein, fat, vitamins, and minerals. But since there is a limit to the amount of protein you can take in—and most people are trapped by the belief that fat is evil—carbohydrates have become the de facto source of dietary energy.

The Nutrition and Metabolism Society, an independent, nonprofit health organization, is trying to spread the word that the high carbohydrate intake resulting from the promotion of low-fat diets could be to blame in the recent rise in obesity, heart diseases, and type 2 diabetes and that higher-fat carbohydrate-restricted diets could actually be the solution for many people. Well-formulated carbohydrate-restricted diets have been shown to be a valid option, often more effective than low-fat, low-glycemic, and Mediterranean diets, to address obesity, cardiovascular disease, and diabetes. Some studies even show the benefits of restricting carb intake to inhibit cancer growth, control epileptic seizures, and even improve neurological conditions such as Parkinson's and Alzheimer's. Digestive problems should also be on the list.

If you have diabetes, hypoglycemia, or other blood-sugar-related disorders, it's important to consult your doctor before cutting carbs from your diet, as is recommended during the elimination phase to reset your digestive system. If you take diabetes medications or insulin, work with your doctor to understand how to adjust your dosage accordingly. You might also need to move into the elimination diet a bit more gradually by slowly reducing your intake of starchy and sugary foods to allow you to keep your blood sugar under control and prevent hypoglycemic reactions. If you want to learn more about how to manage your diabetes by eating a lower-carb, higher-fat diet, consult the book "Dr. Bernstein's Diabetes Solution: The Complete Guide to Achieving Normal Blood Sugars" by Dr. Richard K. Bernstein.

BUT DON'T YOU NEED CARBS FOR ENERGY?

Most nutritional guidelines and dietitians will tell you that you require at least 100 to 130 grams of carbohydrates per day to fuel your brain. While it is true that your brain will use those carbohydrates if you eat a high-carb diet, it doesn't necessarily *have* to.

Your brain doesn't use carbs because it needs them; it uses them because they are available and easy to use. Too much sugar (glucose) circulating in your bloodstream is toxic and causes a lot of damage to the blood vessels in your heart, brain, kidneys, and eyes, so your body burns as much as it can and stores the rest (as glycogen in your liver and muscles if there is room or as fat).

What's important to understand, though, is that your brain can obtain all the energy it needs from other sources. Although your brain corresponds to only two percent of your body weight, it utilizes an impressive *25 percent of the calories you eat.* Even if your brain requires a lot of energy, it doesn't need this energy to come exclusively from carbohydrates.

> It's wrong to say that your brain *needs*
> 100-130 g of *carbohydrates* per day.
>
> It's right to say that it *can burn*
> 100-130 grams of *glucose* (sugar) per day.

Glucose can be derived from the digestion of carbohydrates, but it can also be synthesized from certain amino acids derived from protein and from the glycerol part of fatty acids. The body is clever, and it would have been foolish of Mother Nature to require you to eat a piece of fruit or a muffin every few hours to fuel your brain. Your brain is your most important organ, and you can't afford to let it starve. That's why your brain has another trick up its sleeve. When you burn fat, your body produces ketones (or ketone bodies). If you eat a high-fat diet, ketones supply the majority of the energy your brain needs and the remainder is provided by carbohydrates from vegetables and the conversion of amino acids from protein into sugar.

Between two thirds and three quarters of the energy your brain needs can be derived from ketones. Ketones can also fuel your heart and muscles—in fact, they're a preferred source of energy for most of these organs.

You don't need to eat bread, fruit, or a granola bar every few hours to keep your brain running. If you did, how would our hunter-gatherer ancestors have survived eating only animals and some foraged berries? Do traditional populations like the Inuit turn to smoothies or performance bars to keep up their energy for fishing and hunting? The human genetic makeup hasn't changed much, and your brain can still thrive without excess dietary carbs.

SHOULD YOU BE WORRIED ABOUT KETOSIS?

The supposed danger of ketosis is a common argument against lower-carb, higher-fat diets. What is ketosis? If you eat a standard American diet and get plenty of carbs from wheat, potatoes, and sugary treats, your body will burn the sugar derived from these carbohydrates. If you reduce your carb intake, though, your body will have to start relying on fat to get the energy it requires, from either your diet or your fat stores. Burning fat produces ketone bodies, which can also be used as a source of energy. To be in ketosis means simply that your body is in fat-burning mode and that you have detectable levels of ketones (a byproduct of fat burning) in your body.

As opposed to the type of ketosis that happens during starvation, the ketosis associated with a lower-carb, higher-fat diet is referred to as *nutritional* ketosis and is *not* dangerous. The worst it can do is affect your breath slightly, but this should improve with time as your body learns to use ketones more efficiently.

Why do some people believe ketosis is bad, then? Because they make the mistake of confusing *ketosis* with the life-threatening condition *ketoacidosis*. Ketoacidosis is an extreme case of ketosis that can only occur in people with uncontrolled insulin-dependent diabetes. With ketoacidosis, blood-ketone levels rise to five to ten times higher than what is seen with nutritional ketosis. There is no doubt that ketoacidosis is dangerous, but ketosis is not.

Now that you know how REAL food can help you recover your digestive health, let's move on to the next piece of the puzzle: the how-to. Are you ready to start creating a diet customized just for you? It's time to finally put everything you've learned into practice.

"I am convinced that digestion is the great secret of life." – Sidney Smith

Chapter 5: Design Your Own Diet

Despite all you learned in Chapters 3 and 4 about potentially problematic foods and ones that should be better tolerated, no doctor or dietitian can tell you exactly what *you* should eat. Only *your body* has the definitive answers. It's probably been trying to relay those answers to you for a while now, but it can be hard to listen when all you hear is chaos. The next chapter will show you how to reset your body with an elimination diet protocol so you can quiet your symptoms and hear the peaceful sound of silence again. Then you'll be ready for the reintroduction phase, during which you'll see how your body responds to different foods. Following this protocol will help you finally get clear answers to your questions to allow you build your own optimal diet.

Despite all the recent advances in medicine and technology, elimination diets remain the gold standard for identifying food sensitivities. This protocol was first described by Dr. Albert Rowe in 1926 and published in his book "Elimination Diets and the Patient's Allergies," but they have existed for much longer than that.

Elimination diets include two main phases: the *elimination* phase and the *reintroduction* phase (also called the challenge phase). This underutilized resource can be complicated to use correctly, but this chapter will show you how to proceed to minimize mistakes and maximize your learning so you can move on to living a healthy, happy life as quickly as possible.

The elimination and reintroduction diet protocol is the most effective way to design a diet that will best address your symptoms. You can get tested for food sensitivities, but these tests are expensive and inaccurate. If you have a leaky gut, the results are likely to suggest reactions to dozens of foods.

If you want your digestive health to improve, you need to first address your intestinal permeability by healing and sealing your gut. Then, you need to work on balancing your gut flora to optimize your digestive health. Most people see their symptoms subside in a matter of weeks by following this approach. As the months go by, your digestive health will continue to improve and your food tolerance should increase slowly. Many food sensitivities (with the exception of true food allergies and probably gluten intolerance) can resolve over time if you treat the underlying causes of inflammation, intestinal permeability, and gut dysbiosis.

The Elimination Diet

The rationale behind the use of the elimination diet protocol is simple. During the elimination phase, you'll remove any foods to which you could react. It's like pushing your body's reset button.

> ## It's time to reset your body.

You need to reestablish a baseline of feeling normal if you want to be able to hear what your body has to say. Without the reset of the elimination phase, you won't know what foods you are sensitive to during the reintroduction phase.

There is no one type of elimination diet. There are *many* different types. Some elimination diets are designed to help you identify gluten intolerance, a sensitivity to dairy, or problems with FODMAPs or food chemicals. These are all valid approaches to help you improve your diet and digestive symptoms.

However, eliminating single food groups or ingredients from your diet may not be the most holistic way to proceed, especially if you have been dealing with *chronic* bloating, abdominal pain, flatulence, diarrhea, and constipation. Choosing to eliminate only gluten, only FODMAPs, or only dairy is like using blinders. By focusing only on one potentially problematic element of your diet, you could be missing the big picture. And how will you know what approach to choose, since all of these potentially problematic foods can induce the same digestive problems?

So many things can go wrong with your digestive system. Although gluten-free diets or low-FODMAP diets can help people get better, most people that are intolerant to gluten or FODMAPs are also sensitive to other foods. The other problem is that eliminating only gluten or FODMAPs may help to alleviate symptoms but does not address the underlying issues to improve your food tolerance.

Most doctors and dietitians, but not all, are familiar with the concept of the elimination diet, but many of them prefer not to go suggest it as a treatment option, which is too bad. Elimination diets take work, and they're not exactly glamorous, but they're the best way to get to the bottom of your digestive issues. And remember, although the term "elimination diet" is used to refer to the strict avoidance of specific foods, the goal of an elimination diet is not to eliminate *foods* but to eliminate your *symptoms*.

> ## The goal of the elimination diet is not to eliminate foods, but to eliminate your symptoms.

A properly designed elimination diet can work very well at eliminating your symptoms. And it doesn't have to be difficult if you understand how it works and are prepared for it. It might be scary to have to say goodbye to some of your favorite foods during the elimination phase, but isn't that preferable to dealing with your digestive problems for the rest of your life? You now have the power to do something about your digestive health. What do you have to lose other than a few weeks of not eating your favorite foods? What would you do with your life if your digestive problems simply vanished? Give yourself a chance to find out.

There's no doubt that you'll need to eliminate many foods from your diet at first, but try to think positively. Don't focus so much on all the foods you'll have to eschew. Focus on the ones you *will* be able to eat and reintroduce as the weeks go by. The elimination diet isn't forever—just for a few weeks, long enough to reset your digestive system.

Since the term "elimination diet" may be depressing, let's tweak it to what it really is: a build-your-own (BYO) diet. You will be eliminating foods just long enough to push the reset button of your digestive system and eliminate your symptoms. Once you start feeling better, the real fun will begin and you will be able to start building your own optimal diet based on easy-to-digest, anti-inflammatory, low-irritant, low-allergen and unprocessed foods. See below for a reminder of the seven important factors for building your optimal diet. Let's start building!

Seven Factors of the BYO Diet
1. REAL, Unprocessed Food
2. Easy to Digest
3. Low in Irritants and Allergens
4. Anti Inflammatory
5. Nutrient Dense
6. Carb Restricted
7. Customized

The Elimination Phase

Some people might tell you that milk, bread, or onions is your problem, but beware of simplistic answers. Instead of drawing a straw to see if you should try a low-FODMAP diet, take a no-dairy approach, or go gluten free, why not try to adopt a more holistic approach and try to tackle as many problems as possible at once?

Chapter 3 described in detail the many food groups, ingredients, and food components that could be problematic for you. Table 52 gives you a quick refresher on what to avoid and why during the elimination phase of your BYO diet.

Table 52: Foods to Avoid in the Elimination Phase

Food Groups	Problematic Compounds	Reasons to Avoid Them
Grains (wheat, barley, rye, oats, quinoa, amaranth, millet, teff, triticale, kamut, rice, corn)	Gluten and similar hard-to-digest proteins	• Can increase intestinal permeability • Can irritate your digestive system • Can trigger food-sensitivity reactions
	Carbohydrates (starches and sugars)	• Can feed a gut dysbiosis*
	Anti-nutrients	• Prevent the absorption of nutrients • Can irritate your digestive system
	Insoluble fiber	• Can irritate your digestive system
	Fructans (FODMAPs)	• Can feed a gut dysbiosis*
	Natural food chemicals	• Can irritate your digestive system
	Processed ingredients	• Can trigger food-sensitivity reactions • Can promote inflammation • Can irritate your digestive system
Dairy (all except ghee)	Casein and whey	• Can trigger food-sensitivity reactions
	Lactose (FODMAPs)	• Can feed a gut dysbiosis*
	Added sugars	• Can feed a gut dysbiosis*
Soy	Soy protein	• Can trigger food-sensitivity reactions
Peanuts	Peanut protein	• Can trigger food-sensitivity reactions
	Peanut lectins/aflatoxins	• Can irritate your digestive system
Legumes (beans and lentils)	Galactans (FODMAPs)	• Can feed a gut dysbiosis*
	Starches	• Can feed a gut dysbiosis*
	Natural food chemicals	• Can irritate your digestive system
	Processed ingredients	• Can trigger food-sensitivity reactions • Can promote inflammation • Can irritate your digestive system
Refined Oils (soybean oil, canola oil, corn oil, etc.)	High omega-6 fat content	• Can promote inflammation (especially if eaten in excess of omega-3) • Can contribute to intestinal permeability
Some Vegetables, Fruits and Tubers	Starches (in starchy vegetables)	• Can feed a gut dysbiosis*
	Sugars (in fruits)	• Can feed a gut dysbiosis*
	FODMAPs	• Can feed a gut dysbiosis*
	Cruciferous vegetables	• Can irritate your digestive system • Can feed a gut dysbiosis*
	Natural food chemicals	• Can irritate your digestive system
	Glycoalkaloids (in nightshades)	• Can promote inflammation • Can irritate your digestive system
	Insoluble fiber (especially in the skin, seeds, or membranes, and/or in raw vegetables)	• Can irritate your digestive system
Processed Ingredients	Sugars, FODMAPs, food chemicals, problematic proteins, etc.	• Can trigger food-sensitivity reactions • Can promote inflammation • Can irritate your digestive system
Sugars	Sugars	• Can feed a gut dysbiosis* • Can promote inflammation • Can slow down your immune system
	FODMAPs	• Can feed a gut dysbiosis*
Nuts and Seeds	Natural food chemicals	• Can irritate your digestive system
	High omega-6-to-omega-3 ratio	• Can promote inflammation
	FODMAPs	• Can feed a gut dysbiosis*
	Protein	• Can trigger food-sensitivity reactions
Spices	Natural food chemicals	• Can irritate your digestive system
Eggs	Egg proteins	• Can trigger food-sensitivity reactions

*Gut dysbiosis includes SIBO, candida overgrowth, and other gut-flora imbalances.

Remember that you won't have to eliminate all of these foods for the rest of your life—just the next month or two. Then you can start designing your BYO diet. Many people are able to reintroduce some of the nutritious REAL foods they removed, such as eggs, some vegetables and fruits, dairy, and nuts.

Most elimination diet protocols will provide you with long lists of ingredients you need to avoid, but let's work in the opposite direction and keep things simple? And it can be very simple if you focus on eating REAL food.

It's always a good idea to check the ingredient lists on the labels of the foods you eat. Of course, on a REAL-food diet, most of what you're eating won't even have a label. But when you do have to scrutinize a label to decide if a food is worthy of eating, instead of trying to memorize dozens of potentially problematic ingredients, all you have to do is to follow this one simple rule: if you don't know what it is, don't eat it.

> # If you don't know what it is, don't eat it!

It doesn't matter whether hydrolyzed vegetable protein, sodium caseinate, thickeners, caramel color, or natural flavorings contain gluten, dairy, or fermentable carbohydrates. These strange, unpronounceable ingredients won't provide any of the nutrients your body needs to heal. None of these mysterious ingredients are REAL food.

If you see anything suspicious on an ingredient list, you're probably hanging out in the wrong section of the grocery store: the middle aisles. This section is filled with cans, boxes, and bottles of "food products." Put them back on the shelf and make your way to the perimeter of the store, where you'll find all the REAL food you need. Better yet, make a run for the nearest farmers' market!

GETTING STARTED

Ready to give this a try? Remember that the worst thing that can happen is you have to say no to your bowl of breakfast cereal or your chocolate treat for a few weeks. And the best thing that can happen is that you regain your digestive health and eliminate your GI issues. Sound fair?

Pull out your calendar and put a big circle around the date you want to start your BYO diet. Next week, perhaps, or even better: tomorrow. Until then, you have a little bit of work to do to prepare yourself.

TAKE A DIGESTIVE SNAPSHOT

The first step is to take a snapshot of your digestive health as it is right now. Trust me: It's easy to forget how bad you used to feel once you get better! Humans have a protective ability to let our memories of unpleasant things seem less harsh as time passes.

Use the table below to track your symptoms (you'll also find two copies of this chart for your before-and-after evaluation in Appendix 1). You can add other symptoms to the chart. Don't forget to add details about non-digestive symptoms, too. Consider your skin (acne, eczema, etc.), respiratory problems, mood swings, joint pain, and any other health problems that could be related to your suboptimal digestion. This table will be a good tool for you to evaluate your progress after a few weeks on the elimination diet.

Table 53: Symptom Chart

Symptoms Date: _____	Before							
	Frequency				Severity			
	Daily	Almost daily	3-4 times a week	1-2 times a week	Rarely	Mild	Moderate	Severe
Bloating								
Abdominal pain								
Flatulence								
Belching								
Feeling of urgency								
Acid reflux								
Fatigue								
Depression								
Brain fog								
Bowel movements	Average frequency: per day / week Appearance on the poop chart (circle): 1 2 3 4 5 6 7 a b							

CLEAN YOUR KITCHEN

If you still have bread, crackers, commercial yogurt, beers, or soy milk in your kitchen, it's time to get rid of them. There's no point in sugar-coating reality: the first two to three weeks can be difficult, and having your former favorite foods around is just asking for trouble.

You'll need to be on the elimination phase of your BYO diet for at least three to four weeks, eating no gluten, dairy, soy, corn, sugar, or any problematic foods the whole time. If you succumb to temptation, you may have to start this period all over again. The effects of some of these problematic foods on your digestive health can unfortunately last a little while (a few days to even a few weeks in some cases), and you can't move on to the reintroduction phase before they are fully out of the picture. Bottom line: Clean your kitchen!

Get rid of anything that isn't REAL food. Anything that comes from a food-manufacturing plant or packaged in a can or box is out. To make it easy, pretty much all the so-called "foods" with long ingredient lists should be discarded. You can give them to friends, family or colleagues… but only if you don't like those people, because most of these foods aren't healthy for anyone. Another option if you don't want to waste these "food products" is to put them in a big box. Seal it and hide it, ideally in a difficult-to-reach spot where its contents will be out of your mind for the duration of your elimination diet. The advantage of processed foods is that they can keep for a *long time* without spoiling since they contain very few nutrients and a generous dose of preservatives.

Try not to use this kitchen makeover as a "last meal" opportunity to binge on potentially problematic foods. It can be scary to have to eliminate so many foods at once. But remember that it's just a few weeks, not necessarily forever.

Many foods that can trigger reactions and induce symptoms can actually have an addictive effect on your body, making them very difficult to give up. It may be hard to believe that your body could be addicted to something that makes you feel bad, but it's true. This is also one of the reasons it's so difficult to identify a food sensitivity. It's not uncommon to be unknowingly sensitive to the favorite foods you eat on a daily basis—the ones you might least suspect. When you eat a food to which you are sensitive, your body can respond by releasing feel-good endorphins to counteract the adverse food reaction. After a few days, or even a few hours in some cases, the decrease in your endorphin levels and the appearance of withdrawal symptoms can trigger cravings that push you to eat the food again. And the cycle of feeling "not too bad" then awful continues.

Think positive. You're not depriving yourself of these foods to punish yourself. Don't focus on the foods you are giving up. Remember why you're doing this: because you want take your health into your own hands. You're giving yourself a chance to feel better, to live without worrying about your intestines. It will be challenging, but your efforts will pay off.

WHAT IF YOU DON'T LIVE ALONE?

Living with someone else who is not willing to make the same dietary changes can make things difficult but not impossible. Let the people you live with know that you are trying a dietary experiment to help you feel better. To avoid being confronted with the foods you're trying hard to avoid, ask your spouse, roommate, friends, or children to put these foods in a separate cupboard or section of the fridge to help you at first. In a few months, you probably won't even consider bread, pasta, and cookies deserving of the label "food" after not eating them for so long. Things *will* get easier as you start feeling better.

An even better solution would be to convince your housemates to join your experiment! Even if they don't have the same digestive issues, going grain-, dairy-, sugar- and processed-food-free for a while is a great way for anyone to detox and understand how their body reacts to different foods. This elimination diet protocol can be useful not only for improving digestive health, but also for skin problems, fatigue, asthma, and blood sugar, hormonal, or autoimmune issues. In any case, there is no risk in experimenting with REAL food, and like you, your friends and family will likely be pleasantly surprised by the results.

STOCK UP ON REAL FOOD

The next step to prepare for building your optimal diet is to make sure you have all the ingredients you need—and enough of them. Unlike processed foods like pasta, canned sugary tomato sauces, and breakfast cereals that can last for weeks or months (if not years), REAL food can spoil more easily. This means you may have to go to the grocery store or farmers' market a bit more often to always have the animal protein, vegetables, and healthy fats you need.

If you plan well, you can buy everything you need once a week. You may have to freeze some of your animal protein and thaw it at the end of the week to keep it fresh. Table 54 gives you an idea of what you'll need to have on hand and the approximate amount you'll need per week. Many people fail to eat enough when they eliminate processed foods from their diet. They just don't know how much REAL food they need. It's an elimination diet—not a starvation diet.

Table 54: Stocking up for the Elimination Phase

Food Groups	Shopping List for the Elimination Phase	Weekly Amount for One
Animal Protein**,***	☑ Meat (beef, bison, venison, lamb, wild boar, pork) ☑ Organ meat and offal (liver, tongue, kidneys) ☑ Poultry (chicken, turkey, duck) ☑ Fish (salmon, sardines, herring, mackerel, sole) ☑ Seafood (scallops, oysters, crab, lobster, mussels)	Around 4-8 oz (120-240 g) per meal (and possibly some at snack time) = 5-10 lbs (2.5-5 kg) per week
Traditional Fats	☑ Extra-virgin coconut oil ☑ Ghee ☑ Butter (to make your own ghee) ☑ Extra-virgin olive oil (or macadamia oil or avocado oil) ☑ Duck fat, tallow, or lard	At least 1-3 tbsp (15-45 ml) per meal (and possibly some at snack time) = 1.5-4 cups (300 ml to 1 l) per week
Bones	☑ Ideally from grass-fed cows, pastured chicken, or wild-caught white fish to make homemade bone broth	1 large or 2 small chicken carcasses or about 1-2 lbs of bones per week
Vegetables (always cooked at the beginning)	☑ Carrot ☑ Zucchini ☑ Spinach ☑ Green beans	Between ¼-¾ cup (60-175 ml) per meal (and possibly some at snack time) = 5-21 cups (1.2-5 l) per week
Seasonings (all optional, with the exception of unrefined salt)	☑ Unrefined salt**** ☑ Chives ☑ Asafoetida powder ☑ Cinnamon ☑ Lemon juice ☑ Lime juice ☑ Apple cider vinegar ☑ Fresh herbs ☑ Green part of green onions ☑ Garlic-infused oil ☑ Herb-infused oil	Between ½-1 tsp. (2-5 ml) of unrefined salt a day = 3.5 to 7 tsp (18 to 35 ml) per week The other seasonings can be purchased as needed or desired
Beverages (optional)	☑ Sparkling water ☑ Lemon or lime juice to add to water ☑ Fresh herbs to add to water ☑ Rooibos tea	As needed or desired

*The ideal is to eat organic produce and animal protein, ghee, and butter from healthy, happy, pastured animals; **Avoid shrimp, smoked fish, and aged/cured meats (bacon, sausage, ham) at the beginning; ***Avoid animal proteins that are marinated, in a sauce, or breaded, ****Unless you have been medically advised to avoid salt

BUT REALLY: WHAT WILL I EAT?

During the first phase of the elimination diet, you won't be eating a large variety of foods—just simple REAL food. There's no need for complex recipes; just assemble allowed ingredients from each food category. Keep things simple. You'll find plenty of recipes and meal ideas in Chapter 10 as well as a sample meal plan in Chapter 11.

Here's the magic formula to remember when preparing each of your meals to make sure they are nutritious and complete:

Animal Protein	Traditional Fats	Safe Vegetables	Seasonings
4-8 oz per meal (120-240 g)	1-3 tbsp per meal (15-45 ml)	1/4-3/4 cup per meal (60-175 ml)	Salt + others as desired at least 1/2 tsp. (2 ml) of salt per day

The serving sizes are just a *guideline*. Don't eat less than the lower suggested range, though, even if you're trying to lose weight. It's the minimum amount of food you need to get the basic nutrients you need to heal, but some people might need more. If you're hungry or underweight, eat larger servings (especially of fat and protein) or eat more often (four to six times per day if needed).

a REAL-food meal

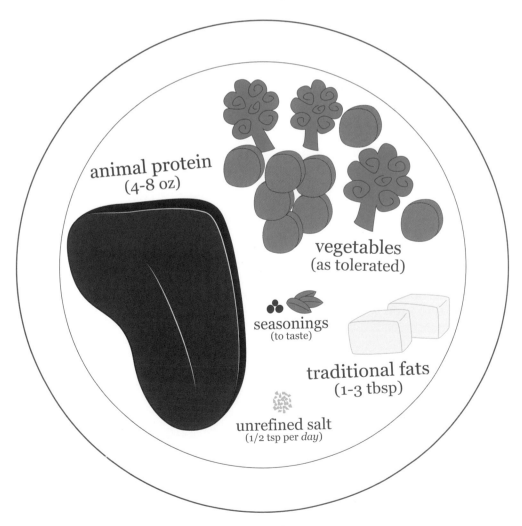

animal protein
(4-8 oz)

vegetables
(as tolerated)

seasonings
(to taste)

traditional fats
(1-3 tbsp)

unrefined salt
(1/2 tsp per *day*)

Still not sure what you'll eat? Table 55 shows a few examples, and there are more ideas in the meal-plan chapter. Even though you'll be eating the same foods often, you don't need to be eating the same meals all the time! Use your imagination and you'll find lots of ways of combining these foods to come up with tasty, creative meals.

Table 55: Quick Meal Ideas

Meals	Menu
Breakfast	• Chicken soup with zucchini [chicken + bone broth + zucchini + chives + salt] • Rooibos tea with coconut oil
Lunch	• Salmon salad [salmon + cooked spinach + olive oil + lemon juice + salt]
Dinner	• Lamb stew [lamb/beef + green beans + ghee + salt + rosemary]
Snacks (as needed)	• Rooibos tea with coconut oil • Leftover soup or stew • Homemade bone broth • Puréed carrots mixed with cinnamon + coconut oil

DINNER FOR BREAKFAST?

Chicken soup for breakfast? Most people are used to having cereals, oatmeal, toast, pancakes, and smoothies for breakfast, but this is a recent practice. These foods were introduced at the beginning of the last century and promoted as a healthy way to start the day, but this was not the main objective behind their invention. Food manufacturers weren't really interested in making your grandparents healthier; they were interested in profit. Processed foods like breakfast cereals are simply more profitable than meat, traditional fats, and vegetables.

It's time to stop thinking of breakfast as a special meal at which you need to eat special foods. Many cultures around the world have long eaten the same foods for breakfast, lunch, and dinner. Kicking off the day with satiating protein, nourishing healthy fats, and nutrient-dense vegetables is the best way to ensure stable energy levels and optimize your digestion. Though it might seem a little strange at first, you'll soon wonder how you once started your day with that high-carb, grain-packed feast.

GETTING ENOUGH ENERGY

One of the most common mistakes people make when starting on this kind of protocol is not eating enough. Some simply remove the processed foods but fail to replace the lost calories with REAL food! When not eating the foods you used to eat, it can be difficult to know what your serving sizes should be. You should get a decent amount of protein at each meal (four to eight ounces or 120 to 240 grams), but most of your calories should come from fat. Remember the magic formula?

Animal Protein	Traditional Fats	Safe Vegetables	Seasonings
4-8 oz per meal (120-240 g)	1-3 tbsp per meal (15-45 ml)	1/4-3/4 cup per meal (60-175 ml)	salt + others as desired at least 1/2 tsp. (2 ml) of salt per day

You will naturally have some fat as part of your animal protein, but that won't be enough. You *need* to add more. You can use the extra one to three tablespoons (15 to 45 milliliters) of fat you need at each meal for cooking your meat, fish, or poultry, or to prepare your vegetables. Use it as a dip for your food, or just add it to your soups and stews or on top of your vegetables. Just make sure you get at least one to three tablespoons at each of your meals.

You can also include some fat at snack time if you feel hungry. Another good way to make sure you get enough fat is to mix it with puréed vegetables, add some to your tea, or even eat it by the spoonful. It might feel strange at first, but you'll soon get used to it as you see how much better this way of eating makes you feel. Don't be afraid of eating too much fat, but increase it gradually so your liver has time to adjust and start secreting more bile, especially if you used to eat a low-fat diet. If you're still worried about the effects of eating more fat on your heart health, reread the fat section in Chapter 4 and have your doctor check your cardiovascular risk markers to be reassured.

THE IMPORTANCE OF JOURNALING

If you don't have a food journal, start one now. A journal is an invaluable tool as you are trying to build your optimal diet. Use whatever form you prefer: a notebook, an Excel spreadsheet, or an online journal. Take a few minutes to write down what you eat and how you feel, ideally after each meal. Doing it at the end of the day is better than not doing it, but try to be as meticulous as you can since it's easy to omit important details.

The following items may not seem to mix well, but they are your best cues to monitor your digestive health:

- Your foods
- Your supplements
- Your symptoms
- Your bowel movements

Write down what you eat at each meal. It's also a good idea to note your serving sizes, especially when it comes to vegetables. The four vegetables you'll include at the start of the elimination diet (unless you have a known intolerance to any of them) are relatively safe, but eating too much at once could still trigger your bloating and other digestive symptoms.

Take note of your symptoms, indicating the severity from 0 to 10, for example, or by classifying them as benign, mild, moderate, or severe. Also write down the times of your bowel movements and what type each one corresponds to on the poop chart. You can even add notes about your sleep and stress. Table 57 shows you an example of a digestive-health journal.

Table 56: Digestive-Health Journal

Day	Food and Supplements	My Health

May 15 (day 4 of the elimination diet)	8am: Chicken soup with ½ cup zucchini and chives, rooibos tea with coconut oil (digestive enzymes, probiotics)
	
	11am: Spoonful of ghee
	
	Noon: Lamb stew with rosemary, ¾ cup pureed carrots mixed with coconut oil and cinnamon (digestive enzymes)
	
	3pm: Cup of bone broth
	
	6pm: Meat patties mixed with the green part of spring onions, ½ cup spinach sautéed in coconut oil (digestive enzymes, probiotics, zinc)
	
	8pm: ½ puréed carrots mixed with cinnamon and coconut oil (cod liver oil)
		Sleep 6 hours, stress 7/10
		
		Abdominal pain between 9-10 am (moderate)
		
		Cravings around 11am
		
		Bloating (moderate) most of the day, but better as the day went by
		
		Headache in pm (moderate)
		
		Skin rash on thighs (moderate, slightly better than yesterday)
		
		4 bowel movements
		
		    7am: type #7
		
		    8h15am: type #6
		
		    3h30pm: type #7
		
		    4pm: type #5
		
		    * saw undigested food

May 16 (day 5 of the elimination diet)
 	
First good day!!!
	8am: Chicken with 12 green beans, ghee and chives, rooibos tea with coconut oil (digestive enzymes, probiotics)
	
	12:30pm: Salmon mixed with ½ cooked spinach, olive oil and lemon juice, spoonful of ghee (digestive enzymes)
	
	2:30pm: Cup of bone broth
	
	6:15pm: Lamb stew with rosemary and carrots (digestive enzymes, probiotics, zinc)
	
	7:30pm: Puréed carrots mixed with cinnamon and coconut oil (cod liver oil)
		Sleep 7 hours, stress 5/10
		
		Abdominal pain between 9-10 am (but very mild)
		
		Bloating (very mild) only after carrot snack
		
		Skin rash on thighs (improving, almost gone)
		
		3 bowel movements
		
		    7 AM: type #6
		
		    7:15 AM: type #5
		
		    8 AM: type #5

Circle, highlight, or put a sticker on each day your symptoms improve significantly so you can see more easily how many days in a row you have been symptom free (or nearly so) and help decide when you're ready for the reintroduction phase.

It can sometimes be hard to see a connection between what you eat and how you feel by looking only at a couple of days, but once you have collected data for a few days or weeks, you'll better discern patterns and identify problematic foods. It's also important to keep in mind when writing and analyzing your journal that your symptoms are not necessarily caused by what you ate at your last meal. Some reactions may be delayed by a few hours or even days, and some foods can have a cumulative effect. And it's not just about food. Sleep and stress play a huge role in your digestive and overall health, as you will see in Chapter 6.

HOW LONG SHOULD I FOLLOW THE ELIMINATION DIET?

In most cases, three to four weeks is sufficient. Your digestive system will start to heal quickly if you give it a chance. Remember that the goal is to reset your digestive system and improve most of your unpleasant symptoms. If your digestive problems are related to your diet, you should see improvement within the first month. And even if each day isn't perfect, you should start to notice a *trend* in the right direction, in which the bad days get better and further apart.

> **Follow these two criteria to gauge how long to stay on the elimination phase:**
>
> - Follow the elimination diet for a *minimum of three to four weeks* and
> - Be *mostly symptom free* for at least *five consecutive days*.

Being symptom free doesn't mean having *perfect* digestive health, but you should experience at least five consecutive days of significant improvement in your symptoms before moving on to the reintroduction phase. For some people, this can happen right at the three-week mark, but others may need as long as six to eight weeks to get there. The severity and duration of your digestive problems may affect how long it takes to reset your digestive system. People with autoimmune conditions may also need more time to reset their system before moving on to the reintroduction phase.

Your food journal will help you keep track of your symptom-free days so you know when you're ready for the reintroduction phase. Once you're ready for the reintroduction phase, the rest will be a walk in the park. It's the first two to three weeks that are the most difficult. Be ready because the elimination phase may make you feel worse before you feel better.

The Storm Before the Calm

This plan is designed to make you feel better, but you might to have go through a little discomfort before things start looking up. But why would eliminating "bad" pro-inflammatory foods and allowing only "good" easy-to-digest, nourishing ones make you feel bad?

> **There are actually three main reasons for feeling worse before feeling better:**
>
> - Withdrawal symptoms
> - Die-off symptoms
> - Low-carb flu (or keto-adaptation)

Depending on where you start and what your current diet looks like, the transition to the elimination diet may be a breeze, a storm, or anywhere in between. Not everyone experiences withdrawal, die-off, or low-carb-flu symptoms, but they're common. Don't give up hope: Once this storm clears, you'll see it was worth weathering.

WITHDRAWAL AND DIE-OFF

Withdrawal and die-off symptoms are somewhat mysterious, but they exist. It's possible to actually be addicted to certain foods that contain gluten, caffeine, dairy, sugar, and other processed ingredients, and giving up these foods can be—pun intended!—no piece of cake.

Withdrawal symptoms generally occur within the first two weeks after eliminating addictive foods and foods to which you are sensitive. They seem to be more common toward the end of the first week but can also happen as soon as within a few hours or as late as the second week.

Withdrawal can cause headaches, fatigue, drowsiness, depression, difficulty concentrating, flu-like symptoms, and even muscle pain and stiffness. You may have experienced a withdrawal reaction if you've ever tried to quit caffeine. The same can happen with bread, yogurt, sugar, and many other foods. Natural food chemicals found in tomatoes and fermented foods, as well as processed foods containing MSG, flavorings, and dyes have been shown to have pharmacological properties that can cause withdrawal symptoms.

Die-off. Sounds ominous, right? A change in your diet can result in big shifts in your gut flora. The elimination diet can help you starve undesirable microorganisms in your intestines. When some of the bacteria, yeast, or parasites die, they can release toxins that are absorbed into your bloodstream. If many of these bugs die at once, your liver's ability to clear these toxins from your body may be overwhelmed, making you feel unwell for a little while. This die-off reaction is also sometimes referred to as the Herxheimer (or Jarisch-Herxheimer) reaction.

It's also possible to experience a die-off reaction if you take regular or herbal antibiotics. Die-off symptoms usually don't last more than three to five days. The die-off reaction tends to appear only at the beginning, but you can experience it later on if you make significant changes to your diet (such as going back to eating sugar then stopping again).

So what are the symptoms of withdrawal and die-off reactions? Almost anything! For most people, it involves a worsening of their usual digestive symptoms, such as bloating, cramping, diarrhea, or constipation. It's also possible to experience headaches or migraines, skin rashes, fatigue, brain fog, fever, cravings, irritability, nausea, vomiting, flu-like symptoms, sleep disturbances, stuffiness, joint pain, and muscle stiffness. If you feel bad when starting the elimination diet, take this as a good sign! Withdrawal or die-off symptoms mean that some of the foods you eliminated are indeed problematic for you.

LOW-CARB FLU (KETO ADAPTATION)

Low-carb flu is another thing that might make you feel worse before you feel better. Low-carb flu is more frequent in people used to consuming a significant amount of carbohydrates, but anybody can experience it when starting on the elimination diet.

For some people, the low-carb flu only lasts a couple of days, but it can linger as long as four weeks for some. Someone reading up on low-carb diets may also come across the terms "fat adaptation" or "keto adaptation," coined by low-carb researcher Stephen D. Phinney, MD, PhD, to refer to this transition period. When your body switches from a higher-carb to a lower-carb intake, it needs some time to adjust. It can no longer burn carbohydrates as its primary source of energy and now needs to rely on fat (from both your diet and body-fat stores) for fuel. Your body is naturally efficient at burning fat for energy, but it can forget how to do so if you've been eating a high-carb diet for a while. Your body is also smart, though, and will re-learn how to favor fat, but in the interim you may feel tired, irritable, dizzy (especially when standing up), or headache-y.

Going through withdrawal, die-off, or the low-carb flu is no fun, but understanding what's happening inside your body can make things easier. These symptoms aren't a sign to give up. Give your body a few more weeks to adjust and see if this approach is working for you.

> ## "After the rain there's a rainbow, after a storm there's calm, after the night there's a morning, and after an ending there's a new beginning."
>
> – Anonymous

ALLEVIATING THE TRANSITION

Although you can't completely avoid the unpleasant symptoms associated with withdrawal, die-off, and fat-adaptation, you can certainly try to minimize their intensity. Here are a few tips to help ease things (see more tips in the troubleshooting chapter):

- **Take warm Epsom salt baths**. Epsom salt is a form of magnesium (magnesium sulphate) that originates in the town of Epsom in England. Its medicinal properties help the release of toxins and metabolic wastes through the skin. The mineral magnesium can also be absorbed into your body through your skin, providing a calming and relaxing effect. Add about two cups (500 milliliters) of Epsom salts to a hot bath and soak for 15 to 20 minutes. Rest for at least 15 minutes after the bath for maximal effect.

- **Try activated charcoal capsules**. Activated charcoal may sound like a strange supplement, but it has been used for a long time, especially to treat poisoning. Activated charcoal can reduce the absorption of poisonous substances, such as the toxins released by dying microorganisms, and lessen side-effects associated with die-off reactions.

- **Eat enough**. Many people make the mistake of not eating enough. Remember: you *need* to eat more fat. You can't be on a low-carb and a low-fat diet at the same time. Your body still needs the same amount of energy and fat is the safest way to provide it during the elimination diet without causing digestive issues. Eating enough fat will also help your body become keto adapted more rapidly. Without sufficient fat, you're likely to experience cravings and feel tired and irritable.

- **Hydrate properly.** Your body needs enough fluids to help it detox. Drinking enough water is also important to prevent the mild dehydration often associated with low-carb flu. You also need enough fluids to normalize your bowel movements and prevent constipation during the elimination diet.

- You should also make sure you add at least one half teaspoon (two milliliters per day) of unrefined salt to your food. Without enough sodium, your body won't be able to retain the right amount of water, leaving you at risk for dehydration. Dehydration can cause fatigue, headaches, irritability, dizziness, and constipation. Drinking bone broth seasoned with unrefined salt is another good way to get a variety of electrolytes and enough fluids into your body.

- **Rest**. Now is the time to take care of yourself. Skip the jogging or your regular exercise routine. Stay home from work or school for a few days if you can. Your body needs all the energy it has to go through this transition period and start the healing process. Be kind to yourself and don't overdo it.

A Strict and Restrictive Approach

The primary goal of this plan is to make you feel better as *quickly* as possible so you can start designing your own optimal diet. It's like putting your broken digestive system in a cast to reset it. You need to eliminate residual symptoms and go through the potential side effects of the elimination diet as quickly as possible so you can move on to the reintroduction phase. Remember: The goal is not to eliminate foods, but to eliminate your symptoms.

If you prefer, you can try a gluten-free diet for a month to see how it makes you feel. Then, if that doesn't work, try a low-FODMAP approach the following month. If your digestion isn't improved, you could then try eliminating dairy, nightshades, or nuts for another month. You get the picture. With such an approach, it could take many months before you start to feel better and understand what foods are best for *your* digestive system. This doesn't mean that some people can't get complete relief by eliminating only grains and sugar or by removing dairy and gluten from their diet. That might be enough for some, but not necessarily for you. Since there is no way of knowing before trying, taking a more holistic approach that accounts for all possible factors at the same time is the best way to help you get better more quickly.

You can use a less restrictive or more gradual approach if you prefer. Cutting out grains, sugar, and processed foods is a good place to start. In many cases, these changes alone can make a big difference in the way you feel. The only problem is that this less-restrictive approach is less likely to make you feel 100-percent better. Is 75 percent enough? It's sure better than the way you feel now, but would you say no to the opportunity to feel *completely* better? The choice is yours.

There's one major exception to this strict approach: If you've been diagnosed with SIBO and were treated successfully with antibiotics (or will be in the near future), you may be able to include a bit more carbohydrates from winter squashes, fruits, and even roots and tubers. This exception may even be appropriate for people with only mild symptoms. You can try to make these higher-carb REAL foods part of your elimination phase if you want. If your symptoms fail to improve after three to four weeks, though, you probably need to return to the stricter fruit-free, starch-free version of the elimination diet.

WOULD A GRADUAL APPROACH WORK?

A step-down approach can work, but will take more time. For example, you could start by eliminating gluten, then all grains. After a few weeks, remove dairy and soy from your diet, then artificial ingredients, then sugar. This tack will probably help you mitigate the side effects associated with withdrawal, die-off, and the low-carb flu, but it will take more time before you feel better and can move on to the reintroduction phase. Keep in mind, too, that you'll need to be on the strictest phase of the elimination diet for at least three weeks before moving on to the next step.

> No matter what path you choose, it will probably lead you to something better. You decide if you want to do the hard, quick hike up the mountain or take the longer, panoramic route.

If you only have occasional indigestion symptoms, the protocol suggested in this book may be overkill. Mild bloating or constipation once or twice a month can probably be avoided simply by eliminating the most common culprits: gluten, sugar, and processed foods. But if you're experiencing digestive symptoms on a daily or almost daily basis, it's time to get serious.

STICKING TO THE PLAN

First, let's be clear: Nobody's perfect. Of course, it's important that you try your best to resist cravings as much as possible, which I know can be quite difficult during the first days and weeks. What will happen if you give in and eat something that's not on the list of foods suggested for the elimination diet? The answer is, it depends: on what you eat; on what your body is most sensitive to; on how much you eat. It also depends on how much you sleep you had and even your attitude toward the "cheat." The most likely consequence, however, of eating foods that are not part of the protocol (such as ice cream, chocolate, or chips) is that you will feel sick if your body is sensitive to one or more of the ingredients they contain.

Another problem with straying from the protocol is that it can make you go through withdrawal and die-off symptoms again. If it was not a pleasant experience the first time, it won't be the second time. Be prepared for more cravings in the days after eating foods to which you are sensitive or that could result in excessive fermentation in your intestines, especially gluten, grains, dairy, FODMAPs, and sugar.

"Guilt is one of the worst foods for the intestines." – Bill Tims

In addition to the return of your previous symptoms, eating the wrong foods can delay your readiness for the reintroduction phase. Remember that you need to be symptom free (or almost symptom free) for at least five days in a row before you're ready to try adding back more foods to your diet. You are probably looking forward to eating a larger variety of foods, but this won't happen if you can't properly "reset" your digestive system. Don't think of this protocol as a "diet" that you must follow. This is a way of eating that you are adopting to feel better. You are *choosing* to avoid foods that make your tummy unhappy and choosing to give your body what it needs to heal and become healthier.

"Never confuse a single defeat with a final defeat." – F. Scott Fitzgerald

It's almost impossible not to make mistakes or succumb to temptation at some point. Consider it *part* of the process and try to learn from it. If you can't resist the muffins at the office meeting or the cake when eating out, what can you do to keep it from happening again? Maybe you can bring something safe to eat next time, or write a list of the symptoms these foods induce on an index card and carry it with you.

"It does not matter how slowly you go as long as you do not stop."

– Confucius

Sometimes, making a mistake and eating something that triggers your symptoms can actually be good for you. Although you might feel sick for a few hours or days, it can be a good reminder of your motivations. When you start to feel better, it can be easy to forget how miserable you used to feel. A quick reality check can help you remember how you don't want to let your bowels run your life anymore. It's also a good reminder that food truly *is* powerful and that it can make you feel bad or good. It's up to you and only you to choose the right foods for your body.

"Fall down seven times; get up eight." – Japanese proverb

FOCUS ON TAKING CARE OF YOU

It can be difficult to change your eating habits and eliminate many foods at once, especially since food is often used as a way to reward or comfort yourself, to fight boredom, to celebrate, or to manage stress. Despite the strong emotional and psychological relationships you may have with food, try changing your mindset. Use food as fuel only in the next several weeks. Find non-food alternatives to get the comfort or reward you deserve.

Try a warm bath with candles. Treat yourself to a massage. Read a book. Rest. Listen to music. Watch a funny movie. Go outside. Take the focus off using foods for the wrong reasons and place it back on taking good care of you. Try to end each of your meals with something positive. You may not eat a dessert in the traditional sense, but you still deserve a treat, so take 10 or 20 minutes after each meal to do something that makes you feel good. Lie down on the couch, dance to your favorite music, or even soak up some vitamin-rich sunlight in a nearby park.

Not only will this help you eliminate the habit of using food to feed your emotions rather than satisfy your body's requirements, but the relaxing effect of taking time for yourself will also help you digest better. See Chapter 7 to learn more about the importance of stress management in digestive health. And remember to think positive. The objective of your *elimination* diet is to eliminate your *symptoms*!

Moving on to the reintroduction phase too quickly could backfire. Even if you are starting to feel great after a week, it is best to wait a bit longer to ensure the effectiveness of the elimination protocol. If you don't follow the elimination diet for a minimum of three weeks, it is still possible to start experiencing withdrawal or die-off reactions in the second or third week, which could make you believe falsely that you are reacting to the some of the foods you are trying to reintroduce.

For example, if you have been on the strict phase of the elimination diet for a week and feel a lot better, you may decide to trial avocados to see how you tolerate them. But if your symptoms return, it will be *impossible* to know whether they're due to the avocado or the appearance of withdrawal or die-off symptoms. Be patient if you don't want to make things more complicated than they already are. Push the reset button *completely*.

"I am a slow walker, but I never walk back." – Abraham Lincoln

Elimination = Nutrient Deficiencies?

Conventional nutritional recommendations insist that variety is essential to obtain all the nutrients your body requires. Of course, having a varied diet is important to maximize your exposure to all the minerals, vitamins, and other important nutrients in different foods. But is the standard American diet really varied?

Most people who follow conventional nutritional recommendations are fooled into thinking they eat a varied diet when they are *not*. Food manufacturers turn a few ingredients like wheat, soy, corn, and sugar into hundreds of different foods that may look different but are all extensively processed and nutrient poor. These processed foods that constitute the foundation of many people's diets contain only the nutrients added to them by food manufacturers. Pasta, tortillas, breakfast cereals, breads, and granola bars all contain about the same ingredients and have poor nutrient density. They contain a lot of carbohydrates and few added vitamins and minerals (often in synthetic, less-bio-available forms).

Even though the elimination diet phase is limited in terms of food variety, it is based on REAL, nutrient-dense food. Animal protein and vegetables are some of the densest sources of nutrition, and you can maximize your nutrient intake by emphasizing the quality of your food, choosing meat from pastured animals, wild-caught fish, ghee from grass-fed cows, and organic vegetables. And remember that you're at risk of nutrient deficiencies anyway if you don't take care of the most important organ responsible for nutrient absorption: your intestines. Also, the stricter phase of the elimination diet only lasts a few weeks. During the reintroduction phase, you'll be able to add a lot more variety to your diet.

Table 57 shows you how the elimination diet can provide you with a lot more nutrients than a standard American one. You can get over 100 percent of eight of the 17 essential vitamins and minerals even in the elimination phase (left column). For the nine nutrients that are lacking, the elimination diet still provides over two thirds of your requirements for five of them. Even if you don't eat a lot of vegetables at first, the generous amounts of fat in your diet will help better absorb the nutrients they supply.

Simply adding a small weekly four-ounce serving of liver and a one-cup serving of broccoli, as well as replacing salmon with sardines (with the bones) in the first week (right column) of the reintroduction phase is enough to help you meet your dietary requirements for 15 of the 17 essential vitamins and minerals.

Table 57: Nutrition in the Elimination and Reintroduction (First Week) Phases

Meals	Elimination Phase (foods)	Nutrient	Value	First Week of Reintroduction Phase (foods)	Nutrient	Value
Breakfast	½ cup bone broth	Calories	1,936	½ cup bone broth	Calories	1,948
	5 oz. chicken	Protein	119 g	5 oz. chicken	Protein	127 g
	2 tbsp. coconut oil	Fat	149 g	1 tbsp. coconut oil	Fat	142 g
Lunch	½ cup zucchini	Carbs	31 g	1 cup broccoli	Carbs	45 g
	5 oz. salmon	Fiber	12 g	4 oz. sardines	Fiber	18 g
	½ cup spinach	Vitamin A	421%	½ cup spinach	Vitamin A	634%
	2 tbsp. olive oil	Vitamin B1	106%	2 tbsp. olive oil	Vitamin B1	122%
	1 tbsp. lemon juice	Vitamin B2	111%	1 tbsp. lemon juice	Vitamin B2	193%
	1 tbsp. fresh chives	Vitamin B3	260%	1 tbsp. fresh chives	Vitamin B3	247%
Dinner	½ cup bone broth	Vitamin B5	88%	½ cup bone broth	Vitamin B5	144%
	6 oz. ground beef and pork	Vitamin B6	209%	6 oz. ground beef and pork	Vitamin B6	207%
	½ cup carrots	Vitamin B12	418%	½ cup carrots	Vitamin B12	700%
	2 tbsp. ghee	Vitamin C	45%	½ cup zucchini	Vitamin C	213%
		Vitamin D	0%	2 tbsp. ghee	Vitamin D	125%
Snack	½ cup puréed carrot mixed with cinnamon and coconut oil	Vitamin E	79%	½ cup puréed carrot mixed with cinnamon and coconut oil	Vitamin E	105%
		Calcium	35%		Calcium	72%
Other	-	Copper	86%	4 oz. of liver per week	Copper	125%
		Iron	61%		Iron	100%
		Magnesium	85%		Magnesium	96%
		Manganese	105%		Manganese	135%
		Potassium	66%		Potassium	74%
		Selenium	243%		Selenium	289%

Nutritional analysis conducted with data from the USDA food database; the nutritional value of organic vegetables, grass-fed ghee, extra-virgin olive oil, pastured chicken and beef, and wild-caught fish is likely to be higher; the nutritional value of bone broth is not taken fully into account here since preparation methods may vary.

IRON

Even though iron, calcium, and potassium intake are slightly lower than what is recommended, the lack of anti-nutrients found in grains, legumes, nuts, and seeds will allow you to absorb more of them. Not getting too much iron may actually be a good thing too, especially at first, since some bacteria can feed off this mineral.

CALCIUM

Calcium intake appears low but it is important to consider that the amount provided by homemade bone broth is not taken into consideration in this table (because of a lack of available data). Homemade broth, traditionally prepared by boiling it for several hours with a little vinegar to allow more minerals to leach out of the bones, is rich in calcium, magnesium, and potassium. It is therefore very likely that you will obtain more of these minerals than the amount shown in this table.

Also, don't forget that you can have healthy bones even if you don't meet the high calcium requirements established by the Institute of Medicine. Many cultures and populations around the world have proven that you can grow and maintain strong bones without dairy, provided that you get enough vitamin D, vitamin K_2, and other bone building minerals, in addition to doing weight-bearing exercises.

VITAMIN D

Sardines are a good source of vitamin D, but it's difficult to obtain enough of the "sun vitamin" from food alone. Vitamin D supplements are often required to get enough of this fat-soluble vitamin, as explained in the supplement chapter.

FIBER

The elimination phase is low in fiber, providing about 12 grams of fiber per day compared to the 25 to 38 grams recommended for healthy adults. This is actually done *on purpose*. Remember that you can't digest fiber, and it can be irritating to damaged intestines. It stays intact in your GI tract and can act like a scrub brush on your intestines, especially if they are already compromised. Fiber that stays undigested in your intestines can also become food for microorganisms in your gut. This is usually a good thing *if* you have a healthy gut flora, but if your gut flora is unbalanced, as is the case for most people with digestive disorders, eating too much fiber can worsen your symptoms.

Removing hard-to-digest whole grains and nuts and limiting your vegetable and fruit intake in the first weeks will help give your gastrointestinal tract a well-deserved break. As you start to feel better, you'll be able to reintroduce more fiber, mainly from non-starchy vegetables, winter squashes, fruits, and nuts (as tolerated). In the previous example, the simple addition of a daily cup of broccoli in the first week of the reintroduction phase helped increase fiber intake by six grams. As you progress, you'll be able to get a significant amount of fiber from plant foods, although individual tolerance can vary. Go back to the table on page 127 (or in Appendix 12) to remind you of all the best grain-free sources of fiber.

In addition, it's important to remember that you don't necessarily need fiber to move your bowels. It might take your body a few days to adjust, but you shouldn't be constipated as long as you drink enough water and eat plenty of traditional fats. If that doesn't seem to be enough, taking probiotics or magnesium supplements in the form of magnesium citrate can be just what you need to stimulate regular bowel movements. Learn about more tips to beat constipation in the troubleshooting chapter.

FOOD QUALITY

Remember that you can also get more nutrition by paying attention to the quality of your food. Free-range chicken, pastured pork, grass-fed beef, wild-caught fish, ghee from grass-fed cows, and extra-virgin olive oil are more nutritious than conventionally raised meat, regular butter, and regular olive oil.

As you progress with the reintroduction phase of your elimination diet, you should be able to meet your nutritional requirements as your food tolerances improve. If you are still worried about nutrient deficiencies, consult the supplement chapter to learn about options to cover all your bases.

What If the Elimination Phase Isn't Working?

What if you've been on the elimination phase of the diet for six to eight weeks, without eating any of the problematic foods from Chapter 3, and still aren't feeling better? The elimination diet is usually very effective at helping people with digestive issues get better. If it doesn't, there are a few possibilities that you should look into:

- GI infection
- Candida infection
- Supplements
- Fat intake
- Stress

GI INFECTION

Did you decide not to have a stool test to check for harmful microorganisms squatting in your intestines? Maybe it's time to take that test. If your stool culture was regular, consider taking a more accurate DNA stool test to make sure you get diagnosed properly and treated accordingly. If you have a parasite infection, for example, you won't be able to get better even if you change your diet. You will need to take the appropriate measures, with the help of a qualified health practitioner, to eradicate the infection before returning to the elimination diet to help heal your intestines.

CANDIDA OVERGROWTH

A DNA stool test can also help you determine if you have excess yeast, such as candida, living in your GI tract. While a very low-carb diet is usually a good tool to get rid of the excess bacteria and yeast in your intestines, it does not always work with candida. In some cases, candida and other yeasts can learn to feed on ketones, the byproducts of fat burning. If this is your case, increasing your carb intake to prevent ketosis and the formation of ketones that feed candida may be helpful. Of course, you don't want to get your carbohydrates from sugar or grains, since these foods are pro-inflammatory, irritating, and nutrient poor, and can also feed yeast. Instead, try adding small servings of sweet potatoes and winter squashes, such as pumpkin, butternut squash, spaghetti squash and acorn squash, to your diet. Try these foods one at a time, every three to four days, to see which ones you can eat without getting symptoms. A serving of one half to one cup (125 to 250 milliliters) at most of your meals should be sufficient to keep you out of ketosis. Try this approach for three to four weeks to see if it helps.

SUPPLEMENTS

Another common problem that can prevent you from seeing improvements in your symptoms is supplements. Some supplements can definitely be helpful for your digestive health, but they can also be counterproductive in some cases. Always read the ingredient lists of any supplements you take. Avoid those containing sorbitol, sugar, rice flour, gluten, dairy, fructooligosaccharides (FOS), or other potentially problematic ingredients. Even if the amount is very small, supplements containing these ingredients could be problematic. In case of doubt, discontinue all of your supplements for a few days to see if your symptoms subside (consult your doctor first to make sure it's safe to do so). Read Chapter 6 to learn more about supplements.

FAT INTAKE

Eating too much fat can also be a problem. Although the elimination phase of your BYO diet is *meant* to be high in fat, your body may not be ready to handle it. The best way to know if your fat intake is problematic is to look at your stools. Frequent diarrhea, especially accompanied with steatorrhea (fatty stools that look greasy, float, and have a pale color and a foul odor), is a good indicator that your body isn't digesting fat properly.

You can try replacing most of your fat with coconut oil or MCT oil, since their fats don't require bile to be digested and absorbed. Also consider taking ox bile or digestive enzymes. Taking betaine HCl supplements to make your stomach more acidic can also help stimulate bile production. Drinking a bit of water with apple cider vinegar or lemon juice right before your meals can also help you better digest fat and control your digestive symptoms. Consult Chapter 6 for more info.

STRESS

Although the foods and supplements you put in your mouth make a huge difference in your quest for good digestive health, you shouldn't neglect non-dietary factors. Even if you're doing everything right diet-wise, not sleeping enough or feeling stressed can be enough to perpetuate your digestive issues. Stress does not cause IBS or digestive problems per se, but it can definitely contribute to making them worse. You've probably already experienced abdominal discomfort or even diarrhea in periods of stress, such as before speaking publicly or taking an exam. Remember that your gut is like your second brain, and don't underestimate the importance of your emotions. See Chapter 7 for more about stress management in relation to digestive health. You can also consult Chapter 9 to discover other factors that could be interfering with your progress on the elimination diet.

Ready to Move On?

If, on the other hand, the elimination phase has worked well for you so far, here are two questions to ask yourself to make sure you're ready to move on to the next stage:

- Have you been on the elimination phase for at least three to four weeks?
- Have you been mostly symptom free for at least the last five days in a row?

If you answer yes to these two questions, it's time to move on to the reintroduction phase. You will now be able to experiment with new foods and expand your BYO diet!

The Reintroduction Phase

The reintroduction phase is where the fun begins! Hopefully, you're now starting to feel better than you have in a long time. Reintroducing foods you haven't eaten for a few weeks is a special and memorable experience, especially once your taste buds have detoxed from processed foods. Rediscovering the taste of REAL foods like eggs, broccoli, and butter can be uniquely pleasurable. Pay close attention to their flavor and texture and enjoy every bite! Even though you may be looking forward to eating a wider range of foods, it's important to heed two pieces of wisdom about the reintroduction phase: *go slow* and *be systematic*.

It's exciting to challenge yourself with new foods and expand your culinary horizons, but many people make the mistake of going overboard and experimenting with too many foods at once. What happens, for instance, if you try adding eggs, avocado, and bacon all at once? One of two things: If you're lucky, you'll keep feeling good and won't notice any changes in your symptoms or bowel movements.

But in many cases, playing around with too many new foods at once can backfire. If you start experiencing bloating, diarrhea, lack of energy, cramping, headaches, insomnia, or constipation, you'll know to suspect eggs, avocado, and/ or bacon—but which one(s), exactly? It could be the eggs, the eggs and avocado, the bacon and eggs, the bacon only, the avocado only, or all of them! How can you figure it out? You'll have to take a big step back and avoid all three foods for four to five days until your symptoms subside. Try again once you have two to three symptom-free days in a row, but with only *one* food at a time.

How Does Reintroduction Work?

Every three to four days, you can reintroduce *one* new food. It's wise to choose foods that are less likely to provoke a reaction, but you can also base your choices on personal preferences (such as foods you miss the most). Let's look at an example to better understand how the reintroduction phase works. Let's say that you just completed the elimination phase and have been almost symptom free for the past five days. The key is to go slow and introduce new foods gradually, in a systematic manner. Let's pretend that the first food you want to trial on Monday is avocado. Continue eating the foods you've been eating, but add one quarter avocado at one of your meals that day. If you're still symptom free on Tuesday, try adding one half avocado. If you still don't notice any changes in your bowel movements or digestive symptoms, try a whole avocado on Wednesday. If you feel fine on Thursday, your digestive system is happy to welcome this new REAL food back into your diet. Table 58 sums up the reintroduction protocol.

Table 58: The Reintroduction Protocol

Progression	Reintroduction Protocol	
First Day	• Eat a small serving of a new food	e.g. ¼ avocado
Second Day	• Double the serving size	e.g. ½ avocado
Third Day	• Double the serving size again	e.g. whole avocado
Fourth Day	• Eat the same serving again (optional)	e.g. whole avocado
If Symptoms	• Stop eating the new food if you start experiencing symptoms • Remove the new food and go back to your safe foods • Reset your body until you get two to three symptom-free days	
If No Symptoms	• Keep the new foods in your diet and try a new food	

It's important to make sure you've been symptom free (or nearly so) for at least two to three days before trying a new food. If you experience symptoms at any time, stop eating the new food. If the symptoms started on the same day or the day after, it is likely that you can't tolerate avocado, at least right now. This doesn't mean you won't be able to tolerate it for the rest of your life, and you can do another avocado trial in a few weeks or months if you like.

If the symptoms start on the third or fourth day, it probably means you can handle small amounts or have the food occasionally, but can't tolerate large servings. It could also mean you have a delayed response to that food and can't tolerate even small amounts. How can you know for sure? You'll need to do another trial. Make it your next trial if you really want to know if you can handle avocado, or wait until later.

SERVING SIZES

The reason to start with a small serving and increase gradually over three to four days is to minimize any potential negative reaction. Your digestive system and gut flora may need to adapt to new foods you are reintroducing and going gradually can help smooth the transition.

Also, most people react within a few hours of eating a food, although it's possible for a reaction to be delayed by over 48 hours. For most people, starting with a small serving will allow them to quickly see how they handle a new food. If you react within a few hours, the reaction will at least be smaller with only a few slices of avocado than with a whole avocado. Smaller servings don't guarantee you won't experience unpleasant side effects, but they're a good strategy to lessen that possibility.

WHAT SHOULD YOU LOOK FOR?

How will you know if you can tolerate a new food? Listen to your body. Any changes in your bowel movements, such as diarrhea or constipation, or a worsening of your digestive symptoms, including bloating, abdominal pain, or gas, are a sign that this food isn't right for you, at least not right now.

But the symptoms you look for shouldn't be limited to your digestion. If you experience systemic symptoms, such as fatigue, brain fog, joint pain, headaches, insomnia, nausea, or skin rashes, you should keep this food out of your diet for a little while. An increased heart rate (10 to 20 beats per minute faster) after eating is also a sign that you don't tolerate a food. If you have an autoimmune condition such as rheumatoid arthritis, multiple sclerosis, or Hashimoto's thyroiditis, a worsening of your autoimmune symptoms is another sign that this food isn't right for you.

Don't forget to use your food journal to keep track. It's easy to remember after trialing only one or two new foods, but it can become very confusing as you add more foods in the reintroduction phase of your elimination diet. Appendix 2 provides a journal template to help you record your food-trialing experiences.

RESET YOUR DIGESTIVE SYSTEM

It doesn't make sense to try adding eggs to your diet if you're still experiencing symptoms from trialing avocado. How will you know if your digestive problems are due to the avocado or the eggs? Anytime you experience symptoms that appear to be due to the reintroduction of a new food, eliminate that food from your diet and go back to your previous safe list of foods. Eat only the foods you know your body can handle until you are (nearly) symptom free for at least two to three days in a row to reset your digestive system. Make sure you have your daily dose of homemade bone broth and that you rest and relax as much as possible to promote intestinal healing and get you ready to trial new foods.

CHOOSING THE RIGHT TIME

You don't *need* to be trialing new foods every three to four days. If you're happy with your food variety, there's nothing wrong with sticking to that diet. You're free to take a break from the food reintroduction phase if you want to keep feeling good without the risk of new symptoms from reintroducing foods.

> Your own optimal diet will always be a work in progress. You're in charge of determining if you're ready to experiment with new foods or if you'd rather keep sailing smoothly for a little while.

It can actually be a good thing to follow a diet that helps you remain symptom free most of the time, because that's when more healing and gut flora rebalancing can occur. However, you shouldn't avoid trialing new foods for that reason alone. It's important to build a diet that provides enough variety to make it easier to stick to this way of eating and be successful in the long term.

The timing of your food trials is also important. If you're going through a stressful situation in your life, such as a move, a tight deadline at work, or exams at school, it might be best to postpone the reintroduction of new foods. Mental or emotional stress can make you less likely to tolerate any new foods. Physical stress like a cold or back pain can also affect the results of your reintroduction experiment. Even positive stressors, like getting married, traveling, or competitive sports can compromise your food tolerance and digestive health. It's best to wait until things have calmed before playing with new foods. If you're going away on vacation or a business trip and can't afford to get sick again, you should also take a break from the reintroduction phase and stick with your safe foods.

Some people decide to try one new food per week instead of every three to four days. If you work full time during the week and don't want to feel bad at work, try your new food at dinner on Friday so you have the whole weekend to recover if you experience a bad reaction. Choose the timing and pacing that work for *you*.

INDIVIDUAL FOODS VS. FOOD CATEGORIES

Wouldn't it be nice if you could assess your tolerance to more than one food at once? You could save a lot of time by challenging entire food groups at once instead of just individual foods. Some IBS and diet books suggest that if you can successfully reintroduce a few foods in a specific category, you're good to go with all the other foods in that category. For example, if you tolerate a couple of polyol-containing foods like mushrooms and watermelons, you can assume that you'll handle *all* other foods within the same FODMAP category, such as apples, apricots, blackberries, pears, avocado, celery, and cauliflower.

It would be convenient if this were the case, but unfortunately, it's not. The problem is that foods are complex and contain many different compounds. With the polyol example, many foods in that category also contain other potentially problematic compounds. Besides containing polyols, blackberries are also high in insoluble fiber and seeds, pears and apples contain fructose, and watermelon contains fructans. Cauliflower is also a cruciferous vegetable, while mushrooms are a fungus, and avocado, mushrooms, blackberries, and apricots are all high in natural food chemicals, especially salicylates.

And that's only counting what we know about these foods. FODMAPs were only recently identified and it's likely that there are other unknown compounds in foods that have similar effects. The bottom line is you can't extrapolate. That you tolerate mushrooms and watermelon only means you tolerate mushrooms and watermelon. Stick to individual food challenges if you want to get clear answers about the foods your body can tolerate at any given point. It may take a bit more time and patience, but it is more accurate and can help you prevent mistakes that can set back your healing process.

Getting Started Reintroducing Foods

You'll be happy to know that there's no specific reintroduction order to follow. Just make sure to keep avoiding hard-to-digest, inflammatory, irritating, allergenic, and processed foods as much as you can.

When deciding which foods to reintroduce first, base your decision on your personal food preferences. Try reintroducing foods that will help make your diet more varied and easier to follow. Choosing to reintroduce nutrient-dense foods that will help you improve your nutritional intake is another factor to keep in mind. And if you want to make sure you continue feeling as good as you have since the elimination phase, prioritize foods less likely to cause a food reaction. Finally, please make sure you never reintroduce foods to which you know you are allergic.

Table 59: Factors of Food Reintroduction Order

Factors To Consider to Establish Your Reintroduction Order	
1. Personal Preference	Choose foods you miss the most and that will help you make your diet more enjoyable and easier to follow.
2. Nutrient Density	Choose nutrient-dense REAL foods that will help you improve your nutritional intake.
3. Reaction Potential	Choose foods that are less likely to provoke a food reaction.

THE ONLY RULES TO FOLLOW WHEN REINTRODUCING NEW FOODS ARE:

- Reintroduce only one new food at a time, and
- Space the reintroduction of new foods by at least three to four days.

If you ever experience side effects from reintroducing a new food, stop eating it and reset your digestive system for at least two to three days before reintroducing another new food. Ready to add more variety to your diet?

EGGS

One of the first foods you can try reintroducing is egg yolk. While some people may react to eggs, they most often react to the proteins found in egg whites. Egg yolks are rich in many important nutrients that can be hard to obtain in other foods (especially choline, for which liver is the only other food source).

You can add egg yolks to a soup, stew, or puréed vegetables, or use them raw as a sauce for your animal protein. If you eat your egg yolks raw, make sure they come from a source you can trust. Don't eat raw egg yolks from the supermarket. You can also hard boil your eggs and separate the yolk carefully from the white. Snack on your hard-boiled egg yolks or mash them with puréed carrots and cinnamon. Once egg yolks are back in your diet, try making hollandaise sauce or homemade mayonnaise with approved extra-virgin or cold-pressed oils (see recipe in Chapter 10).

If you tolerate egg yolks without any symptoms, you can then try whole eggs. If you don't tolerate yolks, though, don't even bother with the whites. Wait a few weeks or months and try again with the yolks once you believe your food tolerance has improved.

It's also important to keep in mind that some people are sensitive to eggs only if they come from a hen that was fed soy or corn. To increase your chance of tolerating eggs, get your hands on some from pastured hens on a completely wheat-free, soy-free, and corn-free diet. You may need to ask a few more questions at the supermarket or farmers' market to find a reliable source, but it could be worth the effort considering the nutrition, versatility, and great economic value of eggs.

VEGETABLES

If you're tired of eating the same vegetables all the time, consider experimenting with new options. You can trial any vegetables you like, whether nightshades, cruciferous vegetables, or high-FODMAP vegetables.

Always start by cooking the vegetables thoroughly. Deseeding, peeling, and puréeing vegetables can also increase your chance of success. It doesn't mean that you will always have to eat your cauliflower puréed, but it can help your body better tolerate it at first. If cauliflower doesn't work, try well-cooked tomatoes, onions, or asparagus.

After a few weeks or months, depending on how you feel, you can try having your vegetables al dente and eventually raw. Keep taking notes to record your trials and symptoms. You can also experiment with vegetables with a slightly higher carb content, but still low in starches, such as winter squashes, pumpkin, and beets. Butternut squash makes a great addition to soups or can be puréed and mixed with cinnamon and butter (if tolerated) for a delicious treat. Spaghetti squash can be used to replace grain-based pasta. You can use beets to make low-starch baked fries. See the recipe chapter for more ideas on how to use these different foods if you're unsure what to do with them.

ANIMAL PROTEIN

Remember that you omitted shrimps, cured and aged meats, and smoked fish during the elimination phase. It's now time to add back these foods, one at a time, if you choose to do so. Some of these foods are a bit more processed, so always read the ingredient list to make sure they don't contain added sugar, MSG, gluten, wheat, soy, or other nasty ingredients. If you see anything you don't like, can't recognize, or can't pronounce, don't eat it. Always try to find a cleaner alternative if possible.

Commercial bacon, ham, and sausages almost always contain added nitrites or nitrates, which are used to preserve the pink color of the meat. Keep in mind that these preservatives are natural food chemicals and can trigger all sorts of symptoms depending on your personal sensitivity and the amount you eat at one time. You can experiment with these foods to see how you tolerate them if you wish. Most people can eat them safely, on an occasional basis and in reasonable amounts.

You may also notice that some brands of aged and cured meats claim to be prepared with only natural ingredients, but "natural" bacon, ham, and sausages are not necessarily nitrite- and nitrate-free. Food manufacturers often use cultured celery extract, a natural source of nitrites and nitrates, to replace the chemical version. These natural nitrates and nitrites can induce the same side effects as other natural food chemicals if you are sensitive to them. Be careful with "natural" cured meats since their total nitrite and nitrate content may even be *higher* than that of conventional cured meats. It's difficult for food manufacturers to know the exact nitrite and nitrate content of cultured celery extract, and there is no maximal limit regarding the use of this "natural" ingredient.

If you are sensitive to nitrites and nitrates, try making your own cured meats or ask your butcher to prepare some with ingredients you tolerate. Some farmers' markets may also offer safer cured-meat options.

TRADITIONAL FATS

If you want to experiment with different types of fat, avocado and olives are delicious, nutritious options. Coconut milk and coconut butter are other good choices, but make sure you choose a brand with no guar gum to maximize your likelihood of tolerating it. You can also try introducing butter, ideally from the milk of grass-fed cows. Unless you have a dairy allergy or severe casein sensitivity, you should be able to handle the very small amounts of casein found in butter.

DAIRY PRODUCTS

Dairy isn't a requirement, but you can certainly try reintroducing it if you miss it. Different dairy products contain different proportions of lactose and casein, and following a specific order of reintroduction can help you minimize adverse effects if you discover you're still sensitive to one or both of these compounds.

Start with butter. If you can do butter, try heavy cream or crème fraîche. Both of these dairy products contain only trace casein and lactose and are tolerated by most people. The next step would be homemade 24-hour-fermented yogurt (see recipe in Chapter 10). By fermenting it long enough, you'll remove almost all, and possibly all, of the lactose present naturally in the milk. Homemade yogurt still contains casein, so people who are casein sensitive should stay away. Homemade yogurt is also rich in beneficial probiotic bacteria, so it should be introduced slowly to prevent a rapid shift in your gut flora that could result in unpleasant side effects. Start with only one half to one teaspoon (two to five milliliters) per day and increase very gradually to minimize potential side effects.

If you're having trouble tolerating homemade yogurt, try making it from grass-fed milk. Many people report that dairy from healthy and happy pastured cows is easier to tolerate. In addition, pastured dairy is nutritionally superior: it contains more vitamins A, D, E, and K_2, anti-cancer CLAs, and many other important nutrients. Raw dairy products, as opposed to pasteurized, are also easier to digest for most people because of the active enzymes they contain. If you can find raw milk from a farmer you trust in your area, try using it to prepare your homemade yogurt to increase your chance of tolerating dairy.

Even if you have an adverse reaction to the casein in dairy products made from regular black and white Holstein cows, you can still experiment with other types of dairy products. You could be sensitive to the A1 type of casein found in most dairy products, but you might tolerate the A2 casein in dairy from Jersey cows, goats, buffalo, camel, and a few other ancestral ruminant species. Many people can't tolerate yogurt made from regular cow's milk but have no problem with goat's-milk products.

There are many options for you if you want to make dairy part of your diet, but again, it's completely up to you. Even if you can't tolerate yogurt now, it doesn't mean your tolerance won't improve in a few months or next year.

Feel free to focus your attention on reintroducing other foods like vegetables and fruits.

If you do fine with yogurt, you can move on to the next step: cheese and milk. Start with a tiny serving and increase it gradually every day. Keep in mind that the quality of the dairy products can make a big difference in how well you tolerate them. Cheese, especially if aged, contains casein but almost no lactose, while milk contains both lactose and casein. Again, people report better tolerance with raw milk and cheese. Dairy products from goat and Jersey cows that produce the A2 version of casein may also be easier to tolerate.

If you're prone to acne, have blood sugar or hormonal issues like diabetes or PCOS, or suffer from an autoimmune condition, you may find that you do best without protein-containing dairy products (yogurt, cheese, and milk). You can certainly trial these foods after the reintroduction protocol if you like, but many people with these conditions find these foods to be problematic. Butter and heavy cream should be fine, but some people are so sensitive that they can only do ghee.

SEASONINGS

If you want to have a bit more fun in the kitchen, try introducing more safe seasonings (see Appendix 5). Treat them as individual foods and experiment with them one by one to make sure your body accepts them.

Coconut aminos are a good soy-free, gluten-free alternative to soy sauce to flavor your Asian-inspired stir-fries, though many people can tolerate the small amount of soy in gluten-free, wheat-free tamari sauce. You can also try different types of vinegars, though be careful with balsamic vinegar, since cheaper versions often contain added sugar, even if it's not in the ingredient list. Avoid "balsamic glaze" as it's full of sugar. Try to choose real Italian balsamic vinegar. If you see the word "aged" on the label, you'll know it's the real stuff. Real balsamic vinegar may be a bit more expensive, but you don't need as much of it since the flavor is more concentrated. You can add balsamic or red wine vinegar to your stews or drizzle it over your meat and vegetables.

Other spices, like black pepper, curry, chili powder, and hot pepper sauce are also okay to experiment with at this point, but keep in mind that they can trigger symptoms in some people. Many seasonings belong either to the nightshade or seed family. Pay attention to your symptoms to ensure your digestive system can tolerate each new seasoning.

FERMENTED FOODS

Fermented foods are the best option to help you start rebuilding a healthy gut flora. You can choose dairy-based fermented foods (yogurt or kefir) or stick to fermented vegetables if you don't tolerate casein. You will find basic ferment recipes in Chapter 10. Either way, make sure you introduce fermented foods *very slowly*.

Even though fermented foods can be good for your digestive health, taking too much without allowing your gastrointestinal tract time to adjust can cause your gut flora to shift too rapidly and induce unpleasant side effects such as bloating, gas, diarrhea, or any of your other previous symptoms. Take baby steps and increase your dose gradually.

One quarter to one half teaspoon (one to two milliliters) of sauerkraut juice or 24-hour homemade yogurt per day is enough to start. Stay at this dose for a few days, then double your dose every few days or every week. You may experience some digestive symptoms, but stick with it for up to one week. With any other new foods, it's best to discontinue any of them if they cause any symptoms, however mild. With fermented foods, however, be a bit more persistent. If you have a severe gut dysbiosis, it is possible that forcing a shift in your gut flora will be slightly uncomfortable at first. If your digestive symptoms become too severe at any time, decrease your dose for a few days and start increasing it again in a few days. If one type of fermented food doesn't seem to be working well for you, experiment with other options (especially dairy-free ones) or consider taking a good-quality probiotic instead (see Chapter 6).

NUTS AND SEEDS

Nuts can be hard on your digestive system because of their high-fiber and inflammatory omega-6 content, but some people can tolerate small amounts. If well tolerated, nuts and nut butters make a convenient portable snack option. Nut flours can also be used to make grain-free baked goods. Just make sure you don't make nut flour one of your new staple foods because it can displace nutrient-dense REAL foods.

Start with nut butters. Your stomach doesn't have to work as hard to digest them since they are already ground. Also be sure to choose ones without added ingredients like sugar or hydrogenated oils (trans fats). You can also make your own nut butter. All you need are nuts and a blender! Grinding the nuts will first allow you to obtain nut flour, which you can use to make grain-free baked goods. Otherwise, grind your nuts a few more minutes until they turn into nut butter. Add a small amount of coconut oil if you like to make the texture smoother and creamier. If you tolerate nut butters well, see how you do with whole, raw nuts. For some people, soaking and dehydrating nuts can make them easier to digest and tolerate (as explained in the recipe chapter).

And if you're worried about the omega-6-to-omega-3 ratio of your diet, choose nuts with the least inflammatory ratio: coconut and macadamia nuts.

Table 60: Omega Ratios of Nuts and Seeds

| Ratio | Omega-6-to-Omega-3 Ratio of Nuts and Seeds | | |
	Ideal	Moderate	High
Recommended Consumption (if tolerated)	Every day	No more than a few times per week	Only occasionally
Nuts	• Coconut* • Macadamias	• Hazelnuts • Cashews • Almonds	• Walnuts • Brazil nuts • Pistachios • Pecans • Sunflower seeds • Pumpkin seeds • Sesame seeds

*Coconut is not a tree nut but a drupe.

Trial macadamia nut butter and whole macadamias first to see how you tolerate them. Cashews, hazelnuts, and almonds have a moderate omega-6-to-omega-3 ratio and can be part of your diet if you tolerate them. However, you should be careful with walnuts, Brazil nuts, pistachios, pecans, and seeds because of their higher omega-6 content. Regardless of nut variety, remember to keep the serving size small. Even those with a more favorable omega ratio are harder to digest than most other REAL foods.

Coconut butter, also called coconut manna or coconut cream concentrate, is a delicious nut butter that you can eat by the spoon, use in sauces, or mix with puréed carrots, winter squash, or avocado for a sweet but sugar-free treat. If you try coconut milk, choose a brand that's free of added gums if possible. Unsweetened, dried coconut flakes also make a good addition to omelets or sprinkled over vegetables. Some dried coconut flakes also come in larger flakes and can be eaten as is like chips. Coconut flour is another option for baking grain-free muffins and cookies, but be careful because not everyone tolerates it well because of its high-fiber content.

BEVERAGES

Any new beverage you want to add back to your diet should be treated as an individual new food. Follow the same protocol, introducing the beverage on its own and allowing your body three or four days to assess your tolerance.

Teas are a great way to vary your beverage options, especially since you can drink them hot or iced. Make sure to check ingredient lists to ensure they don't contain added sugars, artificial sweeteners, or other problematic ingredients. Single-ingredient teas are best. Beware of ingredients such as chicory root or inulin because they are FODMAPs. Stick to teas that are lower in caffeine and resist the allure of caffeine-rich black tea or coffee, hot chocolate, or any alcoholic beverages for a little while to speed up your healing.

Coconut milk and almond milk are also acceptable dairy-free options to drink on their own or use in smoothies or other recipes. Again, read the ingredient list to find brands that contain single ingredients, avoiding those with sweeteners, flavorings, thickeners or gums. Or learn to make your own coconut milk and almond milk. If you don't want to make coconut milk from scratch, you can mix coconut butter (also called coconut cream concentrate or coconut manna) with an equal amount of water for a gum-free, sugar-free coconut milk (see Chapter 10).

GRAIN-FREE CARB OPTIONS

The reintroduction of higher-carb options sometimes needs to be postponed by a few months or even years, especially if you know or suspect you have SIBO. The starches in potatoes, sweet potatoes, and other grain-free roots and tubers, as well as the sugars in fruits and sweeteners, are a ready source of food for the excess bacteria living in your small intestines. To correct the gut dysbiosis and get this chronic infection under control, the GAPS and SCD nutritional protocols, which have been followed successfully by thousands of people, both recommend that starches be avoided for at least one year past no symptoms. If you don't have SIBO, have received antibiotics to treat SIBO, or have been following a low-carb version of your BYO diet for a while, though, you can experiment with some of these grain-free carbs.

Start with fruits. Ripe bananas or cooked apples or pears are usually easier to digest. As with any other new foods, introduce them one at a time, in gradually larger amounts, to assess your tolerance. You can move on to trialing raw fruits, such as berries, stone fruits (peaches, nectarines, plums) and citrus, as you prefer. The order doesn't really matter as long as you maintain a systematic approach. Sweet potatoes, rutabaga, peeled white potatoes, yams, plantains, yucca/cassava, beets, and parsnips are examples of starchy foods with which you can experiment when you feel ready. You can even see how you do with small amounts of honey, maple syrup, or stevia if desired.

CAFFEINE AND ALCOHOL

Caffeinated foods such as tea, coffee, and chocolate, as well as alcohol, should be avoided for *at least* three to six months. This may sound like a long time, but it can help you speed up your recovery. Most people with digestive issues also suffer from fatigued adrenal glands, the small but very important glands that sit on top of your kidneys. Worn-out adrenals can contribute to fatigue, insomnia, reduced immunity, slow healing, and food sensitivities. Caffeine can give you and your adrenals a momentary boost, but this can be damaging and counterproductive in the medium to long term. Your adrenal glands are likely overdue for a little vacation. Give them some time off to rest and come back at full strength in a few months.

Avoiding caffeine and irritating foods, managing your stress, and sleeping enough will help give your adrenal glands the break they need. And don't forget that coffee, cocoa, and chocolate actually belong to the seed family and contain proteins to which you could be sensitive, especially if you react to gluten, have multiple food sensitivities, or have increased intestinal permeability (leaky gut).

After a few months without these caffeine-rich foods, you can try adding small amounts of coffee, unsweetened cocoa powder, or dark chocolate back into your diet. If any of these foods ends up making you feel more tired, interferes with your sleep, or affects your intestinal health, quit it completely again. And soft drinks and energy drinks are *not* REAL food, so hopefully you won't even consider trialing them!

The one exception for alcoholic beverages is the use of red or white wine in cooking, since the heat gets rid of all the gut-irritating alcohol while preserving the flavor.

FOODS THAT AREN'T WORTH IT

Some foods should *never* be reintroduced, at least for a few months or (ideally) years, to allow your gut to heal completely. Grains, gluten-containing ingredients, legumes such as beans, lentils, soy, and peanuts, refined oils, and processed ingredients just aren't worth it. These foods don't provide any nutrients you can't find elsewhere and will only end up compromising your intestinal and overall health. Jump back to Chapter 3 if you need a refresher.

Table 61: Foods for the Reintroduction Phase

Food Categories		REAL Foods	
	Egg protein (In order of reintroduction)	Egg yolks Whole eggs	Yolk usually better tolerated than white If tolerated, try making homemade mayonnaise and hollandaise sauce!
	Other animal-protein options	Shrimp Jerky (without sugar and MSG) Smoked salmon and other smoked fish Bacon, ham, or sausage (ideally without sweeteners, MSG, or artificial ingredients; from pastured animals)	
	Fats	Avocado (and guacamole) Butter Olive (and tapenade) Homemade mayonnaise (if egg yolks tolerated) Coconut milk or coconut cream (without guar gum) Coconut butter (also called coconut cream concentrate or coconut manna)	
To Trial	Dairy — Casein (From least to most)	Butter Cream Yogurt cheese Milk	A2 casein (goat, Jersey's cow, buffalo) is usually better tolerated than A1 casein (regular cows) Dairy products made from raw milk are sometimes better tolerated than pasteurized dairy Dairy products made from the milk of grass-fed animals is sometimes better tolerated than milk from grain-fed animals
	Dairy — Lactose (From least to most)	Homemade yogurt Cream Aged cheese Fresh cheese Milk	
	Vegetables — Cruciferous	Broccoli Cauliflower Kale Cabbage Bok choy More in Table 40	
	Vegetables — Nightshades	Tomato Eggplant Bell pepper Chili powder Paprika Curry Hot pepper sauce (without added sugar or gums) More in Table 39	
	Vegetables — High-FODMAP	Onion Garlic Cruciferous vegetables Asparagus Avocado Mushroom More on pp. 52-67	
	Vegetables — Raw	Lettuce Carrots Celery sticks Any kinds of raw vegetables	
	Vegetables — Moderate carb content	Winter squashes (butternut squash, acorn squash, pumpkin) Beets Rutabaga More in Table 81	
	Seasonings	Black pepper Onion and garlic powder Spices (curry, chili powder, hot pepper sauce, etc.) Balsamic vinegar (sugar free, naturally aged) Red wine vinegar (sugar free, naturally aged) Coconut aminos Tamari sauce (wheat- and gluten-free) Sea vegetables and seaweed (kelp, nori) Sun-dried tomatoes More in Table 50	

Caution		Fermented foods	Fermented vegetables (sauerkraut, pickles, carrots, etc.) Homemade 24-hour yogurt or kefir Kombucha (fermented tea)
		Nuts	Coconut milk (or coconut cream; without guar gum) Nut butter (macadamia, cashews, hazelnuts, coconut, etc.) Nut flour Nuts (ideally soaked and dehydrated) Unsweetened dried coconut (or coconut chips) Coconut flour
		Seeds	Sunflower seeds, pepitas, flaxseeds, chia seeds, sesame seeds Spices (nutmeg, celery seed, cumin seed, fennel seed, mustard seed) More in Table 37
		Beverages	Other varieties of tea Coconut milk (without sweeteners or gums) Almond milk (without sweeteners or gums)
	Grain-free carb options	Fruits (From easiest to hardest to digest/tolerate)	Bananas Cooked, puréed, and unsweetened apples and pears Raw fruits (berries, citrus fruits, melons, etc.) Dried fruits (without any added ingredients)
		Sweeteners	Honey Maple syrup Coconut sugar (or coconut nectar) Stevia Dextrose (glucose)
		Roots and tubers	Sweet potatoes White potatoes (peeled) Plantains Yucca/cassava More in Appendix 14
Watch Out		Caffeine and alcohol (Only after at least 3-6 months without them)	Unsweetened cocoa powder Dark chocolate (at least 85% cocoa) Coffee Alcohol (gluten free and sugar free; dry wine, hard liquor, gluten-free beer only)
Not Worth It		NOT REAL food	Gluten-free grains Gluten-containing grains Legumes (beans, lentils, soy, peanuts) Refined oils Processed ingredients (MSG, artificial sweeteners, etc.) Beer and other gluten-containing alcoholic beverages

Remember the guidelines? Each time you introduce a new food, eat it for three to four days in a row, increasing the serving size gradually, before deciding if it works for you. If you still have no symptoms by the end of the third or fourth day, you can add it to your list of safe foods and move on to trialing a new food. If you experience symptoms, eliminate the food from your diet and reset your body by going back to eating the safe foods that are currently part of your personal BYO diet.

Document Everything

Once you've been in the reintroduction phase for a little while, it can be easy to forget how you once reacted to cabbage, turnip, or cauliflower. Document everything in your food journal to keep track of the foods you tolerate and those you don't. You can also use a table similar to the one below to record your food trials over time (see Appendix 8 for extra copy).

Table 62: Food-Trial Journal

Food Trials	Trial Dates	Serving	Symptoms	Verdict
Avocado (example)	Mon, Sept 10, 2012	¼ avocado	Nothing the first 2 days, bloating on Wednesday after eating whole avocado	Unsure… seem to tolerate small amounts, but need to try again to determine if I tolerate ¼ to ½ avocado
	Tues, Sept 10, 2012	½ avocado		
	Wed, Sept 10, 2012	1 avocado		
Egg yolks				
Whole eggs				
Butter				
Cauliflower				
Onions				
Homemade yogurt				

CREATE YOUR LIST OF SAFE FOODS

As you build your own optimal diet, it can also be helpful to create a list of safe foods to help keep your diet more varied and interesting. It can also be helpful if you eat out at a friend's or if a family member wants to prepare a meal with ingredients you tolerate. You can find a copy of the chart below in Appendix 5.

Table 63: Your Safe-Food List*

Animal Protein	Traditional Fats	Vegetables
☐ Chicken	☐ Ghee	☐ Zucchini
☐ Duck	☐ Coconut oil	☐ Spinach
☐ Beef	☐ Extra-virgin olive oil	☐ Carrots
☐ Bison	☐ Macadamia oil	☐ Green beans
☐ Venison	☐ Avocado oil	
☐ Pork	☐ Palm oil	
☐ Fish	☐ Tallow	
☐ Crab	☐ Lard	
☐ Liver	☐ Duck fat	

Seasonings	Beverages	Non-Grain Carbs (Fruits, tubers, sweeteners)
☐ Unrefined salt	☐ Water	
☐ Chives	☐ Homemade bone broth	
☐ Green part of green onions	☐ Rooibos tea	
☐ Cinnamon	☐ Green tea	
☐ Apple cider vinegar	☐ Sparkling water	
☐ Lemon/lime juice	☐ Water infused with fresh rosemary, mint, or other herbs	
☐ Asafoetida powder		
☐ Fresh herbs		
☐ Garlic-infused oil		
☐ Herb-infused oil		

Other (Dairy, nuts, fermented foods, etc.)		Supplements

*Simply eliminate foods you don't tolerate and add new safe foods you discover during the reintroduction phase.

BE HONEST!

Don't lie to yourself. In some instances, you may subconsciously downplay the negative side effects induced by some foods if you really want to be able to tolerate them. Even though it would be great to be able to eat nuts or yogurt, for example, listen to your body and be honest with yourself. Keeping foods you don't tolerate well in your diet can do more harm than good and compromise your progress in the long term. And don't forget that even if you can't tolerate a certain food now, you may still be able to tolerate it in a few weeks or months. Just give your digestive system a little more time to heal.

Falling Off the Wagon

Don't expect to be 100-percent perfect all the time. Life happens. It's likely that you'll fall off the wagon at some point and eat foods that aren't part of your plan. If you feel a craving, try to use every ounce of willpower you have to at least stay away from grains (especially those with gluten) and other processed ingredients (especially ones to which you're sensitive).

Falling off the wagon almost always means feeling bad, which might actually be a good way to help you find the motivation to hop back on. And the good news is you don't have to start over. All you have to do is go back to your list of easy-to-digest, anti-inflammatory, nourishing safe foods. Stick to the foods you know make you feel good for a couple of weeks, or until you start feeling good again. Once you have been symptom free for at least five straight days, go back to the reintroduction phase and see if you can add new foods to the safe list to vary your diet further and help you resist temptation again.

> "The man who moves a mountain begins by carrying away small stones." – Confucius

Feelings of deprivation are normal. If that's what made you fall off the wagon, try to identify non-food ways to care for yourself. Get a massage, relax and listen to some music, or read a good book. Give yourself a treat that makes both your mind *and* your body feel good.

> "Take care of your body. It's the only place you have to live."
>
> – Jim Rohn

Can Reintroducing Foods Trigger Sensitivities?

Some people worry that following an elimination diet could *trigger* or even *worsen* food sensitivities. Can eliminating gluten or dairy make you more likely to react to these foods when you reintroduce them? It's possible to have a more rapid, severe reaction than before when you reintroduce problematic foods. This doesn't mean that you have become more sensitive to these foods, though, nor does it mean that your body has lost its acquired tolerance to these foods. It simply means your body can now tell you more clearly that these foods *are* a problem for you.

When you consistently eat foods to which you are sensitive, your immune system can become overwhelmed, and the constant inflammation can prevent your body from working as well as it should. Even though you may not have felt at your best before starting on the elimination diet, you may not have noticed any particular reaction when eating potentially problematic foods.

Once you give your body a break from eating those foods, though, you reset your immune system and the inflammation. Once your digestive system has had a chance to reset, reintroducing gluten, dairy, or nuts can sometimes induce a strong reaction. It may just be that your body is now healthy enough to respond appropriately to this assault. Or that you forgot how you used to feel on a daily basis before starting the protocol. Although the specific reason can vary from person to person, what matters is that your body is now able to send you a clear message. Listen to it.

Meal Timing

Your digestive system is working hard most of the day, breaking down food, absorbing nutrients, and removing residual wastes from your body. Rarely does your gastrointestinal tract get a vacation. Allowing your digestive system to take a little time off between meals can help it focus more energy on maintenance and repair and also promote regular cleansing waves to keep your intestines free from debris and excess bacteria.

Remember that these cleansing waves act like the housekeeper of your gut and are a key factor in preventing excess bacteria from growing in your small intestines (SIBO). This housekeeping only takes place every 90 minutes and only if your digestive system isn't busy digesting food. Fasting is not an option because your body needs all the nourishment it can get to heal, but spacing your meals every four to five hours and allowing about 12 hours between dinner and breakfast can help. For example, if you have your breakfast at 7:30 AM, you could eat lunch at 1:00 PM and dinner around 6:30 PM.

Do not attempt to space your meals too far apart right at the beginning when you're transitioning to the elimination diet. Getting rid of grains, sugar, and other undesirable foods constitutes enough of a change at once. Give your body a chance to regulate your blood sugar and energy levels before further spacing your meals.

Don't worry about meal timing at the beginning; just eat when you're hungry. Aim for a minimum of three meals per day and add in snacks as required. Don't attempt to space your meals too far apart if you are underweight, either. Just eat when you're hungry and wait until your weight normalizes before experimenting with this meal-timing strategy. If you prefer eating smaller meals and snacks throughout the day, stick to the meal timing that works best for you. The food you put on your plate is much more important than *when* you eat.

After a few weeks, when you start feeling better and have more stable energy levels throughout the day, you can experiment with eating only three times per day, every four to five hours, and avoiding snacking. Make sure you eat more at each meal since you still need to get the same amount of energy. Make sure you write down your meal times in your food journal to see if this simple change seems to benefit your digestive health. Some people won't see a difference, but others may feel better eating this way. Again, experimentation is the best way of finding out what your body prefers.

THE BOTTOM LINE

The reintroduction phase should be a fun period of discovery. After not eating certain foods for so long, reintroducing them can be a unique experience. In addition to your new appreciation for how REAL food tastes and feels, this diet-building phase will allow you to gain a better understanding of how your body reacts to different foods, and put you on the path to creating your BYO diet. Table 64 below gives you an overview of the three phases of the protocol.

Table 64: Overview of the Elimination Protocol

	Elimination Phase	Reintroduction Phase	Your BYO Diet
Description and Goals	The most restrictive phase, in which you cut out all potentially problematic foods and ingredients to "reset" your digestive system (eliminate your symptoms).	This phase will help you start reintroducing foods and groups of foods you eliminated from your diet to determine the ones you don't tolerate and increase your food variety. Go slow & be systematic.	Your BYO diet will help you manage your symptoms and allow your digestive system to heal to ultimately improve your health and food tolerance.
Rules	Follow this phase for a minimum of 3-4 weeks with at least 5 days in a row symptom free.	Add a new food every 3-4 days. Add to your list of safe foods if tolerated or reset before trying another new food.	Focus on what you can eat and be creative with the food options that make you feel the best.
How Long?	A minimum of 3-4 weeks, possibly 6-8 weeks in severe cases.	You can reintroduce new foods every 3-4 days. If you experience symptoms, keep this food out of your diet and wait until you have at least 2-3 days without symptoms to do a small "reset" before experimenting with another new food.	Forever! Your BYO diet can evolve over time, depending on your health, but you should always eat the foods that you tolerate and eliminate those you don't. Everybody should be on his or her own BYO diet!
Until When?	Until you're mostly symptom free for at least 5 days in a row.	Until you're happy with your food variety. You can switch to your BYO diet if you want to take a break from reintroducing new foods.	Until you feel better or want to experiment with a new food. You can switch between the reintroduction phase and your BYO diet.
What Might Happen?	Withdrawal symptoms, die-off and detox symptoms, and/or the low-carb flu.	You can increase your food variety, but might react to some of the foods you reintroduce.	You will continue feeling good and your digestive system will continue healing.

Your BYO Diet

The goal of this protocol is to construct a diet consisting of foods that are right for you: your BYO diet. The BYO diet is not a static thing, however, and should always be a work in progress. It should provide a "base" of safe foods from which you can experiment and add new ones as you feel ready. This is the diet you'll build by and for yourself, with safe foods that help you feel good and heal. Whenever you feel ready to increase your food variety, just return to the reintroduction phase.

You may read a lot of conflicting information about what people with IBS and digestive disorders should and should not eat. There might even be some studies supporting some of these recommendations, but everyone is different and no studies have been done on *your* body. Following the steps outlined in this chapter to build *your* own optimal diet will allow you to find all the answers you need to feed your body right. No one can argue with your research findings. Your BYO is not a diet you *have* to follow, but one you *want* to follow. It's the way of eating that's right for your body.

"The food you eat can be either the safest and most powerful form of medicine or the slowest form of poison." – Dr. Ann Wigmore

Chapter 6: Supplements

Removing inflammatory foods and choosing foods that are easier to digest are the most important elements in restoring your digestive health, but supplements can also assist the healing process. Supplements are not a substitute for a quality diet, but rather serve as an extra layer of care as you rebuild your digestive well-being.

None of the supplements below are mandatory for digestive health, but some of them can be helpful, depending on your specific situation. Working in concert with a qualified health practitioner familiar with digestive health and non-pharmaceutical modalities can help tailor your supplements to your personal situation and needs. Most medical doctors are unfortunately not comfortable working with supplements, so seeking the help of a naturopathic doctor or integrative-medicine practitioner may be a better alternative.

Although most supplements are not essential to recovering your digestive health, "superfoods" that act as whole-food supplements can play a valuable role in assisting you on your journey toward optimal health. Two such supplements that you should incorporate into your BYO diet have already been discussed: homemade bone broth and fermented foods. In addition to these gut-healing, gut-flora-balancing supplements, Mother Nature's two best multivitamins, liver and fermented cod liver oil, are superfoods that can provide you with precious, hard-to-get nutrients.

Homemade Bone Broth

Homemade bone broth is both a food and a supplement that provides precious compounds such as the glycosaminoglycans (GAGs) that form collagen, to help you heal your gut lining. The glucosamine and chondroitin it also contains can help your joints and tissues stay healthy, preventing joint disease and even improving the appearance of your skin.

Homemade bone broth taken before or with meals can help facilitate digestion and restore your body's ability to secrete sufficient stomach acid. It also provides a variety of important minerals that can help you maintain strong bones and teeth even without dairy in your diet, including calcium, phosphorus, and magnesium. Doesn't it make sense that adding bones to your diet, in the form of broth, would be helpful for your own bones? The minerals in bone broth can also help support your adrenal glands. See the recipe for homemade bone broth in Chapter 10.

Although the nutritional composition of homemade bone broth hasn't been analyzed (and is likely to vary depending on preparation methods and the types of bones used), bone broth has a sturdy track record among traditional cultures the world over.

> **Recommended dosage:** At least 1-2 cups (250-500 ml) per day
> (ideally ½-1 cup before or with each meal)

Homemade bone broth is usually well tolerated by most people, but some people may react to the natural food chemicals it contains. You can minimize the formation of these MSG-like compounds by simmering the broth at a very low temperature. You can also experiment with decreasing the cooking time or using different types of bones to see if you tolerate them better. If you still don't seem to tolerate bone broth, meat broth made with slow-cooked meat can be easier to tolerate at first. During the first weeks, it's best to avoid using onions and garlic in your homemade bone broth, since the fructans they contain are water soluble and will end up in your broth even after filtering it.

Another less time-consuming, easy-to-tolerate way to provide your body with the amino acids it needs to repair your gut lining is to add gelatin to your diet. Unlike homemade bone broth, gelatin is unfortunately not a good source of minerals, but it at least provides the GAGs that can help restore your gut lining. Use gelatin supplements from pastured animals to get the best quality possible (Great Lakes Gelatin is an example). Gelatin is easy to use: Simply mix it with water and drink it, or sprinkle it on your food. If you feel creative, you can prepare Jell-O-like sugar-free treats by using herbal teas to flavor your gelatin (see the recipe chapter).

Fermented Foods

Although your first priorities are to control your symptoms by eliminating irritating, inflammatory foods and to heal your gut with nourishing, easy-to-digest foods, restoring your gut flora is another step that can help you achieve optimal digestive health. The probiotics in fermented foods can also reinforce your immune system and encourage regular intestinal cleansing waves to prevent bacterial overgrowth.

Traditionally fermented foods such as fermented vegetables (sauerkraut, kimchi, pickles), fermented dairy (yogurt, kefir), and non-dairy ferments (coconut milk yogurt or kefir) are the most cost-effective options to accomplish the goal of correcting your gut dysbiosis. Compared to probiotic supplements, fermented foods provide a larger variety and diversity of strains of gut-friendly microorganisms in sufficient numbers to help improve your gut flora over time to enhance your digestion, immune system, and overall health. The next table shows you how fermented foods compare with probiotic supplements and commercial yogurts in terms of probiotic concentration.

Table 65: Sources and Concentrations of Probiotics

Sources of Probiotics	Concentration
Homemade 24-hour fermented yogurt	350 billion CFU* per ½ cup (3 billion CFU/mL)
Raw Sauerkraut	70 billion CFU per ½ cup (1 billion CFU/g)
Probiotic Supplements	1-50 billion CFU per capsule (on average)
Commercial Yogurt	1-8 billion CFU per ½ cup (0.008-0.08 billion CFU/cup)

*CFU = colony forming unit

Making your own fermented foods ensures that you get the best quality possible. Even if you don't tolerate raw or cooked cabbage, you are likely to tolerate sauerkraut since the bacteria fermenting the cabbage get rid of most of the hard-to-digest compounds (including FODMAPs). Avoid heating fermented foods to prevent killing the gut-friendly bacteria.

Unfortunately, no commercial yogurt is fermented long enough to be completely lactose free. Learn how to make your own in Chapter 10. You can find high-quality brands of sauerkraut and pickles, but make sure they're fermented traditionally (not simply mixed with vinegar) and haven't been pasteurized or heated. Good examples of high-quality brands include Bubbies, It's Alive, King Asian Gourmet, Dear Garden, Pleasant Valley Farms, and Farmhouse Culture.

> **Recommended dosage**: ¼ cup to 1 cup (60 to 250 ml)
> a day at least 3-4 times a week (ideally daily)

To ensure you tolerate the probiotics in fermented foods, it's important to introduce them very gradually during the reintroduction phase. Start with just one quarter to one half of a teaspoon (one to two milliliters) on the first day and build up the dose little by little every few days or every week.

Fermented foods can be taken with or without other foods. If you want the probiotics to help your digestion and stomach-acid production, eat a small serving of fermented foods five to 10 minutes before or with your meals. Many traditional cultures use a little bit of fermented foods with their meal as a condiment. For example, you can add a bit of sauerkraut to a meat patty or eggs, serve kimchi with your steak or chicken, or add traditionally fermented pickles to any of your meals to get your daily dose of gut-friendly bacteria.

Liver

Once one of the most prized parts of an animal, liver has unfortunately been relegated to the "nasty" category. Liver is an organ that occupies very important roles, including the storage of many nutrients. It truly is Mother Nature's multivitamin! Eating liver on a weekly basis can help you ensure you get all the nutrients your body needs, including iron, zinc, and selenium, as well as various fat- and water-soluble vitamins (see Table 66). All of the nutrients in liver are found in their natural state, which makes them easier to digest, absorb, and use by your body than the synthetic versions usually found in supplements.

Table 66: Nutrition in a Four-Ounce Serving of Cooked Liver

Nutrients	Nutritional Value		Nutritional Recommendations	
	Beef (4 oz/120 g)	Chicken (4 oz/120 g)	Daily requirements for healthy adults	% found per 4-oz serving of liver
Iron	7.9 mg	14.0 mg	8-18 mg	56% to more than 100%
Zinc	6.4 mg	4.8 mg	8-11 mg	44-58%
Copper	17.1 mg	0.6 mg	0.9 mg	67% to more than 100%
Selenium	43.3 mg	99.0 mg	55 mg	79% to more than 100%
Vitamin A	38,057 IU	15,994 IU	2,333-3,000 IU	More than 100%**
Vitamin D	59 IU	0 IU	600 IU	0-10%
Vitamin E	0.61 mg	0.98 mg	15 mg	4-7%
Thiamin (B$_1$)	0.2 mg	0.4 mg	1.1-1.2 mg	17-36%
Riboflavin (B$_2$)	4.1 mg	2.4 mg	1.1-1.3 mg	More than 100%
Niacin (B$_3$)	21.0 mg	13.3 mg	14-16 mg	More than 100%
Pantothenic acid (B$_5$)	8.5 mg	8.0 mg	5 mg	More than 100%
Vitamin B$_6$	1.2 mg	0.9 mg	1.5-1.7 mg	53-80%
Folate	304 mcg	694 mcg	400 mcg	76% to more than 100%
Vitamin B$_{12}$	84.7 mcg	20.2 mcg	2.4 mcg	More than 100%
Choline	511.2 mg	348.0 mg	425-550 mg	63% to more than 100%
Vitamin C	2.3 mg	33.5 mg	75-90 mg	3-47%

*This is the nutritional composition of regular liver, as found in the USDA Nutrient Food Database; the nutritional composition of liver from pastured animals is likely to be even better; **Vitamin A toxicity risk is reduced if you obtain sufficient vitamin D from diet, supplements, or sun exposure.

For example, many people believe that beta-carotene in carrots is the same thing as vitamin A. However, studies show that no more than three percent of the beta-carotene you eat can actually be converted into vitamin A. Liver is a great way to obtain the active form of vitamin A you need. Some people may be afraid of eating liver because their fear getting too much vitamin A, but there is no reason to worry. The potential for vitamin A toxicity is greatly reduced if you consume adequate amounts of vitamin D (learn more in the vitamin D section). The amount of vitamin D found in liver may not seem very impressive, but this is probably because the data available in the USDA food database is based on liver from indoor animals. Pastured animals with free access to pasture contain more vitamin D because they can synthesize it from sun exposure. Liver truly is an undervalued superfood that everyone can benefit from reintroducing into their diet.

> **Recommended dosage**: At least 1 serving (4-8 oz or 120 to 240 g) a week
> (up to 3 times a week)

Choosing organic vegetables, nutrient-rich fats such as ghee and extra-virgin olive oil, and animal protein from pastured animals can help you maximize your nutrition. Adding a weekly serving of liver, by far the most nutrient-dense food on the planet, is also a wise way to supplement your diet with important nutrients you may be lacking. You can also experiment with other organ meats. Tongue, heart, sweetbreads, kidneys, and other odd bits are also very rich in nutrients (a lot more than the muscle meat we eat most of the time). Not only is eating organ meats a good way to improve the nutrient density of your diet, it lets us pay respect to the animal by using every part of it.

Common Excuse #1: Liver is Full of Toxins

Many people know that one of the main functions of the liver, besides storing nutrients, is to filter, metabolize, and neutralize toxins, but this is *not* an excuse for not eating liver. Yes, the liver is responsible for eliminating some toxins from your body, but it *doesn't store them*. Toxins that it can't get rid of are stored in the fat tissues. Of course, selecting liver from healthy animals, such as grass-fed cows or bison, will help you minimize the risk of exposure to harmful compounds while maximizing the food's nutrient load.

Common Excuse #2: I Don't Know How to Eat Liver

If you've never had liver or you ate it a long time ago and didn't like it, don't be afraid to give it a try. You can mince liver and mix it with ground meat in a patty or meatloaf, or make chicken-liver pâté to use as a dip for your vegetables. Liver also goes well with caramelized onions, balsamic vinegar, and a couple bacon slices. Make sure you don't overcook your liver to avoid ending up with a tough, flavorless piece of meat. Or try frozen liver pills.

FROZEN LIVER PILLS

If you really can't get liver to go down, freeze pill-size chunks of liver (freeze them on a baking sheet first so they don't stick together before putting them in a hermetic container). Use raw liver if you trust your source, but cook it beforehand if you get it from the grocery store. Pop at least five to 10 (the equivalent of about one half to one ounce) of frozen liver pills per day with a little water. You won't taste a thing but will be getting all the potent nutrition liver has to offer.

Fermented Cod Liver Oil

Just reading that subtitle might be off-putting for some, but don't dismiss the benefits of this whole-food supplement. The simple thought of cod liver oil may bring back unpleasant memories, but it really is a superfood that can provide you with hard-to-obtain fat-soluble nutrients.

Don't confuse cod liver oil with regular fish oil, which is rich in omega-3 fats isolated from cold-water fatty fish but does not provide any other nutrients. Thanks to liver's stellar nutritional status, cod liver oil has much more to offer than anti-inflammatory omega-3s. It's one of the best food sources of fat-soluble vitamins, particularly vitamins A, D, and K_2, and its benefits go far beyond that of regular omega-3 supplements and fish oils. If you suffered from diarrhea or steatorrhea (fatty stools) in the past, you're at risk of being deficient in some or many of these essential fat-soluble nutrients.

It's very difficult to get enough vitamin D from diet or even sun exposure alone, so most people need to supplement with this essential vitamin. Not only does vitamin D contribute to bone health, it helps reduce inflammation, strengthen your immune system, and contribute to the integrity of your gut lining. These are benefits you definitely can't say no to, especially if you've been struggling with digestive problems or an autoimmune condition. In fact, many conditions, including celiac disease, inflammatory bowel disorders, and various autoimmune conditions have been linked to low vitamin-D levels.

Although most people equate the beta-carotene found in carrots with vitamin A, these nutrients are not equivalent. Beta-carotene is an important nutrient with antioxidant activities, but very little of it (about three percent) can actually be converted into the active form of vitamin A. The conversion rate is even lower in people with celiac disease, diarrhea, diabetes, hypothyroidism, or a low fat intake. You can't count on plant sources of beta-carotene to get all the vitamin A you need. The roles of vitamin A include reinforcing your immunity and helping with the formation of new healthy cells in your intestines, which can assist in the healing of your gut.

If you're worried about vitamin A toxicity, you should know that taking vitamin D with vitamin A protects against vitamin A toxicity. It's also important to note that vitamin A has only been found to be toxic in its *synthetic* form, in the absence of sufficient vitamin D, or in extremely high doses (100,000 IU per day) taken for many months.

As always, it's safest to get your nutrients from food because Mother Nature has already made sure all the nutrients are present in the right forms and proportions. Isolating individual nutrients or synthesizing them in a lab and putting them in pills doesn't have the same effect. This is why taking fermented cod liver oil is safe, while supplementing with vitamin A or beta-carotene alone is not.

Fermented cod liver oil also contains the omega-3 fats eicosapentaenoic acid (EPA) and docosapentaenoic acid (DHA). Their anti-inflammatory properties can help calm any low-grade inflammation in your gut, in addition to benefiting your heart and brain health.

Fermented cod liver oil is also a great source of vitamin K_2, which helps guide calcium into your bones and teeth to make them strong. One of the reason pure calcium supplements may fail to prevent osteoporosis could be due to a vitamin K_2 deficiency. Without it, the calcium you consume can stick to your arteries and form plaques instead of helping maintain strong, healthy bones and teeth.

Vitamin E, CoQ10, and important cofactors that enhance the absorption of these valuable nutrients are also present in fermented cod liver oil. All of these nutrients work synergistically, making fermented cod liver oil a true superfood. Table 67 gives you a snapshot of the nutritional value of fermented cod liver oil, but keep in mind that this may vary slightly from one batch to another.

Table 67: Nutrients in Fermented Cod Liver Oil

Nutrients	Fermented Cod Liver Oil			Daily Requirements*
	½ teaspoon	1 teaspoon	2 teaspoons	
Vitamin A	3,750-5,000 IU	7,500-10,000 IU	15,000-20,000 IU	2,300-3,000 IU
Vitamin D	750-1,000 IU	1,500-2,000 IU	3,000-4,000 IU	600 IU
Omega-3 fats	750-1,000 mg	1,500-2,000 mg	3,000-4,000 mg	1,000-1,400 mg
Bonus: Vitamin K_2, vitamin E, CoQ10, cofactors enhancing absorption and more				

*For adults, according to the Institute of Medicine.

It's no wonder mothers have been feeding their children this sacred food for generations. Not all cod liver oils are created equal, though. Many commercial cod liver oils are processed using modern techniques that involve refining, bleaching, and deodorizing that can affect the fragile omega-3 fatty acids and other nutrients. Regular cod liver oil actually loses all of its naturally occurring vitamin A and D during processing and manufacturers have to add the synthetic versions of these nutrients back into their products. If you want to make sure the omega-3 you're taking isn't damaged and that you're getting the natural forms of fat-soluble nutrients, fermented cod liver oil is your best option.

Fermented cod liver oil is made according to the old-fashioned traditions of Iceland and Norway, without heat and using the natural fermentation process to extract the nutrient-rich cod liver oil. This process takes at least six months to up to one year. Only one company, Green Pasture, currently makes cod liver oil according to the traditional process, but their products are available worldwide. The Weston A. Price Foundation can help you find it in your country.

How Much Cod Liver Oil Do You Need?

Healthy adults should aim for one half to one full teaspoon per day to maintain optimal nutritional status. If you've been on a low-fat diet, or have a weak immune system or intestinal problems, taking up to two teaspoons per day for the first few months can give you a nutritional boost and help replenish your body's store of fat-soluble nutrients.

> **Recommended dosage**: ½ tsp. to 2 tsp. a day (2 to 10 ml)

How Do You Take Fermented Cod Liver Oil?

The truth is that fermented cod liver oil isn't the most pleasant food to consume, but its healthful properties should provide motivation enough. Fermented cod liver oil usually comes with a plastic syringe that you can use to measure and apply your dose. Simply squirt the oil into the back of your throat and swallow quickly to avoid it touching your tongue. Follow with a glass of water or a bit of food and you'll be just fine.

While surplus B and C vitamins are excreted easily in your urine due to their water-soluble nature, the nutrients in fermented cod liver oil are fat soluble and are therefore stored in your body. You can use this property to your advantage by doubling your usual dose but taking it only every other day if you prefer. There are also flavored versions (such as mint, cinnamon, licorice, or orange) that help hide the taste and smell of fermented cod liver oil. Capsules are another option, but keep in mind that you'll have to take many capsules (five to 10 per day) to get the same dose you would from the liquid form, making it a less economical choice.

Other Supplements

Getting your nutrients from food is best because they are usually more bioavailable (easier to absorb and use) and come in the right proportions to avoid causing nutrient imbalances. However, if you have experienced digestive issues recently, it's possible you have nutrient deficiencies that require special supplements to be corrected.

Most people with poor digestive health will require digestive support (enzymes, betaine HCl, ox bile, digestive bitters) and possibly probiotic supplements (unless taking fermented foods), L-glutamine, zinc, vitamin C, magnesium, omega-3 fats (unless taking fermented cod liver oil), and vitamin D (unless taking fermented cod liver oil). You may not need all of them, and it's important to do your research about each of these supplements, ideally with the help of a qualified health care professional, to determine which are right for you and ensure that they won't interfere with your current medications or health conditions.

Digestive Support: Enzymes, Betaine HCl, and Ox Bile

Enzymes and other supplements that support digestion can make a big difference in your digestive symptoms, in addition to helping your body better absorb the nutrients you need to heal. Undigested food in your stools, frequent belching after meals, bad breath, bloating, and the feeling that food is sitting in your stomach for a long time are all signs that you could benefit from digestive support.

Of course, you should consider the basics first. The first steps to facilitate the digestion process are chewing and eating in a relaxed environment as much as possible. Chewing your food properly seems obvious, but too many people just gobble down their food. It takes conscious effort to chew long enough. You should chew until your food turns to liquid. Try it. You'll need to chew each bite around 30 times to get there. Reducing your food to tiny particles will help your digestive enzymes (both your own and the ones with which you supplement) work more effectively.

"There are no teeth in the stomach." – Dr. Steven Sandberg-Lewis

Try not to take too much liquid with your meals, either (with the exception of soups, stews, or bone broth) to avoid diluting your gastric juices and digestive enzymes. Also, make sure you take time to relax and cultivate positive thoughts throughout the day, especially during your meal times, to allow your body to put itself in digestion mode. You can't digest when you're stressed (see Chapter 7 for more on stress management).

If these basic recommendations aren't enough, however, digestive aids such as betaine HCl, ox bile, and digestive enzymes can help further optimize your digestion. Table 68 lists the specific roles of these digestive aids.

Table 68: Digestive Aids

Digestive Support	Roles
Betaine HCl	• Replaces stomach acid (hydrochloric acid) • Helps enzymes and bile work more effectively • Reduces the risk of gastrointestinal infections and prevents SIBO • Facilitates the absorption of various vitamins and minerals
Ox bile	• Facilitates the digestion and absorption of fat • Essential for the absorption of fat-soluble nutrients (vitamins A, D, and K_2, omega-3 fats, coenzyme Q10)
Pepsin, protease, bromelain, papain	• Breaks down protein into peptides and amino acids
Lipase	• Breaks down fat into single fatty acids
Amylase	• Breaks down starches into smaller pieces (maltose)
Cellulase	• Breaks down fiber
Lactase	• Breaks down lactose into glucose and galactose
Maltase	• Breaks down maltose into glucose
Bitter herbs (Digestive bitters / Swedish bitters)	• Improve stomach acid secretion and bile flow (If tasted and taken 10-15 minutes before a meal)
Apple cider vinegar	• Improves stomach-acid secretion and bile flow (If taken with a bit of water 10-15 minutes before a meal)

Betaine HCl

Most people lack enough stomach acid to properly stimulate the secretion of bile and facilitate the action of various digestive enzymes. Having enough stomach acid is also necessary to absorb various important nutrients, minimize your risk of a gastrointestinal infection, and prevent the overgrowth of bacteria or yeast in your small intestines.

You are especially at risk for low stomach acid (hypochlorhydria) if you have previously taken or are still taking antacid medications, if you have been vegetarian for a period of time, or if you're older than you used to be. In other words, most people are at risk for low stomach acid. If you suspect this may be the case, you can ask your doctor to be referred for the Heidelberg Stomach Acid test to make sure.

You can also experiment with taking betaine HCl supplements, but it's important that you first consult your doctor, especially if you are taking anti-inflammatory drugs such as corticosteroids, aspirin, Indocin, ibuprofen, or other non-steroidal anti-inflammatory drugs (NSAIDs). Since these medications are known to damage the lining of your stomach and gastrointestinal system, supplementing with extra HCl could further damage your already impaired GI lining. You should also stop using betaine HCl or reduce your dosage if you experience any burning sensations or discomfort.

If you decide to experiment with betaine HCl, it is important to always take it with food. The ideal time is after a few bites or toward the middle of your meal. Just make sure to always take a few bites of food *after* taking betaine HCl to make sure it mixes well with your stomach contents. Only take betaine HCl with a meal that contains some protein and fat (which should be all of your meals). Do not take betaine HCl or digestive enzymes if you eat only carbohydrates. Dr. Jonathan Wright, an expert on stomach acid and author of "Why Stomach Acid is Good for You," reports that the average dosage required by his patients ranges between 3,250 and 4,550 milligrams per meal. Follow the instructions in Table 69 to determine the right dosage for you.

Table 69: Betaine HCl Protocol

Timeframe	Betaine HCl Protocol	Important Notes
First Day	Start with 1 pill per meal (after a few bites of food or toward the middle of your meal).	• Betaine HCl can be combined with digestive enzymes and ox bile to optimize digestion.
Following Days	Increase by 1 pill at each of your meals every other day and pay attention to how you feel after your meals.	• Take 2 pills per meal on days 3 and 4; • Take 3 pills per meal on days 5 and 6; • Take 4 pills per meal on days 6 and 7; • Etc.
Warm or Mild Burning Sensation	When you feel a warm or mild burning sensation in your chest, decrease your dosage by 1 pill at the next meal. This should be just the right amount for you at this time.	• If you experiment a warm or mild burning sensation at 5 pills, your dose will be 4 pills per meal for now.
Caution	• If you feel a warm or burning sensation right away with only 1 pill, it probably means that your stomach acid levels are adequate. • Always take betaine HCl with food (protein and fat). • Do not exceed 5 pills per meal. • Your dosage may need to be adjusted if your body naturally starts producing enough stomach acid again. • Ask for your doctor's supervision if you take anti-inflammatory drugs (corticosteroids, aspirin, Indocin, ibuprofen, or other NSAIDs).	

If you don't want to use betaine HCl, there are gentler methods to stimulate proper stomach-acid levels. Bitter herbs are herbal blends that have been used for hundreds of years by Native Americans, Europeans, and the Chinese as a digestive aid. The most popular blend is called Swedish bitters and includes but is not limited to aloe, manna, senna leaves, rhubarb root, angelica root, zedoary root, theriac venezian, carline thistle root, myrrh, camphor, and saffron. Bitters can stimulate stomach-acid secretion, adequate bile flow, and the release of digestive enzymes from the pancreas. You can dilute the bitters in some water, but don't dilute them too much. You need to *taste* their bitterness for them to be effective. You also need to consume foods within the following 10 to 15 minutes for the bitters to work. A German study of 205 patients with various digestive problems showed that bitter herbs helped the patients get relief from symptoms of constipation, flatulence, loss of appetite, nausea, vomiting, acid reflux, and abdominal pain.

Other methods to augment your stomach acid include taking one to two tablespoons (15 to 30 milliliters) of apple cider vinegar, lemon juice, or lime juice mixed in warm water 10 to 15 minutes before your meals. Raw sauerkraut or fermented pickles taken before the meal can also have a similar but milder effect.

Ox Bile

Bile is produced naturally by your liver, stored in your gallbladder, and released into your intestines whenever you eat fat. If you've been on a low-fat diet for a while or had your gallbladder removed, you may not be able to secrete enough bile to digest the fat portion of your meals. If you notice that you have fatty stools that look pale, float, or smell bad, you have a problem digesting fat. Diarrhea and a feeling of urgency can also result from a fat intake that exceeds your body's ability to digest it.

This is why most people with gallbladder issues are advised to adopt a low-fat diet. But if you have digestive problems like IBS or other similar disorders, you *mustn't* go on a low-fat diet, since low-fat diets are by definition higher in carbohydrates. Many carbohydrates contain gluten, starches, sugars, and FODMAPs that can trigger unpleasant symptoms. And you can't be on both a low-fat and a low-carb diet at the same time—because that would be a starvation diet. So you *need* to eat a high-fat diet.

If you can't digest fat, you can simply add extra bile from supplements. Ox bile is a completely natural supplement with no recognized side effects or contraindications. All you need to do is take it with your meals that contain fat. You should notice a rapid improvement in your energy levels, since your body will now be able to absorb this rich source of energy, along with important fat-soluble nutrients. The appearance (and odor) of your stools should also improve.

Digestive Enzymes

Digestive enzyme supplements provide you with enzymes very similar to those your own body produces; pepsin and protease digest protein and lipase digests fat, while amylase, maltase, lactase, and cellulose digest carbohydrates and fiber Taking additional digestive enzymes can be beneficial for a period of a few months to support your digestive system while it is recovering.

> "We must never forget that what the patient takes beyond his power of digestion does harm." – Dr. Samuel Gee

Probiotics

There's no doubt that probiotics can be helpful for restoring your gut flora and improving your digestion. Besides strengthening your immunity, probiotics can promote cleansing waves to prevent the appearance or recurrence of SIBO. Although some people may react negatively to the introduction of probiotics and experience a worsening of their symptoms, starting slowly, increasing your dose gradually, and experimenting with different types of probiotics is likely to pay off in the long term. If probiotics only seem to aggravate your situation, whether they are in the form of fermented foods or supplements, give your body a break and concentrate on other aspects of your gut-healing protocol. You can always try them again, in a few weeks or months.

Fermented foods are probably the best and cheapest way to get a good dose of live bacteria from a variety of strains. If for some reason you can't or don't want to include fermented foods in your diet, probiotic supplements are your best bet. It's important to take the time to compare different probiotic supplements because their quality varies widely. The exact amount you need also has to be individualized and your dosage should be ramped up slowly to allow your gut flora to adjust. While a small dose of one to two billion CFU may be sufficient to maintain good gut health in *healthy* people, those with intestinal problems will likely need more. Most people with IBS, IBD, and other digestive disorders will require *at least* 20 to 25 billion CFU per day and up to 500 billion in some cases.

If you have to take antibiotics, taking probiotics at the same time may help prevent some of the antibiotics' side effects, especially diarrhea, while keeping your intestines from becoming colonized by harmful bacterial strains like *Clostridium difficile* (*C. difficile*). Taking a yeast-based probiotic like *Saccharomyces boulardii* (*S. boulardii*) may be especially useful since yeasts are not killed by antibiotics. Even though this gut-friendly yeast doesn't colonize the human GI tract and is cleared from your intestines within four to six days of stopping the supplement, *S. Boulardii* still has positive effects such as enhancing your immune system and protecting you from infections. Studies actually show that taking *S. Boulardii* (commonly sold as Florastor in North America or SB Floractiv in Australia) reduces antibiotic-associated diarrhea by 81 percent in children and by 51 percent in adults. Be aware that these formulations contain traces of lactose (30 milligrams or the equivalent of what is found in one teaspoon or five milliliters of milk).

With probiotics more than other supplements, quality matters. You can ask a qualified health care practitioner for help selecting a good probiotic, but remember that people can react differently to different probiotics. It's also preferable to change brands regularly to expose your gut flora to a variety of strains. Refrigerated supplements tend to be of higher quality. You can see and compare various examples of supplements in Table 70. These are not recommendations, but merely examples to help you better understand the differences between probiotic supplements.

Table 70: Probiotic Supplements

Probiotic	Concentration	Strains	Cost		Other Ingredients
			Total	Per 10 Billion CFU	
Align	1 billion CFU per capsule	**1 strain:** Bifidobacterium infantis	$43 (42 caps)	$10.23	Microcrystalline cellulose, hypromellose (vegetarian capsule shell), **sugar**, magnesium stearate, **milk protein**, titanium dioxide, sodium citrate dehydrate, propyl gallate, FD&C Blue #1, riboflavin
VSL#3 capsules	225 billion per 2 capsules	**8 strains** Streptococcus thermophilus, Bifidobacterium breve, Bifidobacterium longum, Bifidobacterium infantis, Lactobacillus acidophilus, Lactobacillus plantarum, Lactobacillus paracasei, Lactobacillus delbrueckii subsp. Bulgaricus	$52 (60 caps)	$0.08	Microcrystalline cellulose, stearic acid, magnesium stearate, vegetable capsule (hydroxypropyl methycelluluse), silicon dioxide.
VSL#3 sachets	900 billion CFU per sachet		$86 (30 sachets)	$0.03	Maltose, silicon dioxide
PB8	14 billion CFU per 2 capsules	**8 strains** Lactobacillus acidophilus, Bifidobacterium lactis, Lactobacillus plantarum, Lactobacillus salivarus, Bifidobacterium bifidum, Bifidobacterium longum, Lactobacillus rhamnosus, Lactobacillus casei	$13 (120 caps)	$0.15	Microcrystalline cellulose, capsule (gelatin, water), **inulin**, magnesium stearate, silica
Bio-Kult	2 billion CFU per capsule	**14 strains** Bacillus subtilis, Bifidobacterium bifidum, Bifidobacterium breve, Bifidobacterium infantis, Bifidobacterium longum, Lactobacillus acidophilus, Lactobacillusdelbrueckii ssp. Bulgaricus, Lactobacillus casei, Lactobacillus plantarum, Lactobacillus rhamnosus, Lactobacillus helveticus, Lactobacillus salivarus, Lactococcus lactis ssp. Lactis, Streptococcus thermophilus	$42 (120 caps)	$1.75	Cellulose (bulking agent), vegetable capsule (hydroxypropylmethyl cellulose)
GutPro	200 billion CFU per ¼-tsp serving	**8 strains** Lactobacillus plantarum, Lactobacillus gasseri, Lactobacillus salivarus, Bifidobacterium bifidum, Bifidobacterium infantis, Bifidobacterium longum, Bifidobacterium breve, Bifidobacterium lactis	$155 (60 servings)	$0.13	None
Florastor or Floractiv	5 billion CFU per capsule	**1 strain of yeast** Saccharomyces boulardii	$42 (50 caps)	$1.68	Magnesium stearate, hydroxypropyl methylcellulose, titanium dioxide, **33 mg lactose**
SCDophilus	3 billion CFU per capsule	**1 strain** Lactobacillus acidphoilus	$18 (100 caps)	$0.60	Cellulose, vegetarian capsule, L-leucine and water
	10 billion CFU per capsule		$29 (100 caps)	$0.29	
Ther-Biotic Complete	25 billion CFU per capsule	**12 strains** Lactobacillus rhamnosus, Bifidobacterium bifidum, Lactobacillus acidophilus, Lactobacillus casei, Lactobacillus plantarum, Lactobacillus salivarus, Bifidobacterium longum, Streptococcus thermophilus, Lactobacillus Bulgaricus, Lactobacillus paracasei, Bifidobacterium lactis, Bifidobacterium breve	$31 (60 caps)	$0.21	**Inulin base derived from chicory root**, proprietary polysaccharide complex, vegetarian capsule (hydroxypropyl methylcellulose, water) and L-leucine
Jarro-Dophilus EPS	5 billion CFU per capsule	**8 strains** Bifidobacteria longum, Bifidobacterium breve, Lactobacillus rhamnosus, Lactobacillus casei, Lactobacillus plantarum, Lactobacillus helveticus, Lactococcus lactis ssp. Lactis, Pedicoccus acidilactici	$24 (120 caps)	$0.40	**Potato starch**, magnesium stearate, ascorbic acid, hydroxypropyl methylcellulose, water, less than 0.1% **soy** and less than 0.01% **casein (milk)**
Bio-K+	50 billion per bottle	**2 strains** Lactobacillus acidophilus Lactobacillus casei	$40 (12 bottles)	$0.67	Water, **skim milk powder**, modified **milk ingredients**
	12.5 billion CFU per capsule		$19 (15 caps)	$1.01	Cellulose, hypromellose, ethylcellulose, medium-chain triglyercides, sodium alginate, ascorbic acid, magnesium stearate, silicone dioxide and titanium dioxide
Yakult	8 billion CFU per bottle	**1 strain** Lactobacillus casei Shirota	$3 (5 bottles)	$0.75	Water, **sugar, skim milk powder, glucose, natural and artificial flavors**

*Ingredients in bold may be problematic

Pay attention to the ingredient list, since many *probiotic* supplements are also enriched with *prebiotics*. Prebiotics feed the bacteria in your gut and are usually derived from FODMAPs and short-chain fermentable carbohydrates such as inulin or fructooligosaccharides (FOS). Avoid probiotic supplements in which these ingredients appear as part of the main ingredients (i.e., in which the amount in milligrams is listed). If these ingredients are listed as part of the base (in the "other ingredients" category), they are usually present in very small amounts and won't cause problems unless you are very sensitive to them. Note that some probiotic supplement can contain sugar, starch, lactose, or milk-derived ingredients. Consult your doctor before taking probiotics if you have a suppressed immune system or short-gut syndrome.

Other Helpful Nutrients

L-GLUTAMINE

L-glutamine is an amino acid found naturally in protein. What makes it special is that it is one of the preferred sources of fuel for the cells lining the insides of your intestines. Getting extra L-glutamine in your diet, between 1,500 milligrams and five grams per day for adults, can help repair a damaged gut lining more quickly. You can find L-glutamine in capsules or powder. The powder form is usually easier to absorb, but both can work. Doses of up to 14 grams per day have been shown to be safe.

Recommended dosage: 500 mg, 3 times per day (to up to 5 g per day)

Another benefit of L-glutamine is that it can help curb carb cravings. If you experience strong carb cravings when starting on the elimination diet, this is probably due to the fact that this way of eating is lower in carbohydrates than your previous diet. A gut dysbiosis can also worsen your cravings. Taking three daily doses of 500 milligrams of L-glutamine between meals can help you prevent cravings. You can also take an additional dose of 500 milligrams or a double dose of 1,000 milligrams in the case of sudden or strong cravings. You can carry L-glutamine capsules with you in case you experience sugar cravings. If you do, simply break it open in your mouth and keep the powder under your tongue until it absorbs. This is the best way to ensure that the L-glutamine goes into your system as quickly as possible to attenuate your cravings. Most people feel a difference in as little as 10 minutes. Try it for yourself to see if it helps you better stick to your elimination diet protocol.

ZINC

Zinc is an important mineral that plays a big role in controlling inflammation and boosting your immune system. One study found that people with fructose malabsorption, one of the many possible causes of IBS, were found to have lower levels of zinc in their blood. Researchers found that giving the equivalent of 75 milligrams of elemental zinc per day, divided into three doses, for a period of eight weeks helped patients with Crohn's disease improve their intestinal permeability.

Zinc can also help inhibit the release of histamine, which can be responsible for unpleasant symptoms after the consumption of histamine-releasing foods such as fish, shellfish, wine, strawberries, banana, tomato, avocado, fermented foods, cheese, and cured meats.

Zinc is essential to maintaining the integrity of your skin as well as your mucosa (your intestines and gut lining are a mucosa). Zinc supplementation can also be helpful in some cases of diarrhea. A REAL-food-based diet that includes animal protein at most meals, the best dietary source of zinc, is likely to provide you with all the zinc you need. However, this mineral is not as well absorbed in people with GI disorders or who suffer from chronic diarrhea. Taking extra zinc for a few months can help you replenish your zinc levels and assist you with your gut-healing protocol. Since zinc can inhibit copper absorption, it can be a good idea to choose a zinc supplement that contains small amount of copper (copper requirements correspond to 0.9 milligrams per day for both male and female adults).

VITAMIN C

The vegetables allowed during the elimination phase are not particularly rich in vitamin C. As your tolerance improves you can reintroduce more vitamin C-rich vegetables (bell pepper, broccoli, cauliflower, Brussels sprouts, kale, and tomato) and possibly vitamin C-rich fruits (citrus, strawberries, kiwi, papaya, pineapple, mango, and cantaloupe), and your vitamin C intake should be in line with the current dietary recommendations. Despite getting enough vitamin C in your diet to cover the minimum of 75 milligrams and 90 milligrams women and men require (respectively) on a daily basis, vitamin C supplementation can sometimes be helpful.

Your adrenal glands hold the highest amount of vitamin C in your body, so getting extra vitamin C can help support their function. The more stress your body faces, the more of this antioxidant you need. Adrenal fatigue, or hypoadrenia, is a common situation affecting people dealing with the chronic stresses of life, which include not only financial stress and emotional stress but also physical stressors like gastrointestinal conditions and food sensitivities. Even caffeine, sugary foods, refined carbs, inadequate sleep, and a lack of relaxation time can contribute to adrenal fatigue.

You have two adrenal glands, each about the size of a walnut, located above each of your kidneys. These glands are responsible for modulating your stress response by influencing the utilization of energy and controlling inflammation and pain in your body. There are various levels of adrenal fatigue, from mild to exhaustion. Of course, it's best to address this issue before it progresses to a more serious stage.

Besides fatigue, symptoms of adrenal fatigue include difficulty getting up in the morning, salt cravings, decreased libido, inability to handle stress, light-headedness upon standing, and memory and concentration problems. These symptoms are all very general and non-specific. If you want to verify whether adrenal fatigue is a concern for you, you can take the online questionnaire at www.adrenalfatigue.org/take-the-adrenal-fatigue-quiz and working with a qualified healthcare practitioner to get a saliva cortisol test. This test checks your salivary cortisol levels at four different times throughout the day, from the moment you wake up to bedtime.

If your bowel movements become too loose, cut down slightly on your dose of vitamin C until they normalize. As with many other dietary supplements, it's best to increase your dosage slowly over the course of several days when getting started and decrease it gradually when you want to stop taking it. Consult your doctor if you are on blood-thinning medications or any other drugs because your dose may need to be adjusted.

B VITAMINS

All B vitamins play a role in the production of energy and the proper utilization of carbohydrates, fat, and protein in your body. Some of the B vitamins, including B3, B5, and B6, are also essential to support adrenal function.

Many people with gastrointestinal disorders or gut dysbiosis can become deficient in vitamin B12 due to suboptimal absorption, inadequate stomach acid, or excess bacteria in the small intestines. If you have been diagnosed with SIBO or suspect you have low stomach acid, ask your doctor to have your blood B12 levels tested to determine if you need to supplement more or less aggressively with this crucial water-soluble vitamin. Taking antacids and diabetes drugs can also deplete your B12 levels. Vitamin B12 deficiency is very serious and can result in severe and irreversible nerve damage. The symptoms include neuropathy (pain, tingling or numbness in your nerves), cognitive problems (memory loss and dementia; often confused with Alzheimer's disease), fatigue, a type of anemia called pernicious anemia, tremors (often confused with Parkinson's disease), and difficulty walking (often confused with multiple sclerosis; some people end up in a wheelchair, and damage is often irreversible once it gets to this point). Vitamin B12 deficiency is more common than you think, so get tested.

Taking a vitamin B complex can help you make sure you get the right balance of all of these important vitamins. Another good way to get a good balance of B vitamins without taking supplements is to eat liver at least once a week.

MAGNESIUM

Magnesium is the fourth most abundant mineral in your body and is involved in over 300 biochemical reactions, including muscle function, nerve function, heart rhythm, bone health, and immunity. Unfortunately, soil depletion from unsustainable agricultural practices has decreased the amount of magnesium we can obtain naturally from fruits and vegetables. Magnesium deficiency is common and can cause constipation, disturbed sleep patterns, and anxiety. Try taking your magnesium supplement at bedtime. Its relaxing and calming effect can help you sleep better and normalize your bowel movements the next morning.

> **Recommended dosage**: 400-600 mg a day (up to 1,000 mg in some people);
> increase gradually and adjust with stool consistency.

Magnesium citrate, as found in the supplement Natural Calm®, is a good supplement for people prone to constipation since it helps draw more water into the colon. It helps promote easier and more regular bowel movements by making your stools moister and easier to pass, but it does not stimulate the contraction of your bowels in the same way laxatives do. Start with a small dose and increase it gradually. Once you get loose stools, cut back slightly on your dose to help you maintain normal, regular bowel movements.

If you're prone to diarrhea, you can either divide your dose throughout the day or choose a form of magnesium that is better absorbed to prevent drawing too much water into your colon and worsening your condition. Magnesium glycinate and magnesium malate are better forms of magnesium if you're not constipated. These forms are better absorbed and therefore less likely to affect the consistency of your bowel movements. Epsom salt baths, discussed earlier, are another option to replenish your magnesium levels.

MARINE OMEGA-3 FATTY ACIDS

Omega-3 fatty acids are an essential nutrient because your body can't synthesize them, so they must be obtained from food. If you suffer from diarrhea or steatorrhea, it's likely you are malabsorbing these essential fats, so supplementing may be helpful. Omega-3 fats are recognized for their role in brain and heart health. Not only do they help maintain optimal cognitive function and mood, they also contribute to healthy triglyceride levels. In addition, omega-3 fats are well known for their anti-inflammatory effects and can help soothe your inflamed intestines.

Not all omega-3s are the same, though. Omega-3s of vegetable origin, such as those from flaxseeds, chia seeds and walnuts, are not used as efficiently in humans as those of marine origin. The omega-3 fats found in plant foods are called alpha-linolenic acid (ALA), but your body prefers the omega-3s EPA and DHA. You can use ALA to synthesize EPA and DHA, but the conversion rate is estimated to be lower than 0.5 percent. In other words, you'd need to eat five cups of flaxseeds per day to cover your omega-3 requirements! This corresponds to a *huge* amount (over 200 grams) of fiber, which is definitely not a good idea for your digestive health.

Get EPA and DHA directly, instead. Cold-water fatty fish (see Table 71), especially wild-caught ones, are excellent sources of omega-3. Fermented cod liver oil is another good way to get EPA and DHA in addition to a variety of precious fat-soluble nutrients. Eggs from pastured hens and meat from grass-fed animals also provide small amounts of EPA and DHA.

You can get all the omega-3s you need by eating fish two to three times per week and mostly grass-fed meat the rest of the time. This will help you maintain an optimal omega-6-to-omega-3 ratio and reduce low-grade systemic inflammation.

Table 71: Omega-3s in Fish

Fish		Omega-3s (DHA + EPA) per 3.3 oz (100 g)
Cold-Water Fatty Fish	Mackerel	2.2-2.6 g
	Sardines	1.4 g
	Salmon — Chinook	1.5 g
	Salmon — Canned	1.4 g
	Salmon — Pink	1.0 g
	Salmon — Farmed	1.3 g
	Trout — Lake	2.1-4.6 g
	Trout — Rainbow	0.6 g
	Tuna, albacore	1.5 g
	Herring	1.7-1.8 g
Lean Fish	Halibut	0.5-0.9 g
	Cod	0.3 g
	Catfish	0.3 g
	Flounder	0.2 g
	Sole	0.1 g

If you feel like you're not getting enough omega-3s, you can supplement with small to moderate amounts of fish oil. Even though omega-3 fatty acids are essential to health, taking too much can also be problematic. Omega-3 fats are polyunsaturated fats and are susceptible to oxidation, so choose a good-quality fish oil and avoid large doses. Check the expiry date and beware of discount fish oils that have been sitting on the shelves for too long, since they are likely to be oxidized. To prevent the fragile omega-3 fats in your fish oil from being damaged, store your liquid fish oil or fish oil capsules in a hermetic container in the fridge, away from light, heat, and oxygen. Taking rancid omega-3 fats can do more harm than good.

Recommended dosage: 1 to 2 grams of omega-3 fats (EPA and DHA)
(which should correspond to about 2 to 4 grams of fish oils a day; check the
label to make sure) or 2-3 weekly servings of cold-water fatty fish

---

Consult your doctor before taking omega-3 supplements if you have a clotting disorder or take blood-thinning medications. If you're having surgery, be sure to ask how long in advance you should stop supplementing with omega-3 fats to decrease your risk of hemorrhage or excessive bleeding.

VITAMIN D₃

The sunshine vitamin, which acts more like a hormone than a vitamin, has been found to do more than contribute to bone health. Many studies conducted in the last decade have shown a role for vitamin D in reducing systemic inflammation, strengthening the immune response, and even maintaining normal intestinal permeability. Vitamin D deficiencies have been associated with an increased risk of cancer, cardiovascular disease, depression, cognitive impairment, dementia, fibromyalgia, autism, Parkinson's disease, stroke, diabetes, multiple sclerosis, and many other autoimmune conditions.

Unfortunately, more than half of the world population is deficient in vitamin D. If you have a digestive disorder such as celiac disease, IBS, IBD, or SIBO, you are at particularly high risk of insufficient vitamin D levels. The current daily dietary recommendations from the Institute of Medicine are 600 IU of vitamin D for adults, but many researchers believe this recommendation to be insufficient. The Vitamin D Council actually recommends that healthy adults take at least 5,000 IU per day. Fermented cod liver oil is probably the best food source of vitamin D, with around 2,000 IU per teaspoon. Fatty fish is also a good source, especially if caught wild. Wild-caught salmon has been show to contain 75 to 90 percent more vitamin D than farmed salmon. Eggs from pastured hens also have three to six times more vitamin D than regular cage eggs. Table 72 lists the vitamin D content of different foods and the amount you can synthesize from sun exposure.

Table 72: Sources of Vitamin D

Sources of Vitamin D		Serving Size	Vitamin D Content
Food Sources	Sardines with bones	1 cup (250 ml)	288 IU
	Canned salmon with bones	3 oz. (90 g)	328 IU
	Regular eggs	2 large	82 IU
	Pastured eggs	2 large	246-492 IU
	Liver	4 oz. (120 g)	59 IU
	Fermented cod liver oil	1 tsp. (5ml)	2,000 IU
	Enriched milk	1 cup (250 ml)	115-124 IU
Sunshine (UVB exposure)	Face, arms and hands exposed	20-30 minutes	10,000-25,000 IU
	In a bathing suit	15 minutes	

Sunlight is the quickest way, besides supplements, to boost your vitamin D intake. A few minutes outside with little clothing and no sunscreen two to three times per week, especially between 10 AM and 2 PM, provides enough vitamin D for most people. Although the levels in the table above may seem very high, don't worry, since it's impossible to develop vitamin D toxicity simply from sun exposure. There are also three factors that can interfere with your ability to synthesize and utilize vitamin D: dark skin pigmentation, obesity, and aging. If one or more of these factors applies to you, you might need more sun exposure or require vitamin D supplementation.

Also keep in mind that you *can't* produce vitamin D from UVB rays during the winter months if you live above the 35th parallel. This parallel corresponds to a line between Los Angeles, CA, Columbia, SC, Rabat, Morocco, Kabul, Afghanistan, and Tokyo, Japan, in the Northern Hemisphere and between Buenos Aires, Argentina, Cape Town, South Africa, Auckland, New Zealand, and Adelaide, South Australia, in the Southern Hemisphere. See Table 73 to identify the months for optimal vitamin D synthesis in your location.

Table 73: Optimal Vitamin D Synthesis by Location

	Latitude	Approximate Location	Optimal Vitamin D Synthesis Time
North America	From the equator to 35° North	Below the line between Los Angeles, CA, and Columbia, SC	Year-round
	40° North	Above the line between the northern border of California and Boston, MA	Mid-March to November
	50° North	Above the line between Vancouver, BC, and north of Quebec City, QC	Mid-April to September
Europe	40° North	Above the line between Barcelona, Spain, and Istanbul, Turkey	Mid-March to November
	50° North	Above the line between London, UK, and Prague, Czech Republic	Mid-April to September
Oceania	From the equator to 35° South	Above the line between Adelaide, SA, Canberra, ACT, and Auckland, NZ	Year-round
	40° South	Below the line between the Bass Strait (between Melbourne and Tasmania) and Wellington, NZ	September to May

Different experts have different opinions on optimal vitamin D levels. The best way to determine exactly how much you need is to ask for a blood test. Your doctor can help you check your blood 25-hydroxyvitamin D levels (also called 25(OH)D or calcidiol), which is the best indicator of vitamin D deficiency or sufficiency. Home test kits are also available in some countries. Levels between 50 and 80 nanograms per milliliter (125 and 200 nanomol per liter) are considered optimal.

Recommended intake: 1,000 to 5,000 IU (to keep your blood levels of 25-hydroxyvitamin D between 50 and 80 ng/mL or between 125-200 nmol/L)

If your 25(OH)D levels are below 50 nanograms per milliliter, consider increasing your sun exposure in the summer, taking fermented cod liver oil, and possibly taking a vitamin D supplement. If you choose to supplement with vitamin D, make sure it is in the D_3 form, not the less-effective D_2 form. To enhance the absorption of this fat-soluble vitamin, always take it with a meal or snack that contains fat. Once your blood level of vitamin D is in the optimal range, you can decrease your supplementation dosage slightly, but make sure to get your levels tested regularly.

Supplementing for Gut Health: Overview

Different supplements may be useful for different people in different situations. Whole-food supplements, such as homemade bone broth, fermented foods, fermented cod liver oil, and liver, should definitely be part of your diet if you want to speed up your recovery. You don't need to have them with every meal, but do your best to incorporate them as part of your routine and you'll feel the difference. Table 74 gives you an overview of the different whole-food supplements that could be helpful in conjunction with your BYO diet.

Table 74: Whole-Food Supplements

Whole-Food Supplements	Benefits	Dose	Notes
Homemade Bone Broth	• Gut-healing properties (GAGs, gelatin) • Facilitates digestion • Stimulates stomach-acid production • Joint and skin health (glucosamine, chondroitin, gelatin) • Bone health (calcium, phosphorus, magnesium)	1 to 2 cups a day (250-500 ml) ideally right before or with your meals to facilitate digestion	• You can drink your bone broth or use it in soups, stews, or sauces. • Make large batches and freeze extra to always have some on hand.
Fermented Foods	• Glut flora balance • Facilitates digestion • Stimulates stomach-acid production • Prevents gastrointestinal infections • Increases immunity • Promotes cleansing waves (to prevent SIBO)	¼ to 1 cup a day (60-250 ml) at least 3-4 times a week (ideally daily)	• With dairy (24-hr homemade yogurt or kefir) or without (raw sauerkraut or fermented carrots). • Don't heat fermented foods to preserve their probiotics.
Liver	• Provides minerals (iron, zinc, selenium, copper) • Important source of choline • Rich in B vitamins (especially folate and B_{12}) • Fat-soluble nutrients (vitamin A and K_2)	At least 1 serving a week (1 serving = 4-8 oz or 120 to 240 g) up to 3 times a week	• Mother Nature's multivitamin. • Choose liver from pastured animals to get even more nutrition.
Fermented Cod Liver Oil	• Fat-soluble nutrients (vitamin A, D, and K_2, omega-3 fats) • Strengthens your immune system • Contributes to the integrity of your gut lining	½ to 2 tsp. a day (2 -10 ml)	• Better than regular cod liver oil because the manufacturing process preserves the natural nutrients. • Can be found mixed with butter oil and/or flavored.

Some people may require additional supplements, at least for a few months. Table 75 summarizes the additional digestion-supporting nutrients you might consider including. If you're unsure which supplements are right for you, seek guidance from a qualified naturopathic doctor or functional-medicine practitioner.

Table 75: Additional Nutrients to Support Digestion

Nutrients		Roles	DRIs*	Recommended Intake	Food Sources
Zinc		Immune function, protein synthesis, wound healing, gut-lining integrity, cell division, sense of taste and smell, over 100 enzymatic activities, inhibition of histamine release	Females: 8 mg Males: 11 mg UL: 40 mg	7.5 to 15 mg per day and/or 6 to 12 oz of oysters per week	Oysters, liver, beef, crab, lobster, pork, chicken
Vitamin D$_3$		Immune function, bone health, reduction of inflammation, maintenance of normal intestinal permeability	Females: 600 IU Males: 600 IU UL: 4,000 IU	1,000 to 5,000 IU and/or ½-2 tsp fermented cod liver oil/day	Sunlight (except during winter), fermented cod liver oil, wild-caught fatty fish, pastured eggs, liver
			*UL of over 10,000 IU a day, according to the Vitamin D Council *Goal = blood 25(OH)D levels between 50-80 ng/mL (125-200 nmol/L)		
Vitamin A		Immune function, vision, formation and maintenance of the heart, lungs, kidneys, and other organs, essential for gut-lining integrity	Females: 2,333 IU (700 mcg RAE) Males: 3,000 IU (900 mcg RAE) UL: 10,000 IU (3,000 mcg RAE)	½-2 tsp fermented cod liver oil a day and/or liver 1-3 times/week	Liver, fermented cod liver oil, grass-fed butter, grass-fed ghee, herring, egg yolks, salmon, fat from grass-fed & pastured animals
			*Beta-carotene is converted poorly to vitamin A (real vitamin A is only found in animal foods).		
Vitamin C		*The vitamin A toxicity threshold (UL) is increased by adequate vitamin D intake.	Females: 75 mg Males: 90 mg UL: 2,000 mg	500 to 2,000 mg/day split into smaller doses (according to stool consistency)	Red bell pepper, citrus fruits, broccoli, Brussels sprouts, tomato, cantaloupe, cabbage, cauliflower
B Vitamins	B$_3$ (niacin)	Energy production, conversion of carbohydrates to energy, fat and protein metabolism, sex and stress hormone synthesis, adrenal support	Females: 14 mg Males: 16 mg UL: 35 mg	Vitamin B complex with small amounts of each B vitamins and/or 1-3 weekly serving of liver	Liver, kidney, fish, brewer's yeast, beets
	B$_5$ (pantothenic acid)	Energy production, conversion of carbohydrates into energy, fat and protein metabolism, adrenal function support, red-blood-cell production, synthesis of sex and stress hormones, digestive tract maintenance	Females: 5 mg Males: 5 mg UL: not set	Vitamin B complex with small amounts of each B vitamin and/or 1-3 weekly servings of liver	Liver, meat, fish, avocado, cauliflower, kale, broccoli, tomato, brewer's yeast
	B$_6$ (pyridoxine)	Protein and amino acid metabolism, cognitive development, immune function, blood sugar regulation, adrenal function support	Females: 1.3-1.5 mg Males: 1.3-1.7 mg UL: 100 mg	Vitamin B complex with small amounts of each B vitamin and/or 1-3 weekly serving of liver	Liver, meat, fish, chicken, banana, winter squash, nuts, onions, spinach, watermelon
	B$_9$ (folate)	Produce and maintain cells, synthesis of red blood cells (prevent anemia), prevent neural tube defect in early stages of pregnancy, prevent heart disease, stroke, and Alzheimer's (by keeping homocysteine levels down)	Females: 400 mcg Males: 400 mcg UL: 1,000 mcg	Vitamin B complex with small amounts of each B vitamin and/or 1-3 weekly serving of liver	Liver, spinach, asparagus, avocado, papaya, broccoli, oranges, strawberries, eggs, brewer's yeast
			*Folate is the natural form while folic acid is the synthetic form usually found in enriched foods and supplements.		
	B$_{12}$ (cobalamin)	Red-blood-cell formation (prevent pernicious anemia), nervous system function, prevent heart disease, stroke, and Alzheimer's (by keeping homocysteine levels down)	Females: 2.4 mcg Males: 2.4 mcg UL: not set	Vitamin B complex including small amounts of each B vitamins and/or 1-3 weekly serving of liver Clams, liver, fish, beef, dairy products, eggs (active form only found in animal foods; algae or vegetarian sources are not bioavailable)	
			*Methylcobalamin is the best vitamin B$_{12}$ source in supplements		

Nutrients	Roles	DRIs*	Recommended Intake	Food Sources
Vitamin K$_2$	Appropriate calcification (promote calcification in bones and teeth and prevent it in arteries and soft tissues)	Not set	½-2 tsp fermented cod liver oil/day	Liver, egg yolks, grass-fed butter and ghee, animal fat, fermented cod liver oil/butter oil blend
L-glutamine	Wound healing, gut-lining integrity, brain function, immune system, carbohydrate-craving reduction	Doses up to 14 g/day appear safe	1,500 mg (separated into 3 doses) to up to 5 g a day	Beef, pork, poultry, dairy
Magnesium	Needed for over 300 biochemical reactions, muscle and nerve function, heart rhythm, immune system, bone health	Females: 310-320 mg Males: 400-420 mg UL: 350 mg for suppl. magnesium (not food sources)	400-600 mg at bedtime but up to 1,000 mg in some people (adjusted according to stool consistency)	Vegetables, nuts and tubers (vary depending on soil quality), chocolate, banana
Marine Omega-3 Fats (EPA and DHA)	Brain and cognitive function, mood, reduction of inflammation, heart health	Not set for EPA and DHA	1-2 grams/day from fish oil and/or fermented cod liver oil and/or 2-3 weekly servings of cold-water fatty fish	Fish oil, fermented cod liver oil, cold-water fatty fish (sardines, salmon, herring, mackerel, rainbow trout, albacore tuna)

*EPA and DHA from marine sources are more bioavailable than the ALA in vegetable sources (flaxseeds, chia seeds, walnuts)

*DRI = dietary recommended intake (amount needed daily for healthy adults); UL = tolerable upper intake levels (maximal amount tolerated for healthy adults).

READ THE INGREDIENTS

Always read a supplement's ingredient list before taking it. As with food, it's important to know what you put in your mouth. You'll probably be surprised to find that some supplements contain unnecessary ingredients and fillers that could hinder your digestive health. Avoid any supplements that contain gluten, dairy, or other ingredients to which you know you are sensitive, as well as other non-optimal ingredients. You may find that some vitamin D supplements are encapsulated with corn or soy oil, while B vitamins can be mixed with sorbitol or sugar. Try to find cleaner alternatives whenever possible.

Avoid supplements containing aloe, licorice, and slippery elm for the first months if you have been diagnosed with SIBO or have a gut dysbiosis. Although these supplements are great at soothing gastrointestinal pain and inflammation in some cases, they contain a type of carbohydrate that can feed and exacerbate a bacterial overgrowth.

JOURNALING

Most whole-food supplements can be introduced right away during the elimination phase, especially homemade bone broth, fermented cod liver oil, and liver. Treat any new supplements like food and introduce them one by one every three to four days, paying attention to your symptoms. It is preferable to wait before experimenting with fermented foods and other nutrient supplements, in particular, to minimize the risk of a reaction and avoid delaying your progress on the reintroduction phase. Take notes in your food journal about the supplement, dose, and any side effects. This will help you tweak your supplement regimen to get the most benefit without impairing your digestive health.

MULTIVITAMINS

Are multivitamins a good option to cover all your bases? Unfortunately, not really. Most of them contain fillers, and the synthetic version of vitamins (folic acid vs. folate, for example), don't provide all the nutrients you need, or provide those nutrients in the wrong proportions. It's also not a good idea to supplement with iron or take a multivitamin supplement that contains extra iron if you have a gut dysbiosis, since iron can feed some bacteria. One study that looked at multivitamins found that they don't provide *any* benefits regarding the risk of cancer, heart disease, or mortality. Another study even showed that the synthetic forms of certain vitamins like vitamin A, and vitamin E could actually increase your mortality risk.

Your best bet is therefore to eat REAL nutrient-dense food and use whole-food supplements to get the nutrition you need from natural sources. If you are still worried about developing nutrient deficiencies, you can decide to take a multivitamin to help you feel better. Stressing out about the fear of lacking nutrients is counterproductive if you want your digestion to improve. Just make sure the multi is the best quality possible and introduce it on its own, as you would any other new food or supplement, to assess your tolerance.

Remember that none of the supplements described in this chapter are *essential* to your success. Some of these supplements may be beneficial and speed up your progress while on your BYO diet, but some may not. Eating nutrient-dense foods and avoiding foods that contain anti-nutrients will alone get you most of the nutrition you need. Adding stress management (see next chapter) is another big part of the puzzle. And don't forget that even though supplements are more natural than drugs, they can also have powerful effects. Be careful if you have any health conditions or take medications, and work with a qualified naturopathic doctor or functional-medicine practitioner to create a plan that's right for you.

Chapter 7: The Mind-Body Connection

Your gut health can influence your mental health via the gut-brain axis (as discussed in Chapter 1), but this isn't just a one-way connection. Your mind, your thoughts, and your attitude can also influence your physical and digestive health. If you want to adopt a holistic approach to take your health to the next level, you also need to consider the role of your thoughts. Conventional allopathic medicine unfortunately doesn't really seem to pay attention to this part of the health equation, despite its vital, undeniable importance.

Don't skip this chapter if you want to reach your full health potential. You don't need to adopt an entirely new, esoteric practice to improve your mind-body connection. Little things like better managing your stress, taking time for yourself, laughing, thinking positive thoughts, and sleeping well can make all the difference in the world.

> "There is no question that the things we think have a tremendous effect upon our bodies. If we can change our thinking, the body frequently heals itself."
>
> – C. Everett Koop, M.D.

Stress and Digestive Health

Stress can and will prevent you from progressing on your BYO diet, so don't make the mistake of dismissing its importance. Even if you're doing everything right with your diet, not paying attention to your mental health can be enough to perpetuate your digestive problems and limit your food tolerance.

Stress can be acute (short term) or chronic (long term). It can be emotional or physical. All types of stress can be problematic for your digestive health. Common sources of stress include deadlines, overworking, financial concerns, interpersonal conflicts, and not getting enough sleep or downtime. If you have a type-A personality and are always looking for something to do, you're especially prone to stress. Even positive forms of stress can trigger a stress response in your body. Traveling, beginning a new relationship, getting married, starting a family, or taking up a new job can be equally stressful for your body.

Physical forms of stress can also have negative consequences for your health. Excessive exercise (especially endurance exercise), as well as pain, infection, gastrointestinal problems, or food sensitivities can all compromise your progress. Stimulants like caffeine can also put extra stress on your body.

WHY IS STRESS SO PROBLEMATIC?

Your body has a switch that allows it to work in two different modes: parasympathetic or sympathetic. Your parasympathetic mode should be your default mode. This is the "rest and digest" mode that allows your body to do repair and maintenance work. This mode is also responsible for setting the conditions for healthy digestion. It is only when your parasympathetic mode is activated that you can produce stomach acid, digestive enzymes, and bile to facilitate digestion and help you better absorb the nutrients from your food.

Table 76: The Autonomic Nervous System

Mode	Parasympathetic	Sympathetic
Nickname	"rest and digest" mode	"fight or flight" mode

Functions	• Maintains homeostasis (balance in your body)
	• Stimulates digestion:
	  o Salivation
	  o Stomach-acid production and secretion
	  o Digestive-enzyme production and secretion
	  o Bile production and secretion
	  o Nutrient absorption
	  o Intestinal motility
	  o Cleansing waves
	  o Defecation
	• Promotes the repair and maintenance of the body
	• Promotes sleep
		• Increases heart rate
		• Raises blood pressure
		• Activates sweat glands
		• Stimulates the release of sugar from your glycogen stores and the production of sugar in your liver
		• Inhibits digestion
		• Reduces stomach-acid production
		• Inhibits cleansing waves in your GI system
		• Suppresses the immune system (if stress is chronic)
		• Releases cortisol and adrenaline (which can wear down the adrenal glands over time)
		• Disrupts sleep (insomnia)

Many people have impaired digestion because stress turns their body's switch to sympathetic mode. In this "fight or flight" mode, not only is digestion inhibited, but stress hormones like cortisol and adrenaline are secreted in large amounts. This response is completely normal and even necessary in cases of acute stress to prepare you to face potential dangers. The problem is that our nervous system was built mainly to face short-term stressors like hunting for food or fleeing from predators. The stress response initiated by the sympathetic nervous system makes you ready to face the situation by making you more alert so you can respond by either fighting or fleeing.

The type of stress we tend to experience today is of a more chronic nature, preventing our bodies from returning to their default parasympathetic mode that facilitates proper digestion and healing. The elevated cortisol levels associated with the activation of your sympathetic mode can also:

- Disrupt your sleep
- Fatigue your adrenal glands
- Contribute to blood-sugar regulation problems
- Promote weight gain around your waist
- Alter your gut flora
- Downregulate your immune system
- Promote inflammation
- Inhibit cleansing waves (essential to preventing overgrowth of microorganisms in your small intestines)
- Increase intestinal permeability (causing leaky gut and leading to many digestive and systemic symptoms, as well as multiple food sensitivities).

"Stress is the trash of modern life. We all generate it, but if you don't dispose of it properly, it will pile up and overtake your life."

– Danzae Pace

Everyone deals with stress in his or her daily life. You can't avoid stress, but what you can change is how you react to and cope with it. You can't try to manage your stress only once a month, though. You need to cultivate stress management and relaxation on a daily basis, just like a garden that needs to be tended every day. If you don't keep the weeds under control, your flowers won't bloom.

Remember that your mind and body are intimately connected. Don't ignore your mental health or your physical health may plateau and even relapse instead of reaching its full potential. Cultivating a positive attitude isn't always easy when you suffer from chronic GI issues, but it's important to focus on the positive. While it may be difficult to feel good about bloating, diarrhea, and constipation, focus on the positive changes you're making and feel empowered by what you've already learned about digestive health. You now better understand what is at the root of your symptoms, and you know how to use a REAL-food-based elimination diet to say goodbye to your symptoms and recover your digestive health. You're taking charge of your health, and things can and will get better soon. It will take some work, but you're closer to optimal digestive health than you ever were.

You have the opportunity to overcome your digestive problems, or at least improve them significantly, if you only give yourself a chance. Focus on the relationships and other positive elements in your life, however small they may seem. It doesn't have to be something big: a pet that's always there for you, a sunny day, or the fresh smell of rain. If you can't think of anything positive, make something positive happen. Buy yourself flowers, treat yourself to a massage, or indulge in some quiet meditation.

"Your mind can only hold one thought at a time. Make it a positive and constructive one." – H. Jackson Brown, Jr.

Techniques to Tend Your Inner Garden

What else can you do to manage your stress, besides quitting your job and spending the rest of your life on a desert island? You can implement small strategies as part of your daily routine to cultivate a healthy mind and put your body in rest-and-digest mode. Maintaining a positive attitude alone is already a big improvement, but you can also include a few simple, quick relaxation techniques in your daily routine.

All you need is five to 10 minutes once or twice a day (and if you can dedicate more time, even better). Every minute you take to nurture your mind garden will help keep out the weeds out and allow your flowers to bloom. The following techniques only take a few minutes and can offer big benefits to your mental and bodily health:

- Belly breathing
- Finding a secret "happy place"
- Spending time with Mother Nature
- Body scanning
- Making a gratitude list
- Finding a hobby
- Laughing!
- Smiling

PRACTICE BELLY BREATHING

Lie down on your bed, on your couch, or outside on the grass. You can also sit if you prefer. Close your eyes, place your hands on your lower abdomen, and try to breathe only with your belly by making it inflate and deflate like a balloon as you breathe in and out. Your chest shouldn't move too much. It might feel a bit awkward at first but you'll get used to it. While breathing in, count from one to seven, in your head or aloud. Hold your breath for one count then count down from eight to zero while breathing out, trying to push all the air out of your lungs.

Breathe as slowly and as deeply as you can. If you prefer, you can omit the counting and repeat a mantra word or phrase with each respiration. Or simply imagine your breath as a light that fills your body each time you inspire. Try to do belly-breathing exercises for at least five minutes, but 15 to 20 minutes is ideal to get a maximal reinvigorating effect.

"And when I breathed, my breath was lightning." – Black Elk

FIND A SECRET "HAPPY PLACE"

You can do this exercise anywhere. Make yourself comfortable, lying down or sitting as you prefer. Close your eyes and think of a place or moment in your life that made you happy. Imagine the setting in your head, what it looked like, how it felt, what you heard, what you smelled, the people who were with you. It could be a vacation place, a nature spot, or the site of a special celebration.

Try to relive the moment you chose, as if you're watching a favorite movie. You can even adjust your memory to make it more interesting or enjoyable—or create one from scratch! Just make sure you imagine every detail to make it as real as possible. Do this for as long or as short as you like. Anytime you feel stressed, close your eyes for a minute or two and conjure this happy place to help you feel more relaxed and address your stress.

"Memory is a way of holding on to the things you love,
the things you are, the things you never want to lose."

– From the TV show The Wonder Years

SPEND TIME WITH MOTHER NATURE

Nature can have a powerful, calming effect. Unfortunately, too many people spend most of their lives inside their homes, classrooms, offices, and cars. All you need to experience the invigorating power of nature is a little piece of grass, ideally with a few trees. It could be in your backyard, a city park, or even on a beach. Lie down or sit in the grass and enjoy the nature around you. Try not to think too much, letting your thoughts come and go without focusing on any single one. Instead, pay attention to the sensations you experience, such as the feel of the wind, the sun's warmth on your skin, and the smells and the sounds around you. Feel your body being supported by the strong ground underneath you.

"One touch of nature makes the whole world kin." – William Shakespeare

Try to keep some part of your skin in direct contact with the grass or sand. Earthing, or the practice of being directly in contact with the ground, has been shown in various studies to decrease stress, regulate cortisol levels, lower inflammation, and promote better sleep. You can also get the same grounding benefits by taking a walk barefoot or swimming in a lake or the ocean. Going outside to relax will also give you the added bonus of getting some vitamin D. It may be a bit more difficult to practice earthing during winter in some areas, but you can still enjoy the fresh air and Mother Nature's calming effect by taking a walk or sitting in a quiet park.

"Look deep into nature, and then you will understand everything better."

– Albert Einstein

PRACTICE BODY SCANNING

Lie down or sit somewhere comfortable. Close your eyes and scan your body, body part by body part. One by one, slowly contract each muscle group of your body starting from your face, neck, shoulders, upper arms, lower arms, hands, and fingers, without moving. Move to your chest, back, and abdomen before attending to your glutes, thighs, calves, feet, and toes. Doing the cycle once is enough to feel more relaxed, but you can repeat it as often as you'd like to deepen the relaxation.

"The best cure for the body is a quiet mind." – Napoléon Bonaparte

MAKE A GRATITUDE LIST

Experiencing gratitude is a great way to feel calm and relaxed. Feeling appreciative results in the release of the hormone oxytocin, which activates your parasympathetic nervous system and switches your body into its rest-and-digest mode. You can activate gratitude by creating a "gratitude list" of everything you're thankful for: the meaningful relationships in your life, your ability to take charge of your health by changing the way you eat, and even the restful sleep you had the night before. You can be grateful for things you've done, things that have happened to you, or things you've received. Keep this list on your fridge or bedside table or somewhere else you can see it, and read it as often as you need. Add more items as you think of them. Whenever you feel stressed, focus on one of the items on your list for a few minutes. See Appendix 21 for a template to write your gratitude list.

"Gratitude helps people feel more positive emotions,
relish positive experiences, have better health, deal with adversity,
and build strong relationships."

– Harvard Medical School

Instead of a list, you can also write all the things for which you're thankful on separate pieces of paper and put them in a jar. Whenever you feel down, open the jar and pick one to cheer you up. Hold on to the gratitude as long as you can to help you feel calmer and more centered.

"When you are grateful, fear disappears and abundance appears."

– Anthony Robbins

LAUGH!

Laughing is a serious matter. It oxygenates your body, stimulates circulation, and encourages the release of feel-good hormones (endorphins) that can calm you down and make you feel better quickly. Laughter can even boost your immune system. Most people understand the importance of not taking life too seriously and that laughing is good, but not many make it a regular exercise.

Try simply laughing for three to five minutes straight. You don't have to be laughing at anything; faking it counts. Even if you feel ridiculous during this exercise, do it at least once to experience the powerful effect of laughter. Alternate between vowel sounds and adjust the loudness and quality of your laughter as you like. It can be hard to do at first but you'll feel amazingly relaxed afterwards—and you'll likely want to do it again soon.

Whenever you face a stressful situation, try to respond by—yep—laughing. Laughing can help you detach yourself from the negative emotions associated with the situation. Laugh out the stress!

"Do not take life too seriously. You will never get out of it alive."

– Elbert Hubbard

SMILE ☺

Some researchers believe that emotions are activated by facial expressions rather than the other way around. The simple act of smiling, even a forced smile, can send a message to your body and mind that triggers the release of important calming and relaxing hormones. If you don't feel like laughing, or you're in an environment where laughing wouldn't be appropriate, just smile. You can do this in your car on your way to work, when working on your computer, during a meeting or exam, or while talking to friends.

"A smile is a curve that sets everything straight." – Phyllis Diller

FIND A HOBBY

Most people are too busy, or believe they are too busy, to take the time for hobbies they once enjoyed. Hobbies are a fantastic way to adjust your mind frame and forget about the stresses in your life. If you find you're not as interested in collecting stamps or stickers as you did when you were 11, try taking up a new pastime. It could be dancing, listening to music or playing an instrument, scrapbooking, drawing, photography, jewelry making, wood working, knitting, model building, studying a foreign language, rock climbing, gardening, writing, or reading (ideally not health- or nutrition-related!). Whatever you choose, make sure it's something that helps you feel more relaxed and take your mind off your worries.

"A hobby a day keeps the doldrums away." – Phyllis McGinley

DO WHAT MAKES YOU FEEL GOOD

Experiment with these relaxation methods to see which ones you prefer. Write down a list of your favorite techniques and put it on your fridge to remind you of all the great tools you've developed to help combat stress. You can even try combining the techniques. Try to do some belly breathing while smiling and/or thinking of a special place that makes you feel calm and relaxed. Or take a nature walk while recalling items from your gratitude list. There are no rules, except no stressing about any of it! You deserve to spend a bit of time every day doing what makes you feel good and happy.

ADDRESS STRESSFUL SITUATIONS HEAD-ON

It's important to take time on a regular basis to practice the techniques above, just like you need to tend your garden frequently to prevent weeds from suffocating your flowers. But what should you do when confronted with an immediately stressful situation? Whenever a stressful situation arises, remember to stay calm. This might be easier said than done, but the more you practice the better at it you will become. With any problem, there are always three things you can do to resolve it:

- Change the situation,
- Adapt yourself to the situation, or
- Leave the situation.

"It's not stress that kills us. It is our reaction to it." – Hans Selye

How would this work in practice? Let's say that work is a significant source of stress in your life. What can you do? You can either try changing the situation by talking to your supervisor about making deadlines more reasonable or trying to find ways to make your workload easier to manage. If you can't change the situation directly, you can adapt yourself to it by changing your attitude toward your work. Instead of feeling like your job is a chore or torture, try looking at it as a challenge. Try to adopt a positive attitude by recognizing how your job helps you get the money you need to afford nice things and better appreciate the time you spend outside the office. If neither of these strategies works, and the job is making your life miserable and interfering with your quality of life and your health, try to find another job that would be a better fit for you. You have options. Don't be a victim, and take control of your life.

"Quit giving someone else the job of making you happy." – Joyce Meyer

GET ENOUGH QUALITY SLEEP

Many studies emphasize the importance of sleep for optimal health. Lack of sleep can compromise your learning and memory, mood, weight, cardiovascular health, and immune system, and can even trigger cravings. A single night of poor sleep can induce insulin resistance in healthy people, which constitutes a risk factor and a first step toward developing type 2 diabetes and heart disease.

Not getting enough sleep can also be perceived as a stress by your body and result in the same harmful consequences for your digestive health caused by any other type of stress. Insomnia can be also a sign of adrenal fatigue, and one can worsen the other in a vicious cycle. You need good sleep to allow your body and digestive system to heal and function optimally, so you have to make sleep a priority.

"A good laugh and a long sleep are the best cures in the doctor's book."

– Irish proverb

You need between eight and nine hours of sleep every night, so make sure you go to bed at the right time, ideally before 9:30-10 PM. If you have trouble falling asleep, make sure you turn off the lights or keep them to a minimum one or two hours before bedtime. Turn off the television and stay away from the computer. Too much light interferes with the release of hormones like melatonin that make you naturally sleepy within a few hours after the sun sets. To avoid interfering with these hormones, use the last hour or two before your bedtime to read by a small table lamp, take a bath or shower, or just relax to help your body get ready for a good night's sleep.

Light is what synchronizes your body's natural rhythm. Humans are meant to go to sleep within a few hours after the sun goes down and wake up when the sun rises (varying according to the time of the year). Artificial light disrupts this normal cycle by causing insomnia or preventing you from getting restorative sleep. Try to get some natural sunshine during the day to help your body knows it's daytime, and make your room as dark as you can at night so your body gets the message that it is nighttime. Cover up your windows as best you can and remove any night lights, alarm clocks, or other light sources in your room, since they can interfere with sleep hormones.

> "Sleep is the golden chain that ties health and our bodies together."
>
> – Thomas Dekker (1577-1632)

EXERCISE

Exercise is another potential part of your plan to improve both your physical and mental health. It can improve circulation, heart health, cognition, body weight, appetite, mental health, and mood. Studies have actually shown that exercise works better than antidepressants, with added benefits on your overall health and no side effects. When you exercise, your body releases neurotransmitters called endorphins that can help you feel less stressed and more relaxed.

Take Care of Your Mind
• Understand how stress affects your health (p. 204)
• Do some belly breathing (p. 207)
• Go to your secret happy place (p. 207)
• Hang out with Mother Nature (p. 208)
• Try the body scan (p. 208)
• Write a gratitude list (p. 208)
• Laugh (p. 209)
• Smile (p. 209)
• Practice a hobby (p. 209)
• Do what makes you feel good (p. 209)
• Allow yourself to rest
• Live in the present
• Surround yourself with people you love
• Avoid caffeine and foods you are sensitive to
• Sleep 8-9 hours per night (p. 210)
• Avoid excessive and endurance exercise (p. 211)
• Address stressful situations (p. 210)
- Change the situation,
- Adapt yourself to the situation, or
- Leave the situation

However, don't think about exercising before first addressing stress management, relaxation, and sleep. If you are still feeling very tired and malnourished as a result of your compromised digestive health, don't sweat it. You don't need to exercise for now. You'll know your body is ready once your energy levels improve and you feel the natural impulse to be a bit more active.

> "Walking is man's best medicine." – Hippocrates

Exercise can help you better manage your stress and improve your health, once your body is ready for it, but not all kinds of exercise are the same. Avoid high-intensity and endurance forms of exercise since they can raise the stress hormone cortisol and contribute to increased intestinal permeability. Jogging and aerobic exercises can actually be stressful for your body. Instead, choose low-intensity exercise. Walking is your best option. Gentle yoga is also good, but avoid high-intensity or hot yoga. Strength training can also provide a lot of benefit. Just make sure you listen to your body. Don't force yourself to exercise and don't try doing too much, especially at first. Start with five to 10 minutes of gentle exercise and increase gradually if you have the energy. As your digestive health improves and your energy increases, you can make exercise a more central element of your stress-management regimen.

> "If you don't like the road you're walking, start paving another one."
>
> – Dolly Parton

Changing the way you eat will help you recover your digestive health, but adopting a holistic approach that includes cultivating a positive attitude, taking good care of yourself, and getting enough sleep can accelerate the healing process. As your digestion improves, your mind will feel better, and working on your mental health will help your digestive health improve simultaneously. Everything is connected, and you will get the best and quickest results by tackling your GI issues from as many angles as possible at once. See Table 77 for a quick list of techniques that can help you take care of your mind.

Chapter 7: The Mind-Body Connection

Chapter 8: Living Life—Eating Out And Traveling!

Eating differently to retake control of your health doesn't mean you have to stop living your life and stay home alone. Although it might be easier to do the elimination phase at home, it shouldn't keep you from having fun and spicing up your routine by eating out, socializing, and traveling. Things will get easier as your build your BYO diet and expand your dietary horizons, but you don't have to wait that long. A little more planning is necessary with special dietary requirements, but it can be done.

For most people, food plays a role far beyond basic nourishment. Food means love, comfort, and celebration. But saying no to someone offering you spaghetti or a piece of cake doesn't mean you don't love and appreciate them. Would you feel guilty saying you can't eat bread, peanuts, or alcohol if you had celiac disease or a peanut allergy or were a recovering alcoholic?

Whether it's at a family dinner, with friends over for brunch, or during a special occasion at work, you can enjoy the company of the people you love and still eat the foods that make you feel good. Most people will understand your new way of eating if you explain that you are simply trying to feel better and improve your health. If you need to, you can mention that this is not a fad diet, but a medical diet. This isn't a lie, since elimination diets *are* the medical gold standard to identify food sensitivities and build an optimal diet. Try to focus on conversations and enjoying your time with loved ones in. It's not the food, but the mood that truly matters.

Family and Friends

If you have a dinner or other special occasion planned with family or friends, take the time to let them know about your new way of eating. If you're inviting them over, it should be easy to provide options that are suitable for you. If the meal is elsewhere, make sure to discuss your situation with your hosts. Explain that you're currently eliminating gluten, grains, sugar, and other foods to improve your health. If they are receptive and willing to make modifications to their menu to accommodate you, make sure to give them a list of foods and ingredients you *can* eat. If your hosts seem to find your diet too complicated, offer to bring a dish you can eat and share with everyone or, if the hosts have already planned the menu, simply bring your own meal.

At Work

When colleagues tempt you with bagels and muffins at a team meeting or with cake at a monthly birthday celebration, it's important to be prepared to respond. Think of how you want to handle the situation ahead of time to remove all the guesswork. You can mention that you aren't hungry, that you're allergic to gluten, or that you don't eat processed food. The explanation you give is up to you and depends on how much you're willing to share with your coworkers. The best option is probably to bring something you can eat along with your colleagues and not suffer the consequences of eating something that could compromise your gut health.

Restaurants

Eating out at restaurants can be trickier if you have food restrictions, but it's not impossible. While eating out isn't ideal since you can't control the quality of the ingredients or the risk of cross contamination, if you plan in advance and do your homework, you should be able to eat out without getting sick.

Unfortunately, an alarming majority of chefs (96 percent), including many who offer gluten-free options at their own restaurants, failed a simple four-question questionnaire about gluten knowledge administered by the National Foundation for Celiac Awareness (NFCA). Many chefs don't know that gluten can hide under many ingredients and are unaware of cross-contamination risks. Moreover, other restaurant staff may not have the knowledge required to help you choose the best options, especially if you combine your gluten-free diet with the elimination of all grains, dairy, eggs, nightshades, nuts, and other foods and ingredients.

So how do you survive when eating out? Ask questions! Lots of questions. Start by doing some research about the restaurant. You can often find menus on the restaurants' website. Call ahead of time to explain your dietary restrictions and find suitable options. It's your *right* to know.

Be particularly wary of marinades, sauces, and breading. Many of these can contain gluten, grain-derived ingredients, sugar, soy, or MSG. Don't forget to ask about the preparation methods, too. If your quarter chicken is fried in the same fryer used for breaded chicken, you could be in trouble if you react to gluten. The same cross-contamination problem can occur if your food is prepared on the same cutting board, cooked on the same grill, or manipulated with the same utensils used to prepare gluten-containing foods. If the waiter doesn't provide satisfying answers to your questions, ask to talk directly to the chef. In most cases, they will be happy to assist you and adapt some menu items to accommodate your limitations.

Don't be shy about asking for substitutions, either. Most meals come with some kind of starch or grain, but you can ask to have it replaced with more vegetables or a salad. Steakhouses are usually a good restaurant option, but most restaurants offer a grill selection with chicken, steak, or fish. Choose a protein option and simply asked to have it served plain (unless the sauce contains only acceptable ingredients) with lots of vegetables. Ask for extra olive oil if possible (or butter if you tolerate it). If you want to make sure your meal will be satisfying enough, bring your own healthy traditional fats. Carry a small container of extra-virgin olive oil, coconut oil, ghee, or butter to add to your veggies. If you're going for sushi, order sashimi to avoid the rice. Sidestep the gluten-filled soy sauce by asking for coconut aminos or gluten-free tamari sauce (or bring your own). Be creative! The next table gives you some more ideas about how to make restaurant meals suitable for you. Be polite when discussing your options with the waiter or chef and you might be surprised at the delicious dishes they can create just for you.

Table 78: Restaurant Meal Options

Cuisines	Best Options	Beware of These (ask questions!)
Anywhere	• Ask for a plain serving of protein (chicken, beef, fish, pork; without marinade, sauce, or breading) • Substitute grains/starches (rice, pasta, potatoes) with vegetables and/or extra fat • Ask for salads (without croutons and first check the ingredients in the dressing)	• Omelets, quiches, and scrambled eggs often contain dairy and/or flour • Sauces (many contain flour or gums as thickeners, as well as MSG, soy, or sugar for seasoning)
Burger	• Ask for the burger without the bun and substitute the French fries with vegetables/salad	• Sauces, marinades, salad dressings, cheese
Steakhouse	• Ask for a plain serving of protein (chicken, beef, fish, pork; without marinade, sauce, or breading) • Substitute grains/starches (rice, pasta, potatoes) with vegetables and/or extra fat	• Sauces and marinades (may contain flour to thicken them as well as sugar or MSG to flavor them)
Rotisserie	• Roasted chicken without gravy • Substitute grains/starches (rice, pasta, potatoes) with vegetables and/or extra fat	• Seasonings or stuffing that can contain gluten • Sauces and gravies
Italian	• Look for the grill section and choose chicken, steak, or fish (plain, without sauces or marinades) • Ask for vegetables as a side dish and add extra olive oil	• Sauces (may contain flour as a thickener)
Greek	• Kabobs • Ask to have the rice and potatoes replaced with vegetables/salad	• Sauces, marinades, and salad dressings
Japanese	• Sashimi (sushi without rice) • Ask for or bring coconut aminos or gluten-free tamari sauce	• Soy sauce, edamame • Rice • Tempura • Surimi (fake crab)
Mexican	• Ask for the filling only of the tacos or burritos with ingredients you tolerate • Ask for extra guacamole (if you tolerate avocado)	• Corn-based nachos, tacos, or tortillas • Cheese and sour cream • Rice • Beans

If a restaurant is unwilling to accommodate you, go somewhere else. If you're eating out with others and can't go somewhere else, bring your own meal. Mention that you have food allergies and they will probably be happy not to have to deal with you. Most restaurants will even agree to heat your meal in the microwave. Ask in advance to be sure and make sure to bring a cold meal if they are not collaborative. If you're stuck, eat before going to the restaurant and just have something to drink while your friends eat.

If you have a word to say in the selection of the restaurant, try to find one that offers gluten-free or Paleo-friendly options. Although gluten-free options like gluten-free pasta, rice- and potato-based dishes, and sugary gluten-free treats are not ideal, at least you won't have to worry about cross contamination or hidden gluten in sauces. Paleo menus can make eating out a lot easier since they are 100-percent free of gluten, grains, dairy, soy, and processed foods. Most also eliminate all sugars. Simply search for the keywords "Paleo restaurant" or "gluten-free restaurant" and the name of your city and you might be lucky to discover a great new spot or two where you can eat out safely and deliciously!

Traveling

Many people with IBS and other digestive disorders avoid traveling, fearful that their symptoms might ruin their vacation. Once you've made it through the elimination phase of the protocol described in Chapter 5, you should have more energy and have your symptoms under enough control that leaving home for more than a few hours isn't a daunting prospect. This, plus a little planning will allow you to continue eating the foods that make you feel good and help you make the most of your well-deserved time away from home.

ROAD TRIPS

If you're going on a road trip, you can prepare a few meals in advance and keep your food for a few days in a cooler provided you regularly add ice to keep it fresh. Bring foods you don't mind eating cold. Cook some chicken and vegetables and bring extra-virgin olive oil, coconut oil, or ghee to have complete meals. Other easy combinations include smoked fish with avocado, or hard-boiled eggs and homemade mayonnaise. Jerky, coconut chips, nuts, and fruits, depending on your tolerance, also make great road-trip snacks. Bananas with a bit of almond butter or sugar-free baby purées mixed with coconut butter or oil also make an easy treat if these foods are part of your BYO diet.

ACCOMMODATION

When planning a vacation, try to find accommodations that include a kitchen or kitchenette, such as a budget-friendly hostel with a communal kitchen or a fancier private apartment if you can afford it. Staying with relatives is another good option that enables you to cook your own meals. You can even bring your own pots and pans or an electric skillet to cook meals while on the road. Many hotels will provide a mini-fridge or microwave to store your fresh food and do some basic cooking, but ask beforehand to make sure.

If none of these options are available, you can always bring foods that keep well at room temperature. Canned fish, jerky, avocado, and nut butter make for quick and easy meals and snacks, and you can eat the rest of your meals at restaurants (following the tips above). If you don't want to cook during your vacations, make sure to do your pre-trip research to find suitable restaurant options. If in doubt, opt for the steakhouse! Skip the gravy and sauce and sub the potato, rice, or fries with more vegetables. And don't forget to ask for extra fat. Bring your own ghee, olive oil, or coconut oil with you if you don't want to feel energy deprived. These traditional fats can all be kept at room temperature without issue.

Table 79 gives you a few ideas for foods you can eat easily while on the road. Don't forget to bring a can opener, fork, spoon, and knife, as well as a small plate so you can eat on the go anywhere.

Table 79: Easy Foods for the Road

To Carry with You* (at room temperature)	Easy to Find at Most Grocery Stores* (no cooking required)
• Jerky (without artificial ingredients)	• Whole roasted chicken (without stuffing; check the ingredients)
• Pemmican	• Smoked salmon (without artificial ingredients)
• Canned fish (tuna, salmon, sardines)	• Butter/ghee and extra-virgin olive oil
• Nuts	• Avocado
• Nut butters	• Olives (canned or jarred)
• Fruits (fresh, canned or dried; without added sugar)	• Nuts and nut butters
• Coconut oil	• Jerky (without artificial ingredients)
• Ghee	• Prosciutto and other deli meats (without artificial ingredients)
• Olive oil	• Canned fish (tuna, salmon, sardines)
• Avocado	• Fruits (fresh, canned or dried; without added sugar)
• Pickles (canned or jarred)	• Vegetables (fresh, canned)
• Olives (canned or jarred)	• Puréed baby food (without sugar, starch, or other artificial ingredients)
• Coconut butter	• Coconut milk (without gums)
• Coconut chips	• Cheese and plain yogurt (if you tolerate dairy)
• Coconut milk (without gums)	• Eggs (can be bought hard-boiled or cooked easily in a microwave)
• Puréed baby food (without sugar, starch, or other artificial ingredients)	

* As tolerated

FLYING

If your flight includes a meal, you can usually make a request (in the "manage your booking" section online or on the phone) for a gluten-free, lactose-free, or kosher meal. The advantage of asking for a special meal is that you will be among the first to be served on the plane! Just remember that none of these meals will be 100-percent appropriate for you. The gluten-free meal is probably the best option to choose since gluten can easily sneak into sauces and seasonings and is usually harder to detect visually than dairy or potatoes—and you won't have to worry about cross contamination. You'll probably be able to eat at least the protein choice and some of the vegetables in this meal. Avoid the gluten-free carbohydrate options (rice, gluten-free pasta, or potato) and gluten-free desserts (made with gluten-free grains, dairy, or sugar) if you're unsure about the ingredients. Snacks provided on the plane are rarely gluten free, but ask for fresh fruit if you can tolerate it.

If you don't want to rely on airplane food, though, bringing your own is the best strategy to stay well fed while you fly (see Table 80). You might want to avoid bringing foods with strong odors if you don't want to make enemies. Bring foods that will keep at room temperature, such as jerky, nuts, avocado, canned fish, or fruit. If you want to prepare your meal in advance, add ice packs to your lunch or freeze the protein component of your meal ahead of time so it's safe for a few hours until you're ready to eat it.

Examples of meals that you can eat cold are salads of cooked or raw vegetables mixed with chicken, beef, or fish and coconut oil, ghee, or olive oil. You can also pack your fat separately. You are allowed to carry small bottles containing up to three ounces (100 milliliters) of liquids as long as each label indicates its volume. Pack some olive oil, coconut oil, or ghee with you for a concentrated source of energy. You can also bring an empty water bottle (ideally not made of plastic), which you can fill up as soon as you pass the security checkpoint.

If you're traveling to a foreign country, acquaint yourself with their specific regulations. Some countries like Australia have strict regulations and require you to declare foods you carry with you, especially fresh and dried fruits and vegetables, herbs, spices, herbal teas, snack foods, dairy products, animal products, and nuts. Some of these will be inspected and given back to you, but some may be quarantined. Try to bring food that you can finish during the flight, then just restock at the closest grocery store once you arrive at your destination.

LANGUAGE BARRIERS

If you'll be traveling to a country where you don't speak the language, take some time before you go to translate basic words to help you communicate your dietary restrictions. You can use any online translator tool to look up terms in Italian, German, French, Chinese, Japanese, Spanish, Swedish, or any other language you need. The next table gives you a head start with a few different languages and some words that might be useful when ordering out abroad. You might not be able to stick to your BYO diet 100 percent of the time when traveling, but avoiding the biggest offenders will help you feel as good as possible during your trip.

Table 80: Translated Food Terms for Traveling

Words	French	Spanish	German	Italian	Chinese	Vietnamese	Arabic
Food allergies	allergies alimentaires	Alergias alimentarias	Nahrungs-mittel-allergie	alergie alimentari	食物过敏	dị ứng thức ăn	الحساسية الغذائية
Grains	céréales	granos	Getreide	grani	谷物	các loại ngũ cốc	حبوب
Wheat	blé	trigo	Weizen	frumento / grano	小麦	lúa mì	قمح
Gluten	gluten	gluten	Gluten	glutine	面筋	gluten	الغلوتين
Dairy	produits laitiers	lácteos	Milcher-zeu-gnis	latticini	乳制品	sữa	الألبان
Sugar	sucre	azúcar	Zucker	zucchero	糖	đường	سكر
Soy	soja	soya	Soja	soia	黄豆	đậu nành	فول الصويا
Peanut	arachides	maní	Erdnuss	arachide	花生	đậu phộng	الفول السوداني
Nuts	noix	nueces	Nuss	noce	坚果	Nut	بندق
Meat	viande	carne	Fleisch	carne	肉类	thịt	لحم
Poultry	volaille	carne de ave	Geflügel	pollame	家禽	gia cầm	دواجن
Chicken	poulet	pollo	Huhn	pollo	鸡	Chicken	دجاج
Beef	boeuf	carne de res	Rindfleisch	manzo	牛肉	thịt bò	لحوم البقر
Pork	porc	cerdo	Schweine-fleisch	carne di maiale	猪肉	thịt lợn	لحم خنزير
Fish	poisson	pescado	Fisch	pesce	鱼	cá	سمك
Vegetables	legumes	vegetales	Gemüse	verdure	蔬菜	rau	خضروات
Butter	beurre	mantequilla	Butter	burro	黄油	bơ	زبدة
Olive oil	huile d'olive	aceite de oliva	Olivenöl	olio d'oliva	橄榄油	dầu ôliu	زيت الزيتون
Avocado	avocat	aguacate	Avocado	avocado	鳄梨	bơ	أفوكادو
Coconut	noix de coco	coco	Koko	noce di cocco	椰子	dừa	جوزة الهند
Fat	gras	grasas	Fett	grasso	脂肪	chất béo	دهن
Eggs	oeufs	huevos	Eier	uova	鸡蛋	trứng	بيض
Please	s'il-vous-plaît	por favor	bitte	per favore	请	xin	من فضلك
To substitute	remplacer	sustituir	ersetzen	sostituire	替换	thay thế	استبدل
Thank you very much	merci beau-coup	muchísimas gracias	danke schön	grazie mille	非常感谢	cảm ơn bạn rất nhiều	شكرا جزيلا

With the exception of French, Spanish, and German, most of these translations were done with an online translator.
I cannot guarantee that these translations are 100-percent accurate.

TRAVELING AND PREVENTING GI INFECTIONS

Whether you're traveling within your country or abroad, preventing infections like food poisoning or diarrhea should always be in the back of your mind. Catching a bad bacteria or a parasite could not only make your vacation miserable, it can also set you back in your gut healing. Traveling in developed countries is usually quite safe. Just make sure not to keep perishable foods at room temperature for too long.

If you're visiting any developing countries, however, you'll need to adopt additional precautionary measures. It's usually advised to avoid eating raw vegetables or fruits that you don't wash yourself with safe water, as well as undercooked seafood or meat. Street food is especially iffy, so eat it at your own risk. Tap water or beverages made with tap water, as well as ice cubes, can also carry harmful microorganisms, so stick with bottled water and hot beverages like teas, which are safer since the heat destroys potentially harmful pathogens. Always use bottled or boiled water to wash your food and brush your teeth.

Another good strategy to minimize the risk of a gastrointestinal infection during your travels is to take probiotics. Probiotics and fermented foods should be part of your daily routine before going away to optimize your digestive health and can protect you from GI infections by keeping your immune system strong. A healthy gut flora can also protect you against harmful microorganisms by preventing them from invading your intestinal lining.

In addition to taking probiotics before hitting the road, it may be beneficial to continue taking some on a daily basis while you're away. *Saccharomyces boulardii* (mostly known as Florastor or Floractiv), which is a yeast, is especially convenient since it can be kept at room temperature without altering its efficacy. Studies have shown that starting to take *S. boulardii* (500 to 1,000 milligrams per day) five days before leaving and for the duration of your trip may reduce the incidence of gastrointestinal infections by as much as 25 to 33 percent.

"An ounce of prevention is worth a pound of cure." – Benjamin Franklin

Chapter 9: Troubleshooting

Although you now know what to do and how to eat to recover your digestive health, things don't always go according to plan. Some people feel rapidly discouraged and give up before giving their body a chance to detox itself and start the healing process. If you feel like you're doing everything right but not seeing the results you hoped for, read this chapter to troubleshoot your problems and get your health moving in the right direction again.

Problem #1: Cravings

Most people will experience cravings of some sort, which can make it difficult to stick either to the elimination phase or your BYO diet. Cravings can be due to a gut dysbiosis, a withdrawal or die-off reaction, your body detoxifying, or the keto-adaptation (fat-adaptation) process.

Withdrawal reactions are common after eliminating grains and sugar because these foods can elicit an addiction. Switching from a standard American diet to a lower-carb, higher-fat intake requires your body to learn how to utilize fat instead of carbohydrates for energy. If you have a gut dysbiosis, it is also possible that the bacteria and yeast that are now starving to death are sending signals to your brain begging you to eat something sweet or starchy. And remember that studies have shown that sugar can be more addictive than cocaine!

Succumbing to temptation can delay your progress and prolong your misery while trying to transition to your optimal diet. Giving in to a craving for whole grain bread, honey, or fruit-flavored yogurt in the first weeks of the elimination diet can just make it more difficult for your body to go through withdrawal and keto-adaptation. It can also allow an overgrowth of microorganisms in your intestines to survive a little longer. And if you're the kind of person who can't stop after eating just a small piece of chocolate, you may end up eating the whole bar and craving more, which can bring back the very symptoms you're trying to eliminate.

Although cravings may seem impossible to resist when they strike, being prepared and using some of the techniques below can help you beat them. The good news is that your cravings should decrease and vanish eventually as the weeks go by. It may be hard to believe right now, but your body will sooner or later realize that you're already giving it all the nutrients it needs to function at its best. Here are a few things you can do to curb or prevent cravings:

EAT MORE, ESPECIALLY FAT

Eating more frequently and making sure you get enough protein and fat at each of your meals and snacks can help your body realize it's not starving. Many people make the mistake of simply eliminating sugar and grains from their diet during the elimination phase and forget to compensate for their decreased carbohydrate intake by increasing their fat intake, whether they do so voluntarily or not. Consult the meal-plan section for a better idea of how much protein and fat to eat each day. For most women, at least four to six ounces (120 to 180 grams) of protein and two tablespoons (30 milliliters) of fat are required at each meal, while men should aim for at least six to eight ounces (180 to 240 grams) of protein and three tablespoons (45 milliliters) of fat per meal. Everybody is different, so you should adjust these guidelines according to your hunger and body weight. You can also use an online tracking tool to estimate your daily calorie intake and adjust it as necessary.

Eating more meals and snacks throughout the day can also be useful at first to manage your cravings. If you're still afraid of fat, reread the section about traditional fat in Chapter 5. And remember that fat doesn't make you fat. You *need* to eat more fat to help your body learn how to utilize fat instead of carbohydrates for fuel—especially during the transition period corresponding to the first few weeks on the elimination phase. Don't limit your fat intake and eat extra fat at snacks between meals to reduce cravings and help your body adjust more quickly to your lower-carb, higher-fat way of eating. Try adding a spoonful of coconut oil in a cup of green tea, having a snack of cooked vegetables with ghee or olive oil, or simply drink a spoonful of coconut oil or ghee by itself.

A spoonful of coconut oil can be especially effective at silencing cravings. Its medium-chain triglycerides (MCTs) are easy to digest and utilize as a source of energy. A little bit of coconut oil can help you get the boost of energy you need to avoid eating for emotional reasons such as boredom, fatigue, or comfort.

Hypoglycemia or blood-sugar dysregulation can also trigger sugar and carb cravings. As your body becomes keto-adapted, your blood sugar levels should become more stable throughout the day, helping you avoid cravings completely. If you have diabetes or take medications to control your blood-sugar levels, consult your doctor or diabetes educator before making any dietary changes for help making adjustments to medication dosage and timing. Cutting down on your carb intake should reduce your need for such medications relatively quickly. If your cravings are the result of hypoglycemia (low blood sugar), follow your caregiver's recommendations on dealing with hypoglycemia and make an appointment to discuss your treatment plan in light of your new way of eating.

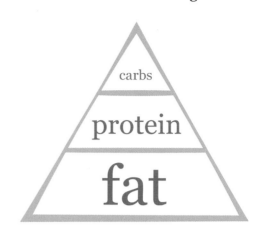

macronutrient balance for digestive health

ADD UNREFINED SALT

A mild state of dehydration or adrenal fatigue can also lead to cravings. You can correct this easily by adding more salt to your diet. Unrefined salt, such as Celtic salt, Himalayan salt, or other minimally processed salt varieties are best because they offer a wide range of minerals without any chemical residues. Eating enough salt will help you stay properly hydrated (since a lower-carb diet can have a mild diuretic effect), as well as support your adrenal function to prevent cravings from occurring in the first place. If you have a craving *right now* and don't know if you'll be able to resist the temptation, have a cup or two of homemade bone broth. The amino acids and minerals found in bone broth should calm your craving within minutes.

AVOID ARTIFICIAL SWEETENERS

Although artificial sweeteners aren't recommended on the elimination phase, some people decide to keep them in their diet to sweeten their tea or sugar-free chewing gum. Even though artificial sweeteners like sucralose, aspartame, and stevia do not provide any calories or carbohydrates, their sweet taste can reinforce your desire for sweet foods and perpetuate your cravings. Not only can these chemicals compromise your progress, they can make your life harder and even ruin your efforts by inducing irresistible cravings.

SLEEP ENOUGH

How well are you sleeping? Are you getting at least eight to nine hours per night? Be honest! If the answer is no, this might explain why you're having difficulty dealing with cravings. A lack of sleep is associated with blood-sugar dysregulation, which can make your body crave carbs and sugars. Make sleep a priority. It's an *essential* component of your gut-healing program.

GET MORE AMINO ACIDS

Certain amino acids, the building blocks of protein, can be particularly helpful for controlling cravings. You can usually get all the protein you need from REAL food, but it's not uncommon for some people to not have enough of specific amino acids to keep their brain chemistry balanced. This is especially true for people who have dealt with food restrictions (particularly vegetarian diets), food malabsorption, and other digestive problems. Two of the amino acids that can help you beat carb cravings are L-glutamine and 5-hydroxytryptophan (5-HTP).

L-glutamine is one of the supplements that can be useful to restore your digestive health since the cells lining your intestines love to feed on it. L-glutamine can also serve as a quick source of energy for your brain cells. Whenever you crave carbs, it can be a signal that your brain is lacking energy. Your brain knows very well that sugar is the quickest source of energy and that's why it makes you crave it. Taking L-glutamine can quickly (within 10 to 15 minutes) provide your brain with the extra energy it needs to make a craving subside. To prevent cravings from happening, try taking 500 mg of L-glutamine three times per day between meals. If you're experiencing a strong craving at any time, try a stronger dose of 500 to 1,000 milligrams whenever the craving hits. You should feel a difference relatively quickly. If you don't feel any change, it's probably not what your body needs. Keep experimenting with different strategies until you find what works best for you.

If your carb cravings usually occur in the afternoons or evenings, or during your PMS period for women, your brain may be deficient in the neurotransmitter serotonin. Many people with low serotonin crave carbohydrates because sugar and starches can boost serotonin levels. The problem is that this effect is not long lasting. Before long, your serotonin levels will drop again and the cravings will return. In order to escape this vicious craving cycle, you'll need to supply your body with better building blocks to keep your serotonin levels more stable. 5-HTP is an important precursor, or building block, for the synthesis and regulation of serotonin. This supplement has the added benefit of helping promoting regular intestinal cleansing waves, an important factor in preventing bacterial overgrowth. You can start with 50 milligrams in the middle of the afternoon and increase gradually to up to 150 mg until you achieve the desired effect. Taking a small dose at bedtime can also help you feel more relaxed and improve your sleep quality.

As always, consult your doctor to make sure that supplementation with these individual amino acids is right for you and won't interfere with your medications, especially if you have liver or kidney problems, lupus, a thyroid disorder, or an ulcer; are pregnant; or suffer from a mental disorder.

Problem #2: Fatigue

Like cravings, fatigue is a common symptom you can experience in the first weeks as you go through the withdrawal, detox, and keto-adaptation periods. Most people with digestive issues often feel tired or lethargic, and these symptoms can sometimes worsen during the elimination phase of the diet as your body is trying to adapt to your new way of eating. Most people feel that their energy levels improve significantly after three to four weeks on the elimination diet, probably because their digestive system has recovered enough to absorb nutrients properly and start the healing process. However, if your energy levels don't improve after a few weeks, it might be because you're not eating enough fat or sodium, that you're too stressed, or you're not getting enough restful sleep.

EAT MORE FAT

For many people, the low-fat mantra is so ingrained that it is hard for them to get past it. If you eat too little fat *and* restrict your carb intake, it will be *impossible* for you to get all the calories you need. Don't be afraid of fat. It won't make you fat or clog your arteries, especially not traditional fats such as ghee, tallow, lard, extra-virgin olive oil, and coconut oil. Aim for *at least* one to three tablespoons (15 to 45 milliliters) per meal and adjust the amount depending on your hunger levels and body weight, but never go below one to two tablespoons of extra fat per meal.

If you have trouble digesting a higher amount of fat, consider taking betaine HCl, ox bile, or digestive enzymes (especially lipase). Coconut oil may also be easier to digest and absorb because it's made of roughly half MCTs. In addition to not needing to be broken down to be absorbed, the MCTs in coconut oil are easier to use as a source of energy and may help you feel less tired.

GET MORE SODIUM AND WATER

Lowering your carb intake by cutting out grains and sugar can have a light diuretic effect, which is a good thing because it allows your body to get rid of extra water it may be holding on to unnecessarily. However, if you don't replenish your electrolytes and fluids, this diuretic effect can result in mild dehydration. Fatigue, headaches, irritability, and dizziness upon standing are common dehydration symptoms. By cutting out processed foods, it's also very likely that you're not getting enough sodium (salt) to help your body retain the right amount of water to stay hydrated.

You can add a little salt back into your diet to help your body maintain its optimal fluid and electrolyte balance. Choose unrefined salt, such as Himalayan or Celtic salt, and add some to each of your meals to get a minimum of one half to one teaspoon (two to five milliliters) per day. Your homemade bone broth is another good way to supply you with a variety of electrolytes. And make sure to drink enough water so that your urine is only lightly colored.

MANAGE YOUR STRESS

Whether or not you're aware of it, stress could be exhausting your body and hindering your energy levels. Read Chapter 7 and make sure you incorporate some of the suggested techniques. Sometimes life gets in the way and we forget our new good habits, but it's never too late to jump back on the wagon.

GET MORE SLEEP

It's obvious that a lack of sleep can lead to fatigue, but sometimes people are so focused finding answers through diet or supplements that they forget about the basics. Your body needs eight to nine hours per night, especially if you've been dealing with digestive and other health problems for a while. Go to bed by 9 PM. If you have trouble sleeping, consider turning down the lights after the sun sets and avoiding computer and television screens for an hour or two before bedtime. If that's not enough, try a small bedtime snack of protein, vegetables, and fat, or consider supplementing with 5-HTP or melatonin to help you fall asleep more easily. See a qualified healthcare provider to help improve your sleep quality as naturally as possible.

TRY INCREASING YOUR CARB INTAKE

Your carb intake during the elimination phase will be low, since many of the foods that can trigger digestive symptoms (grains, sugar, dairy, legumes, starchy vegetables and some fruits) are rich in carbohydrates. If you still feel tired after the elimination phase, despite sleeping well, eating enough fat, drinking enough water, getting enough sodium, and managing your stress, it's possible that your body will function better with slightly more carbohydrates.

The best sources of grain-free, sugar-free, and legume-free carbohydrates are winter squashes (pumpkin, butternut squash, acorn squash), fruits, and honey. Root, tubers, and starchy vegetables like sweet potatoes, peeled white potatoes, yucca, plantains, and parsnips are also excellent sources of safe starchy carbohydrates, but be careful with these carbohydrate-rich foods if you've been diagnosed with SIBO or a gut dysbiosis as they can feed a bacterial or yeast overgrowth and trigger the return of your symptoms.

As with any other foods you want to reintroduce, add them back slowly and one at a time as part of your reintroduction phase. Keep journaling your food intake and symptoms and you should be able to determine if they're right for you within a week or two. If any of these foods seem to trigger bloating, digestive problems, or cravings, try experimenting with different carbohydrate-rich foods. You may find you do better with only a small amount of winter squashes and fruits, but not tubers. Following the reintroduction protocol will help you find the answers your need to optimize both your health and energy levels. See Appendix 14 for more ideas of grain-free, sugar-free carbohydrate sources.

Problem #3: Return of your Symptoms

The elimination and reintroduction protocol detailed in this book is *nearly* foolproof, but little details may still get in the way of making you feel 100-percent better. Don't forget that it's normal for many people to feel worse before feeling better during the first month of the elimination diet due to die-off, withdrawal, and the keto-adaptation process. But if your symptoms return or worsen after the first three to four weeks, consider all the factors below to see what could be triggering them.

PERSONAL MODIFICATIONS

Have you modified the protocol described in this book to include a little bit of banana, a few eggs a week, or occasional nut butter? The elimination phase of the protocol is not easy, but be sure to follow it strictly for at least three to four weeks.

CUMULATIVE EFFECTS

Your food journal is an invaluable source of information: the best scientific study ever conducted on yourself, so use it! It can be difficult to understand what triggers your symptom by looking at just a single day, but analyzing weeks of data can help you detect patterns over time. For example, your journal may show you that during the reintroduction phase you tolerated tomatoes and eggplant separately, but eating them on the same day exceeded your tolerance threshold for nightshades and resulted in bloating and abdominal pain. Or maybe it helped you determine that you can tolerate small amounts of onion, but not on your watermelon days since they both contain fructans. These kinds of food reactions may be tricky to pinpoint, but your food journal is your best tool to identify these patterns. See Figure 14 for a refresher on the concept of the tolerance threshold.

Figure 14

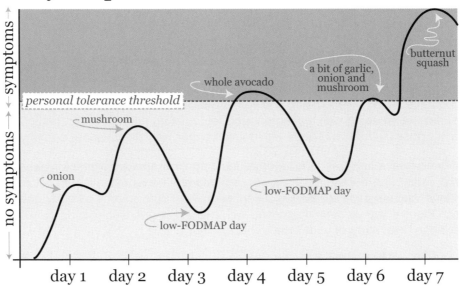

Your symptoms only appear once you exceed your personal tolerance threshold by eating too much of the foods to which you are sensitive within a certain period of time. In this example, you might think only avocado and butternut squash are problematic for you when in fact, the onions, mushroom, and garlic are also contributing to putting you above your tolerance threshold and the triggering of your symptoms. The blame is not always on what you ate last!

GOING TOO FAST

Once you start feeling better on the elimination phase and get tired of eating the same foods, it can become harder to follow the protocol to the letter. You may find yourself reintroducing more than one food at a time or eating larger amounts than you planned, but remember that going too fast could be counter-productive. You might be lucky and not experience any symptoms after trialing more than one food or in larger serving sizes. But if you do have a reaction, you'll need to take a few steps back and reassess each of these foods (in smaller amounts) to see which ones you tolerate.

Not allowing your digestive system to recover fully before trying to reintroduce a new food could also blur the results of your self-experiments. Let's say that you try cheese on Monday and avocado on Tuesday or Wednesday, and you experience symptoms within a few hours of eating the avocado. Since some food reactions can take over 48 hours to develop, it will be *impossible* for you to know if your reaction is due to the cheese, avocado, or both. Slow down to minimize mistakes and get clearer answers from your food-reintroduction challenges.

CROSS CONTAMINATION

No longer eating bread, pasta, cookies, cheese, and soymilk doesn't mean your diet is necessarily free of gluten, grains, sugar, dairy, and soy. Many foods can hide small traces of the ingredients you're trying to avoid, or they may become cross contaminated during the preparation or cooking process. Carefully read the ingredient lists of all the foods you eat. This shouldn't take too long if you are basing your diet on REAL foods, since most of them shouldn't even have labels. If you see anything you're unsure about, don't eat it.

Even if you don't find any questionable ingredients that could be hiding the presence of gluten, grains, dairy, soy, sugar, or other problematic ingredients, it's time to think about the potential of cross contamination. Cross contamination is more likely to occur if you eat out or if you share your kitchen with someone who eats some of the foods you are trying to avoid. This is especially true for gluten. A very small amount of this protein, less than what's found in a breadcrumb, can cause problems in sensitive people. Try washing your utensils, kitchen knives, cutting boards, skillets, and plates thoroughly before using them if they have been or are still in regular contact with gluten-containing foods. Even better, purchase new dinnerware and cooking equipment just for you to minimize the gluten cross-contamination risk.

If you eat out regularly, this could be the reason you're not seeing improvement in your digestive symptoms. Be extremely careful when eating out. Simply removing the croutons from your chicken salad is not enough if you want to keep gluten out of your diet. Ask about preparation and cooking methods. Request that your food be prepared and cooked separately. Use the "A" word if you need to: Mention that you are "*allergic*" to gluten, dairy, soy, and any other ingredients you're trying to avoid. Eating chicken fried in the same fryer used for chicken nuggets or having your steak cooked on the same grill as the burger buns—even if only once or twice per month—can be enough to perpetuate your digestive problems for days and weeks. Try to eat at home as much as you can to prevent exposing your intestines to ingredients that could set you back.

Gluten contamination can also occur from licking the glue of stamps and envelopes. Use a sponge or self-adhesive envelopes and stamps if you know you're sensitive to gluten. And if you're Catholic, make sure you skip the communion wafer because it contains gluten. Some churches offer "gluten-free" versions, but be aware that although they contain a lot *less* gluten, they're *not* completely gluten free.

PROBLEMATIC BODY-CARE PRODUCTS

What goes on your skin can get inside your body. Have you ever taken a look at the ingredients in your lip balm, shampoo, deodorant, toothpaste, or cosmetics? These products may contain hidden gluten and other problematic ingredients. Although most experts don't believe that gluten can be absorbed through your skin, all agree that the small amounts of gluten in lip balm or lipstick can be swallowed and cause symptoms in sensitive individuals. Other products that are close to your face or that can come in contact with your mouth can also induce intestinal problems. Artificial ingredients other than gluten can also be problematic with only skin contact. Try to find natural alternatives with as few ingredients as possible, or find homemade recipes for making your own personal hygiene products. For example, coconut oil makes a great natural lip balm, skin moisturizer, and makeup remover.

PAST EXPOSURE

Even though food should pass through your digestive system within 12 to 24 hours, the consequences of exposure to gluten or other problematic ingredients can last for days or even weeks. Eating some of these offenders, knowingly or not, can also subject you to withdrawal and detox symptoms. If exposure to gluten or other problematic ingredients triggered a reaction that doesn't seem to be going away, go back to the elimination diet for as long as you need to feel better. Eat less vegetable matter and make sure your veggies are cooked, puréed, de-seeded, and peeled thoroughly. Avoid fruits, raw vegetables, and any types of starches and sugars. Once you feel better, simply go back to eating what you were eating before your symptoms returned.

STRESS AND LACK OF SLEEP

It's likely that at one time or another, your digestive issues will resume despite doing everything right. If you haven't changed your diet and are confident that you haven't been exposed to problematic ingredients, it's time to evaluate your stress levels.

Your mind and body are connected, and the two need to work together if you really want to get better. Whether the stress in your life is positive or negative, physical or emotional, it can affect your digestive health. Even if you don't feel stressed, increased physical activity, an injury, travel, or a lack of sleep or rest can be perceived as stress by your body. Return to Chapter 7 for a refresher on the different relaxation and calming exercises you can incorporate into your daily routine. Just a few minutes every day can make a big difference. It can also help to rate your stress levels in your food journal. And make sure to get a minimum of eight to nine hours of sleep per night.

BIOFILMS

Biofilms are mesh-like structures made by bacteria and yeast that allow them to reside, thrive, and multiply safely, on the surface of your gut lining protected from your immune system. Think of biofilms as an armored apartment complex for microorganisms. Hiding in these biofilms also makes them more resistant to antibiotics because of the physical protection the biofilms provide and because they allow bacteria to exchange antibiotic-resistant genes. Biofilms are why many gastrointestinal infections can be so difficult to eradicate. The biofilms also allow microorganisms to survive longer even if you are trying to starve them by cutting your carbohydrate intake. One study actually showed that microorganisms can survive for up to 43 days in biofilms despite not having access to *any* food. Biofilms are present in 90 to 95 percent of people with IBD and 65 percent of people with IBS, but only 35 percent of healthy controls.

If you're still experiencing symptoms, it's likely you have some of these biofilms in your intestines. For your dietary approach to be effective, you'll need to break down the biofilms to expose the microorganisms and make them more vulnerable to antibiotics or starvation. Taking digestive enzymes (*without* betaine HCl) or bromelain (a natural enzyme in pineapple) one hour or so before your meals can help break down these biofilms over time. Do not attempt to take digestive enzymes on an empty stomach if you have gastritis, an irritated gut lining, or any other severe gastrointestinal disorders before talking with a doctor.

An alternative to digestive enzymes is to take one to two tablespoons of apple cider vinegar or lemon juice mixed with a little water about an hour before your meals. Berberine, a compound that can be extracted from the herb goldenseal, can also help disrupt biofilms. Consult a qualified healthcare professional for help choosing the right option for you.

Elaine Gottschall, creator of the SCD, recommended avoiding probiotics in the *Bifidus* family because of their tendency to overgrow and form biofilms. If the other strategies don't help you to get better, it could be worth a try to change your probiotic supplements for a brand that doesn't contain *Bifidus*. It's also preferable to avoid supplementing with minerals, especially calcium and iron, since bacteria can use them to make the biofilms stronger and more resistant.

TOO FEW CARBS

Keeping your carb intake very low for the first weeks of the elimination phase is a good strategy since many people suffering from digestive problems can be sensitive to carb-rich foods. Grains may contain gluten or other hard-to-digest proteins, many fruits contain fructose, polyols, or other FODMAPs, and the carbohydrates in grains, fruits, tubers, and sugars can feed a gut dysbiosis. The return of symptoms after a few months of improvement on your BYO diet may be a sign that your body requires more carbohydrates to function optimally.

A lack of improvement in your symptoms on a very low-carb diet can also indicate a yeast overgrowth or parasite infection. Get tested to make sure. Although these microorganisms love to feed on sugar, they can also adapt to using ketones for energy. In some cases, lowering your fat intake and consuming a bit more carbohydrates may be all you need to get your digestive health moving in the right direction again. Don't eat more carbohydrates than your body can absorb or they could end up feeding these nasty bugs, but eat enough to prevent the formation of ketones that could become another source of food for them. It's a delicate balance. Some people also seem to do better with moderate amounts of carbohydrate in their diet because they can help maintain a healthier gut flora, depending on the specific composition of your gut flora.

You can try some of the other strategies described in this troubleshooting section first, but if nothing seems to work and you keep experiencing digestive problems after three to four weeks, try incorporating grain-free, easy-to-digest carbohydrate sources such as sweet potatoes, peeled potatoes, plantains, yucca, winter squashes, fruits (bananas, cooked apples, cooked pears, blueberries), and even a little honey or maple syrup. Keep in mind that roots, tubers, and fruits are the most nutritious options and that sugar should only be consumed if your diet already provides you with all the nutrients you need. As always, each of these new foods should be introduced one by one. If your symptoms don't worsen with these carby foods, keep including them in your diet. You can aim for up to 100 to 150 grams of carbs per day (see Table 81 below to help you determine your carb intake). If you see significant improvements in your energy levels and symptoms within two to three weeks, you'll know you're on the right track.

Table 81: Carbs and Fiber in Various Foods

		Food	Serving Size	Total Carbs	Fiber
Roots and Tubers	Dense Carbs	Sweet potatoes (skinless)	1 medium (5 oz or 150 g)	27 g	3.8 g
			1 cup (250 ml) mashed	58 g	8.2 g
		Yams (skinless)	1 cup (250 ml), cubed	38 g	5.3 g
		Potatoes (skinless)	1 cup (250 ml)	26 g	1.8 g
			1 medium	34 g	2.3 g
			1 cup (250 ml), mashed	36 g	3.2 g
		Plantains	1 cup (250 ml), mashed	62 g	4.6 g
			1 cup (250 ml), sliced	48 g	3.5 g
			1 cup (250 ml), green, fried	58 g	4.1 g
		Yucca (cassava root)	1 cup (250 ml)	78 g	3.7 g
	Moderate Carbs	Taro root	1 cup (250 ml), sliced	46 g	6.7 g
		Parsnip	1 cup (250 ml), sliced	27 g	5.6 g
		Butternut squash	1 cup (250 ml)	22 g	6.6 g
		Turnip	1 cup (250 ml), sliced	8 g	3.1 g
		Rutabaga (swede)	1 cup (250 ml), sliced	15 g	3.1 g
		Jicama	1 cup (250 ml)	11-12 g	6-6.5 g
		Spaghetti squash	1 cup (250 ml)	10 g	2.2 g
		Pumpkin	1 cup (250 ml), mashed	12 g	2.7 g
		Beets	1 cup (250 ml), sliced	9 g	1.7 g
Fruits		Apples	1 medium (3"), without skin	20 g	2.1 g
			1 medium (3"), with skin	25 g	4.4 g
		Applesauce	1 cup (250 ml), unsweetened	28 g	2.7 g
		Banana	1 medium (7-8" long)	27 g	3.1 g
		Blueberries	1 cup (250 ml)	22 g	3.6 g
		Melon	1 cup (250 ml) cantaloupe	14 g	1.6 g
			1 cup (250 ml) watermelon	12 g	0.6 g
			1 cup (250 ml) honeydew	16 g	1.4 g
		Kiwi	1 fruit (2" diameter)	10 g	2.1 g
		Mango	1 cup (250 ml), diced (1/2 fruit)	25 g	2.6 g
		Orange	1 medium fruit (2.5-3")	15 g	3.1 g
		Peach	1 medium (2.5" diameter)	14 g	2.3 g
		Pears	1 medium or 1.3 cup slices	28 g	5.5 g
		Pineapple	1 cup (250 ml) chunks	22 g	2.3 g
		Strawberries	1 cup (250 ml) whole, ¾ cup (175 ml) whole or about 12 medium	11 g	2.9 g
Sugars		Honey	1 tablespoon (15 ml)	17 g	0 g
		Maple syrup	1 tablespoon (15 ml)	13 g	0 g
		Coconut crystals	1 tablespoon (15 ml)	7 g	0 g
		Coconut nectar	1 tablespoon (15 ml)	13 g	0 g
		Molasses	1 tablespoon (15 ml)	15 g	0 g
		Table sugar	1 tablespoon (15 ml)	13 g	0 g

*Peel your fruits if you know that too much fiber bothers you; you can also cook your fruits to make them easier to digest.

SUPPLEMENTS

When symptoms strike, it can be easy to pay attention to food and forget about the supplements you're taking. Did you add a new supplement to your diet recently? If so, have you examined its ingredient list carefully? It may be that this new supplement just isn't right for you (probiotics can be particularly problematic). Discontinue the supplement for about one week to see if you get relief from your symptoms. Once your symptoms are under control again, you can try reintroducing new supplements, one by one, to assess your tolerance.

MEDICATIONS

Some medications are known to alter your gut flora or even contribute to increased intestinal permeability. Prescription and over-the-counter medications like NSAIDs (acetylsalicylic acid like aspirin, or ibuprofen like Advil, Motrin, naproxen, and ketoprofen), the birth control pill, hormone replacement therapy, and others can prevent your digestive health from improving. Instead of taking NSAIDs to mitigate pain, try acetaminophen (Tylenol) instead. Women should consider alternative contraception methods to the pill. Discuss alternatives with your doctor if you suspect some of your medications are getting in the way of your progress.

PLASTICS (BPA)

Bisphenol A (BPA) is a compound found in many types of plastics, including water bottles, containers, and wraps. BPA has been linked to many chronic conditions, including diabetes, heart disease, PCOS, and cancer. A recent study also found that exposing gut cells to low levels of BPA (10 times lower than the limit considered safe by the government) could contribute to leaky gut. Using a lot of plastic to prepare and store your food could be preventing your digestive system from recovering fully.

To decrease your BPA exposure, avoid bottled water, unless it's in a glass or stainless-steel BPA-free water bottle. The lining of many canned foods, such as canned fish and canned vegetables, also contains BPA. Make an effort to avoid canned foods, especially acidic foods like tomatoes, since the acidity promotes the transfer of even more BPA from the lining into your food. Use fresh tomatoes or try to purchase tomatoes packaged in glass bottles instead. If you bring your lunch to work, try using a Pyrex container instead of a plastic container. If you have to use a plastic container, make sure that the food has cooled before storing it since heat encourages the transfer of BPA and other toxic compounds from the plastic into your food. And never heat your food in a plastic container.

NOT FACILITATING DIGESTION

If you experience bloating, steatorrhea, belching, flatulence, or problems with your bowel movements, or see undigested food in your stools, it's likely you're having trouble digesting your food properly.

The first step to promote healthy digestion is to chew your food properly. Your mouth and teeth have a very important role to play in digestion. Are you shoving down all your food within five minutes at your desk in front of the computer? Remember that your stomach doesn't have teeth and that it can't fully digest whole pieces of chicken and broccoli. Make sure you chew at least 30 times, or until your food is liquidized, before swallowing. Don't forget that eating under stress also prevents your body from releasing enough gastric juices and enzymes to enable the digestion process.

If chewing your food and eating in a more relaxed environment don't help, you may need to rely on digestive-support supplements like betaine HCl (to replace stomach acid), ox bile (especially if you have fatty stools or poor gallbladder function), digestive enzymes, or digestive bitters. See the supplement chapter for more details.

GI INFECTIONS

Taking a stool test before modifying your diet is recommended to ensure the success of your BYO diet. If you skipped this step and your symptoms aren't improving or seem to return randomly, consider getting tested for GI infections (bacteria, parasites, and yeast). Taking a SIBO test may also be useful. If you test positive for any of these tests, you'll probably need antibiotics to get rid of the infection before experiencing the digestive benefits of your new way of eating.

ARTIFICIAL SWEETENERS

Sugar cravings can be hard to resist and some people are ready to make all the necessary changes *as long as* they can keep a little artificial sweetness in their diet, but this could be the mistake that's perpetuating your GI symptoms. Some artificial sweeteners have been shown to alter your gut flora—and you know how important a healthy gut flora is for your digestion and overall health. Other artificial sweeteners are mixed with maltodextrin or sugar alcohols, which can feed a bacterial overgrowth or induce excessive fermentation in your intestines. Some of these chemicals can also irritate the gut lining of some people. The troubleshooting section on cravings has some tips to help you eliminate artificial sweeteners from your diet.

ALCOHOL AND COFFEE

After a few months on your BYO diet, you may have tried reintroducing small amounts of gluten-free alcohol, dark chocolate, or coffee. Some lucky people seem to do fine with these foods, or at least they want to believe this is the case. You may not want to give up these foods and beverages, but if tummy trouble returns, it could be worth leaving them out again for two to three weeks to see if they are the culprits. Alcohol can contribute to increased intestinal permeability, and both alcohol and caffeine (including decaf coffee and chocolate) are irritating for the intestines. Even if you find out that you can't have them for now, it doesn't mean you'll have to avoid them forever. Some people are able to tolerate these foods after giving their GI tract time to heal, although for some people they will always be special indulgences at best.

LARGE SERVINGS OF SAFE FOODS

Once certain foods pass the reintroduction phase and become part of your BYO diet, it can be tempting to eat large amounts of them, especially if they're foods you really enjoy. But too much of even a good thing can be bad for you. You may be able to tolerate a small handful of nuts, but eating half the jar of nut butter could be too much for your digestive system to handle. Your tolerance should improve over time, but you may have to limit your serving sizes of certain safe foods, especially some vegetables, nuts, fruits, and honey, for a little while to keep your symptoms in check.

FOOD QUALITY

Some people are so sensitive that they react to meat, chicken, fish, and eggs that were fed corn, soy, or gluten grains. Since most conventional animal-protein options found at the grocery store are likely to be fed such a species-inappropriate diet, you may have to expend additional effort to get the best-quality food possible. Choosing exclusively grass-fed beef, eggs from pastured hens, and wild-caught fish may be the final tweak you need to optimize your health. Selecting organic produce can also help you decrease your exposure to potentially gut-irritating chemicals.

REMAINING PROBLEMATIC FOODS

Even though the foods recommended for the elimination phase are usually well tolerated, you may still react to some of them. If you're sensitive to carrots or spinach, eating them on a regular basis could be preventing you from getting better. Play around with your vegetable options to see if you do better without some of them. Some people may also have problems with coconut oil or chicken, for example (though a reaction to chicken is most likely due to the soy, wheat, or corn in the chicken's diet). Rotate the different foods in your diet to identify patterns, and think about everything you put in your mouth. Do you chew gum? Sugar-free gum contains artificial sweeteners (such as sugar alcohols like sorbitol, a FODMAP) and flavorings that can be problematic for some people. The real sugar in regular gums can be equally problematic. Scrutinize everything you put into your mouth to find the culprit(s).

HORMONAL CHANGES IN WOMEN

Bloating and changes in your bowel movements can be caused by the hormonal shifts that occur naturally during your menstrual cycle, especially in the weeks before your period (PMS) and during your period. Don't forget this factor when seeking the cause of your digestive symptoms.

NORMAL PROGRESSION OF YOUR CONDITION

In some instances, it's possible that there simply aren't any good explanations for the sudden return of your digestive problems. If they come and disappear on their own within a week or two, it is highly probable they were part of the normal progression of your gastrointestinal condition, whether due to a die-off reaction, the detox process, or something else of which we are not yet aware. If you're doing everything right and have tried the strategies in this troubleshooting section, don't worry too much and continue with your steady approach. If your symptoms don't improve within three to four weeks, consider consulting a qualified health professional, ideally a naturopathic doctor or functional-medicine practitioner, to help get back on track.

Problem #4: Dealing with Symptoms

Although digestive symptoms following a food reaction or resulting from the healing process (die-off and detox reactions) are a normal part of the process, they're certainly not pleasant. Besides trying to learn from what happened (see the troubleshooting tips in the previous pages), you can try to alleviate your symptoms to minimize discomfort and speed up your recovery by implementing some of the following strategies:

EPSOM SALT BATHS

Epsom salts are a form of magnesium (magnesium sulphate) with medicinal properties that help the release of toxins and metabolic wastes through the skin. The magnesium can also be absorbed through your skin, providing a calming effect. Add about two cups (500 milliliters) of Epsom salts to a hot bath and soak for 15 to 20 minutes. Rest for at least 15 minutes afterward to get the maximum benefit. Consult your doctor before trying Epsom salt baths if you have severe varicose veins or high blood pressure.

ACTIVATED CHARCOAL

Activated charcoal can reduce the absorption of poisonous substances, such as the toxins released by dying microorganisms as part of the die-off reaction and the gas produced by excessive fermentation. This supplement can be helpful in cases of bloating or other unpleasant systemic symptoms. Because it can prevent the absorption of other medications and supplements, take it between meals at least two hours before or after taking any other medications or supplements. You can start by taking two to four capsules with a big glass of water three times a day for a few days until your symptoms ease. Be aware that activated charcoal can cause your stools to be darker for a few days.

DIRECT HEAT

Heat can relax your muscles and reduce abdominal pain and cramping. Use a hot water bottle or heating pad to apply heat directly to your abdominal area. Make sure the temperature is just right so you feel a warm sensation without burning yourself. Don't put the hot water bottle or heating pad directly on your skin. Use a piece of clothing in between to minimize the risk of burns, and hold it in place with a scarf or pashmina if you want to sit or stand.

HYDRATION

Hydrate yourself properly to help your body eliminate toxins more effectively. Avoid cold water and try warm water, green tea, or rooibos tea instead. Drinking warm homemade bone broth seasoned with unrefined salt is another good way to get a variety of electrolytes and help you keep the right fluid balance.

REST

Now is not the time to do any kind of physical activity or work too hard. Take a day off if you can or ask someone to help you out with your daily tasks. Your body needs all the energy it has to sustain itself through this period and start the healing process.

TURMERIC

Turmeric is the spice that gives traditional Indian curries their yellow color. Its strong antioxidant and anti-inflammatory properties have been shown to alleviate pain in pilot studies conducted on patients with IBS, ulcerative colitis, and Crohn's disease. Your intestines are likely to be inflamed whenever you experience digestive problems, and turmeric may help soothe the inflammation to alleviate your symptoms. Turmeric should not be taken during pregnancy or chemotherapy, if you have low blood pressure, or if you take medications (especially blood thinners and antiplatelets).

PEPPERMINT OIL, GINGER, OR CHAMOMILE

The anti-inflammatory properties of peppermint oil, ginger, and chamomile can be very soothing if you suffer from abdominal pain or cramping. Experiment with these different herbs to see which gives you the most relief:

- Enteric-coated peppermint oil capsules have the advantage of helping SIBO because of their natural antimicrobial effect.
- Ginger can be added to your food or taken as a tea. Simply grate one to two teaspoons (five to 10 milliliters) of fresh ginger and add it to hot water. Let steep a few minutes, drain, and drink slowly. Take at least one to two cups a day. You can also add a bit of honey if you want (and if you tolerate it, of course). Ginger is also widely recognized for its nausea-reducing potential.
- Chamomile tea can also help improve IBS-related symptoms. Use whole leaves and flowers if possible. If you can only find chamomile tea bags, read the ingredient list carefully to make sure it contains no sweetener, inulin, chicory root, or other ingredients.

AVOID NSAIDS

Medications in the NSAID family, such as aspirin and ibuprofen, are usually not effective at mitigating the abdominal pain associated with IBS and similar digestive disorders. These drugs can even delay your progress by contributing to leaky gut. If you must take something to control pain, acetaminophen (Tylenol) is a better alternative since it doesn't have the same GI side effects as NSAIDs. Or try turmeric, peppermint oil, ginger, or chamomile to alleviate the pain naturally without any side effects.

Problem #5: Constipation

Although constipation is defined as having fewer than three bowel movements per week, skipping just one or two days is definitely not ideal. You should have between one and three bowel movements per day to excrete waste from your body, prevent bloating, and avoid excessive intestinal fermentation. Some people may manage to have a daily "number two," but their stools are dry and hard to pass, resembling type 1 or 2 on the poop chart.

What can you do to regularize your bowel movements and prevent straining? Besides avoiding holding back when you feel the urge to go, you can experiment some of the following strategies to promote more regular elimination and help you feel better:

BE PATIENT

Many people experience constipation during the first days or weeks of starting on the elimination diet, simply because their bodies have to adjust to a reduced fiber intake. It's not that you absolutely *need* fiber to have regular bowel movements (remember the Inuit?), but that your body simply has to go through an adaptation period. If you aren't going daily or your constipation doesn't resolve within a week or two, try some of the strategies below to help move things along.

EAT MORE FAT

Are you skimping on your fat intake? You *need* to be consuming enough fat on your lower-carb diet, not only for adequate calorie intake, but also to maintain regular bowel movements. Many people are unfortunately convinced that fiber is the most important factor to prevent constipation, but fat also plays an important role. Fat stimulates the release of bile from your gallbladder, which triggers peristalsis (the intestinal contractions that keep things moving). Make sure you include at least one to three tablespoons (15 to 45 milliliters) of fat at *each* meal to keep the bile flowing and prevent constipation.

AVOID TRIGGER FOODS

Sometimes, constipation is the only symptom of a food sensitivity. Take a good look at your diet to make sure you haven't reintroduced any foods or supplements that could be causing constipation, especially since it can take one or two days before you notice the constipation side effect associated with certain food sensitivities. Eggs, dairy, gluten, grains, soy, FODMAP-containing foods, and higher-carb choices are a few foods that could be contributing to your problem. If you added a new food to your diet recently, try removing it for four to seven days to see if your bowel movements regularize.

TREAT YOUR SIBO

SIBO can cause constipation. If the bacterial overgrowth is not under control, you might need antibiotics (regular or herbal). Consuming too many carbs from vegetables, fruits, tubers, or honey can also feed a bacterial overgrowth, inducing constipation. The methane gas produced by the large number of bacteria in your small intestines can actually cause reverse peristalsis, which means that your bowel movements start going in the wrong direction! If you haven't been tested for SIBO yet, it may be time to consider taking the breath test. If the result is positive, taking the appropriate steps to eradicate the excess bacteria, by working with a qualified practitioner, should help things start moving normally again.

TAKE PROBIOTICS

A healthy gut flora is a key factor in regular bowel movements. Whether you take a probiotic supplement or eat fermented foods, make sure you get your daily dose of gut-friendly bacteria to encourage your daily number two. Choosing sauerkraut as your probiotic delivery method has the added bonus of promoting good bile flow (because of the cabbage), which is another important factor to keep things moving as they should.

GET ENOUGH FLUIDS

You can't expect to have an easy time passing your stools if you're dehydrated. Aim for a minimum of six to eight cups (1.5 to two liters) of fluids per day, including water, homemade bone broth, soups, stews, and tea. Check the color of your urine to adjust your fluid intake. If you're properly hydrated, your urine should be lightly colored. Dark-colored urine means you're not drinking enough. Keep in mind that some supplements like B and C vitamins can make your urine bright yellow for a few hours.

EXERCISE

Regular physical activity can help your intestines contract to stimulate normal bowel movements. You don't need to go for a run or spend hours at the gym to enjoy the benefits of exercise. Walking a total of at least 30 minutes per day can help you stay regular.

MANAGE YOUR STRESS

Stress can cause either constipation or diarrhea. Even a little change that may seem insignificant, such as a change in your schedule or being away from home for a few days, can disrupt your bowel habits. If you're under stress or facing changes in your life, revisit some of the stress-alleviating techniques and strategies in Chapter 7. Your body needs to be in parasympathetic (rest-and-digest) rather than sympathetic (fight-or-flight) mode to promote regular elimination.

Figure 15: Abdominal Self-Massage

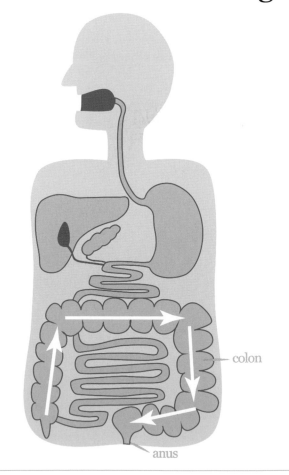

MASSAGE YOUR ABDOMINALS

You can promote the movement of your stools through your colon by self-massaging your abdomen (or having it done by a professional). To perform an abdominal massage, first make yourself comfortable and lie on your back. Use the palms of your hands and gently massage your abdomen clockwise (when looking at your own belly), following the natural flow of your colon. Your *ascending* colon, the part of your colon in which your stools move upward, goes from your lower right abdomen, at your hip bone, up to below your ribs. Your *transverse* colon then goes from the right to the left side of your abdomen just below your ribs. Finally, your *descending* colon goes down from the left part of your abdomen below your ribs down toward your lower abdomen, close to the hip bone, then moves toward the middle of your abdomen. See Figure 15.

Never go counter-clockwise if you don't want to worsen your situation! After massaging with your palms for a little while, increase the pressure gradually and add some palmar kneading, which can also help stimulate normal bowel movements, even if it may feel slightly uncomfortable. Be sure to wait at least two hours after eating and stop if you notice any pain.

TAKE MAGNESIUM

If your stools are dry and hard to pass, supplementing with magnesium can help make them moister and prevent straining. Magnesium does *not* act like a laxative and force contractions, but simply draws more water into your intestines by osmosis. The best time to take a magnesium supplement is at bedtime. You can choose a powered form of magnesium citrate (such as Natural Calm) to dissolve in water and have as a warm tea. Start with 200 to 300 milligrams for the first few days and increase gradually to up to 1,000 milligrams until your constipation is resolved. If your bowel movements become too loose, simply cut back on your dose. Magnesium supplementation is safe and its main potential side effect is loose stools, which you can use to your advantage if you're constipated.

AID YOUR DIGESTION

A healthy digestive system should result in normal, regular bowel movements. Constipation is a sign that your digestion is not working properly, and digestive aids may be what you need to unclog your plumbing. Taking betaine HCl or stimulating stomach-acid production with apple cider vinegar or lime or lemon juice in a little warm water can help stimulate the digestion process and your bowel movements. Having adequate levels of stomach acid is also important to promote bile secretion, which can be very helpful for constipation. Apple cider vinegar and lemon/lime juice also stimulate bile production, as can digestive bitters. If you suffer from constipation and have had your gallbladder removed, you might want to try supplementing with ox bile.

USE CASTOR OIL PACKS

This is an ancient remedy that can be useful for constipation and other related digestive problems such as bloating and abdominal pain. Castor oil is extracted from the castor plant and although very little is understood of it, its unique fatty acid, ricinoleic acid, seems to increase blood flow and draw toxins out of the body. Do not take castor oil orally because it's toxic.

To use a castor oil pack, saturate a piece of cotton flannel with castor oil and put it directly on your abdomen. Cover with a plastic sheet and a heating pad or hot-water bottle. You can start doing the oil packs for about 10 to 15 minutes per day and increase gradually to up to one hour. The ideal time is at bedtime. Just make sure you don't wear your fancy pajamas because castor oil can stain your clothes and linens.

SIP GINGER TEA

Constipation can also be caused by decreased intestinal motility. Besides its anti-nausea effect, ginger can help stimulate the movement of the food through your intestines and encourage bile production. Just put one to two teaspoons (five to 10 milliliters) of fresh, grated ginger in a cup of hot water for a few minutes, drain, and drink it two to three times per day. You can also add one half to one full teaspoon (two to five milliliters) of honey for a touch of sweetness if desired and as tolerated.

EAT MORE CARBS

If you used to have normal bowel movements but recently started suffering from constipation, insufficient carb intake could be at fault. Fruits, winter squash, and unrefined sugars provide prebiotics, nutrients that can feed your gut flora, which in turn helps you be healthier and have regular bowel movements. For many people with digestive problems, though, especially when their symptoms are uncontrolled, eating foods that contain carbohydrates and prebiotics can be problematic since they can feed an intestinal overgrowth of bacteria or yeast. However, some people seem to do better with a little more of these foods in their diet. If other strategies have failed, it could be worth experimenting with adding fruits, winter squash, starchy vegetables, and even a bit of unrefined sugar (honey or maple syrup). Start slowly and introduce these foods one at a time to see if you tolerate them. Use the chart in Appendix 14 to find different safe-carb options to introduce. You should see improvements within two to four weeks if that's really what your body needs for regular elimination.

ADJUST YOUR POOPING POSTURE

Do you know of any other creature that sits to poop? Sitting on a toilet is simply not natural. It changes the anorectal angle, making it more difficult to eliminate your stools. This is simple mechanics. You know you shouldn't strain when going number two. If you do or if you sometimes feel like you have an incomplete evacuation, it could simply be that your posture is not conducive to proper elimination. What happens to the flow of water when you bend a hose? The same thing happens when you sit on the toilet. Leaning forward instead of backward back can improve the anorectal angle. If this is not enough, putting your legs up on a stool will help you get into a squatting position to make your elimination easier and more complete. Or get the Squatty Potty or a similar product to improve your pooping posture.

SEE YOUR DOC

If nothing seems to work for your constipation, it might be a good idea to consult your doctor. Many conditions can cause constipation, including hypothyroidism (low thyroid), diabetes, lupus, and various neurological disorders. Certain gastrointestinal infections, especially with parasites, can also result in constipation, so it might be time to get checked under the hood.

Problem #6: Diarrhea

If your stools are more liquid than solid (types 5, 6, and 7 on the poop chart) or if you have to go more than three or four times a day, things are moving too quickly through your digestive system. Diarrhea reduces your body's ability to absorb the nutrients you eat and therefore puts you at risk for various nutritional deficiencies and dehydration. If your symptoms were improving but you suddenly started experiencing diarrhea, this is a sign that your digestion is not working properly. The following tips will help you address the cause of your diarrhea to improve your digestion, absorption, and quality of life. In the meantime, make sure you stay hydrated by drinking plenty of water, homemade bone broth, or tea. You can drink your bone broth or add it to soups and stews. If you're out of bone broth, make sure you add enough unrefined salt to your food to rebalance your electrolytes.

AVOID TRIGGER FOODS

Diarrhea is one of the most common symptoms of food sensitivities. Examine your diet to make sure you haven't reintroduced any foods or supplements that could be causing your diarrhea. Keep in mind that sometimes symptoms can manifest only after a few days. Eggs, dairy, gluten, grains, soy, and FODMAP-containing foods, as well as starchy or sugary foods, are examples of foods that could be contributing to your problem. If you added a new food to your diet recently, try removing it for four to seven days to see if things get better.

SUPPLEMENTS

Although some carefully selected supplements can be beneficial for your health, some of them can loosen your bowel movements and provoke diarrhea. Magnesium, vitamin C, fish oil, and probiotics containing *prebiotics* are common culprits. If you are taking any of these supplements, discontinue them for one or two weeks to see if your diarrhea improves. If it does, this doesn't necessarily mean you can't take these supplements; you may just need to experiment with a different form or dose. If you want to supplement with magnesium, try the more absorbable forms of magnesium glycinate or malate that don't draw as much water into your intestines. With vitamin C, fish oil, and probiotics, try different brands and lower doses. With all supplements, it's best to start with a small dose and increase gradually. Cut back slightly if you notice loose stools.

WATCH YOUR FAT INTAKE

As you now know, fat is not the enemy. However, it could be contributing to your diarrhea, especially if you recently increased your fat intake. If your body hasn't had time to adjust to your higher intake, the fat you eat will move undigested through your intestines and cause steatorrhea. Fat-induced diarrhea is more common in people with gallbladder issues, without a gallbladder, or who used to consume a low-fat diet.

There are a few things you can do to remedy the situation. The first thing is to cut back on your fat intake and ramp it up slowly over a few days or weeks to allow time for your liver to adjust its bile production. Keep in mind that this option may not be ideal if you really need the calories and energy from fat or have had your gallbladder removed. You can also consume apple cider vinegar or lemon juice in a little water or take a little bit of raw sauerkraut or sauerkraut juice 10 to 15 minutes before meals to stimulate bile production, or try supplementing with ox bile, which will permit you to tolerate a higher fat intake without experiencing diarrhea. Coconut oil and MCT oil are also good options since MCTs don't need to be digested before they're absorbed.

ADJUST YOUR PROTEIN INTAKE

Some people who are afraid of eating fat and who also restrict their carbohydrate intake to better manage their digestive symptoms end up getting most of their calories from protein. An excessive protein intake (over 30 to 35 percent of calories), can result in diarrhea. Your body simply can't handle too much protein at once. If you think this is your case, lower your protein intake and increase your fat intake gradually. Your diarrhea may subside easily.

TWEAK YOUR PROBIOTIC REGIMEN

Probiotics from both supplements and fermented foods can be tricky. The amount you take and the strains of bacteria they provide can influence your digestive health for better or worse. If you recently introduced a new source of probiotics, stop taking it for a few days to up to one week to see if the frequency and consistency of your bowel movements improve. If your probiotics came from fermented foods, it may be that you took too much too fast or that it's not the right probiotic food for you. For example, some people who don't tolerate dairy can experience unpleasant side effects from eating homemade yogurt. In this case, go for fermented vegetables or other dairy-free alternatives such as coconut milk yogurt or water kefir.

If your digestive system is very sensitive, start with very small amounts. With sauerkraut, for example, start with only one half teaspoon (two milliliters) of sauerkraut juice for a few days, then slowly ramp up to one teaspoon (five milliliters) per day, then take it twice a day, then three times a day before starting to double the dose every few days. Once you get to one tablespoon of sauerkraut juice three times per day, you can add a bit of solid sauerkraut, but be careful to build up the amount you take very gradually.

If probiotic supplements seem to have worsened your diarrhea, either switch to a different type or use a lower dose of the same one until you find something that works for you. If you always get diarrhea from probiotics, whether they come from supplements or fermented foods, just exclude them for a few months. Focus on keeping your symptoms under control and allowing your digestive system to recover for now. You can always try reintroducing probiotics and fermented foods later on.

MANAGE YOUR STRESS

Stress can trigger diarrhea. If you are under stress, incorporate some of the stress-alleviating techniques and strategies described in Chapter 7 into your daily routine.

DEAL WITH GI INFECTIONS

If your diarrhea isn't going away or seems to have worsened, you could have a new or lingering gastrointestinal infection. Take a stool test. You can also have a breath test done to check for SIBO. If you test positive in either case, you'll probably require antibiotics (herbal or regular) to eliminate your infection.

USE ACTIVATED CHARCOAL

Activated charcoal can help alleviate diarrhea in some cases. Because it can prevent the absorption of other medications and supplements, it's important to take it between meals, at least two hours before or after taking any other medications or supplements. You can start by taking two to four capsules with a big glass of water three times per day for a few days until your symptoms ease. Be aware that activated charcoal can give your stools a darker color for a few days.

RESET YOUR DIGESTIVE SYSTEM

If you can't get your diarrhea under control, it might be time to give your digestive system a break by going back on the elimination diet and keeping vegetables to a minimum. You can even avoid all vegetables and sources of fiber for a few days until your diarrhea subsides. Remember that fiber can be harsh on your gut lining. Stick to animal protein, traditional fats, homemade bone broth, and seasonings to calm the inflammation and allow your digestive system to reset. Once the diarrhea resolves, you can start adding back small amounts of thoroughly cooked vegetables and other fiber-containing foods slowly and as tolerated.

Chapter 10: Recipes

Still feeling unsure about what you'll eat during the elimination and subsequent phases of this protocol? Giving up grains, dairy, legumes, sugar, starchy vegetables, fruits, eggs, and certain vegetables doesn't mean you won't have anything left to eat.

Of course, you may need to spend a little more time in the kitchen since processed, convenience, and restaurant foods are likely to contain many ingredients you're trying to avoid. Consider it an investment in your health. You can save time and energy by always having REAL-food-based ingredients on hand, as well as cooking in large batches and using your slow cooker.

You should consider the recipes in this chapter as ideas rather than instructions to be followed to the letter. Cooking isn't the same as baking: You don't have to calibrate each ingredient or cooking time. Use the recipes as guidelines and let your inspiration lead you.

"When baking, follow directions. When cooking, go by your own taste."

– Laiko Bahrs

Besides, you don't really need recipes when working with REAL food, since it tastes good naturally. Simply combining a few REAL foods, such as a protein, a fat, a vegetable, and seasonings, can yield a delicious meal every time. If you're an inexperienced cook, just be careful with your seasonings. Add only a little at a time and taste often to get it just right.

There's no need to make recipes; all you need is to assemble ingredients!

The recipes in this book don't have fancy names, but they're all delicious and nutrient dense since they use REAL-food-based ingredients: ingredients that are natural, easy to digest, anti inflammatory, and low in irritants, allergenic compounds, and starches and sugars that could result in excessive fermentation and gut dysbiosis.

Are you ready? It's time to eat outside the box. No more processed junk—only REAL foods to help you improve your digestive and overall health and achieve the quality of life you've always wanted.

"Learn how to cook—try new recipes, learn from your mistakes, be fearless, and above all, have fun!"

– Julia Child

Recipe Chart

Use this recipe chart to quickly find recipes containing only the ingredients you tolerate. There are plenty of recipes you can try, even in the elimination phase, to avoid falling into a food rut. Consult the meal-plan examples in the next chapter for more ideas of how to plan your weekly menus during the elimination phase and subsequent phases.

Table 82: Recipe Chart

Recipes		Page	Elimination Phase	As Tolerated					
				Egg	Coconut	Nuts	Night-shades	New veggies	Other
Basics	Bone broth	244	✓						
	Ghee	246	✓						
	One-size-fits-all stew	248	✓						
	One-size-fits-all soup	250	✓						
	Mix-and-match meals	252	✓						
	One-skillet meal	254	✓						
	All-in-one meal salad	256	✓						
	Sneaky burgers	258	✓						
	Grain-free chicken pesto pasta	260	✓						
	Kebabs	262	✓						
	Meat cupcakes	264	✓						
	Salmon cakes	266	✓						
	REAL-food inspiration	268		✓			✓	✓	✓
Side Dishes	Vegetables	270	✓						
	Vegetable fries	272	✓						
	Mashed cauliflower	274						✓	
	Cauli-rice	276						✓	
Sauces, Dressings and vinaigrettes	Lemon butter sauce	278							
	Pesto	280	✓						
	Herbed ghee	282	✓						
	Garlic-infused oil	284	✓						
	Reduction sauce	286	✓						
	Homemade mayonnaise	288		✓					
	Basic vinaigrette	290							✓
Snacks	Gelatin squares	292	✓						
	Chicken liver pâté	294						✓	✓
	Coconut chips	296			✓				
	Kale chips	298						✓	✓
	Nut bars	300			✓	✓		✓	✓
Ferments	Sauerkraut	302	✓						
	Fermented carrots	304	✓						
	Homemade yogurt	306							✓
Breakfast	Breakfast sausages	308	✓						
	Coconut Oatmeal	310			✓				
Eggs	Deviled eggs	312		✓					
	Frittata	314		✓					
	Egg-drop soup	316		✓					
Treats	Carrot treat	318	✓	✓					
	Carrot cupcakes	320		✓					
	Baked apple pudding	322			✓	✓			✓
	Avocado mousse	324		✓	✓			✓	
	Coconut macaroons	326		✓	✓				
	No-bake frozen cookies	328			✓	✓			
Other Projects	Infused water	330	✓	✓					

Homemade Bone Broth | appropriate for the elimination phase

Homemade bone broth is one of the whole-food supplements that should be part of your diet if you're striving for optimal digestive health. The amino acids in bone broth can help heal and seal your gut to improve your intestinal permeability. The gelatin, glucosamine, and chondroitin in bone broth can also help your joint and skin health, while the minerals calcium, phosphorus and magnesium can keep your bones and teeth healthy even on a dairy-free diet. Avoid commercial broths and bouillon cubes since they don't contain these beneficial nutrients and may contain ingredients that could be harmful for your digestive health (FODMAPs, MSG, gluten, etc.). Only homemade bone broth prepared traditionally is beneficial for your health. Don't forget to add the vinegar to improve the mineral content of your broth.

INGREDIENTS

Ingredients	Chicken Bone Broth	Beef Bone Broth
Bones	1 large or 2 small chicken carcasses (including the bones and skin; add the neck, feet and gizzards if you have them)	1-2 lbs. (0.5-1 kg) of beef bones 1 calf or pig foot (optional)
Essential	4-12 cups (1-3 l) of water 1-3 tbsp (15-45 ml) of vinegar (apple cider vinegar or red wine vinegar) 1 tbsp (15 ml) of salt, adjust to taste	
Optional	3-4 carrots, peeled and coarsely chopped 2-3 celery sticks, coarsely chopped 2-3 onions, peeled and coarsely chopped	2-3 whole garlic cloves 1 teaspoon of whole or crushed black peppercorns A few branches of rosemary, thyme, or parsley

PROCESS

1. Put all the ingredients in a large pot, slow cooker, or crockpot.
2. Add optional ingredients if desired. During the elimination phase, only add carrots and herbs if desired. Wait until you have challenged the other vegetables before using them in your broth.
3. Heat on high until the broth starts boiling. Stay close to avoid an overflow. Remove the foam if desired to improve the taste of your broth.
4. As soon as the broth starts to boil, reduce the heat to low. The heat should be adjusted to allow the broth to simmer (you should only see very small bubbles in the center).
5. Cook at low temperature for at least six to eight hours to up to 24 hours.
6. Once ready, let cool down an hour or two.
7. Strain your broth using a metal colander (and cheesecloth if desired).
8. Discard the bones. You can keep the vegetables if desired.
9. You can keep your bone broth in the fridge for up to four to five days.

IF YOUR BONE BROTH DOESN'T GEL:

High temperatures can denature the gelatin in your bone broth. Make sure the water is *barely* simmering next time. Some slow cookers unfortunately do not have a low enough setting. Use a large pot on the stove or find another slow cooker that allows you to better control the temperature.

It's possible you used too much water for the amount of bones. Try using less water or more bones next time. Adding chicken skin, chicken feet, or a calf's or pig's foot can also help your broth gel more easily.

If your broth doesn't gel, it could simply be because you didn't cook it long enough. Try cooking it longer next time.

"Caldo de gallina, a los muertos resucita." ["Chicken broth resurrects the dead."]

– South American proverb

EXTRA TIPS:

If you have too much bone broth to use in four or five days, freeze part of it. Portion it out into small glass jars, leaving one inch (two to three centimeters) at the top of each jar to allow for the expansion of liquids and prevent your jars from breaking. You can also use ice cube trays to freeze your bone broth into convenient and easy to reheat cubes.

When you want to use your bone broth, heat it in a saucepan (not in the microwave) to avoid damaging its amino acids.

Drink your homemade bone broth by the cup or use it for preparing sauces, soups and stews.

A good-quality bone broth should gel in one to two days once refrigerated. The gelatinous appearance of your bone broth is a good indicator of its high gelatin content. Heat it in a saucepan (no need to dilute it) and it will become liquid again.

A white layer of fat will form at the top of your chilled bone broth. Some people use this fat for cooking. However, keep in mind that even stable animal fats can be damaged after being heated for hours. Discarding it is probably safest.

Use the water you used to boil vegetables to make your broth to make good use of the nutrients lost from the vegetables during cooking (they will be in your broth!).

Every time you have chicken or meat, keep the bones and freeze them. You'll be ready to make a new batch of bone broth once you have enough.

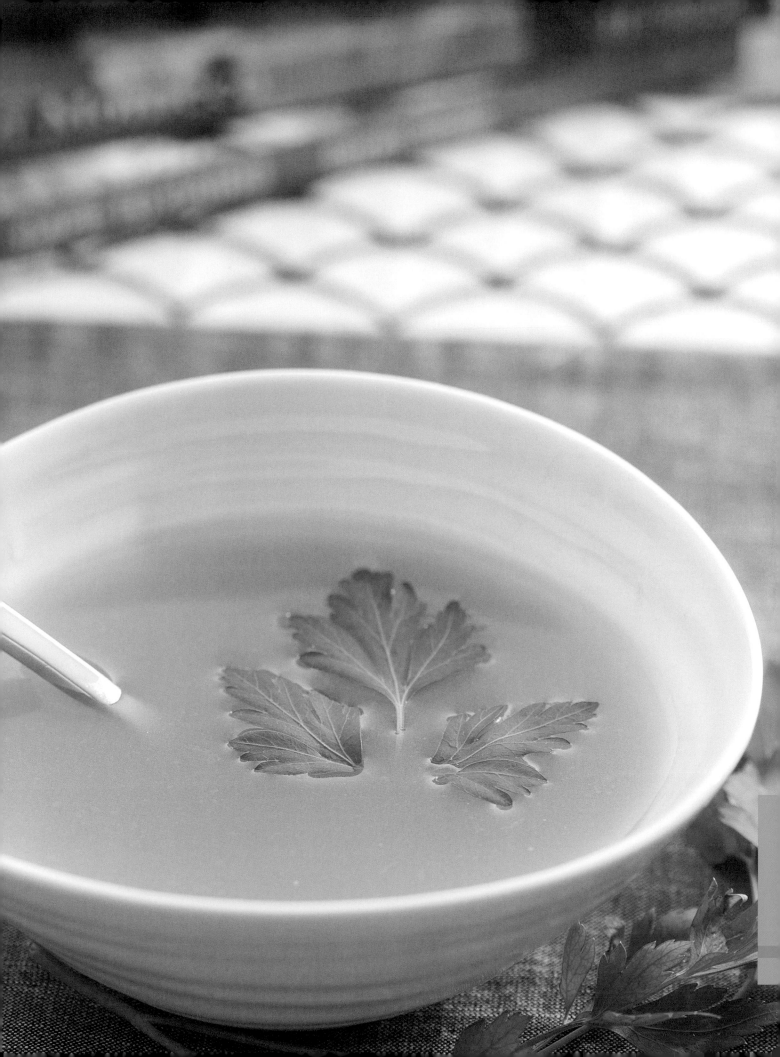

Ghee | appropriate for the elimination phase

Ghee (clarified butter) is a perfect fat option during the elimination phase. It has a unique, caramel-like taste and can accompany any kind of protein or vegetables well to make a complete meal. It's also good by the spoon whenever you feel hungry between meals. Ghee is rich in fat-soluble nutrients, especially if prepared with butter that comes from grass-fed and pastured animals. Ghee can be found in some grocery stores or Indian markets. The process of making ghee removes almost all traces of casein and lactose found in butter, making it a great option even if you're sensitive to casein or lactose.

INGREDIENTS

Yields about 1.5 cups of ghee per pound of butter used:		
1-2 lbs	Butter (ideally unsalted and grass-fed)	0.5-1 kg

PROCESS

1. Melt your butter in a medium pot at medium temperature.
2. Let it simmer at low temperature. Some foam may form at the top. Don't worry and just make sure that your butter keeps bubbling gently. While the butter simmers, the water evaporates and the casein will cook and stick to the bottom of the pan.
3. Check on your ghee every five to 10 minutes to make sure it continues to simmer. You can use a metal utensil to push the foam that forms at the top and check the color of your ghee.
4. After 20 to 25 minutes, the ghee will become clear and transparent. You should be able to see the bottom of the pot. Your ghee is ready!
5. Turn the heat off and let it cool down an hour or so.
6. Once your ghee has cooled, strain it using a metal colander and a piece of cheesecloth. Be careful as it may still be hot.
7. Store your ghee in glass jars.

VARIATIONS:

Add lemon zest and lemon juice to the boiling butter to obtain a lemon-flavored ghee.

Infuse your ghee with garlic by adding grated or chopped garlic to the boiling butter (the garlic flavor will infuse the ghee, but not its FODMAPs since they are water-soluble). You can keep the caramelized garlic that served to infuse your ghee for other people that tolerate garlic in your household. Or use ghee to make your garlic-infused oil (p. 284).

Mix your melted ghee with equal amounts of coconut oil for an interesting fat blend to cook with or add to your meals.

You can season your ghee with dried herbs (basil, thyme, rosemary, etc.) or with spices (cinnamon, ginger, cardamom, turmeric, etc.).

TIPS:

Unlike butter, you can keep your ghee at room temperatures for months. It will be more or less solid depending on the room temperature. You can keep some in the fridge if you prefer a harder consistency to spread on your veggies.

Ghee can be used for cooking at higher temperatures than butter, which can burn more readily because of its casein.

The quality of the butter you use will influence the quality of the ghee you make. Butter from grass-fed and pastured cows or goats is best.

GRASS-FED BUTTER?

Butter from Ireland and New Zealand is almost always grass fed. Brands like Kerrygold, Anchor, Smjör, and Organic Valley guarantee you high-quality butter. You can also find grass-fed butter at your local farmers' market. Your local chapter of the Weston A. Price Foundation can also help you find good sources in your area. The yellower the butter, the more likely it is to be grass fed and high in fat-soluble nutrients. Pure Indian Foods and Ancient Organics also offer ready-to-eat ghee prepared from the organic milk of grass-fed cows.

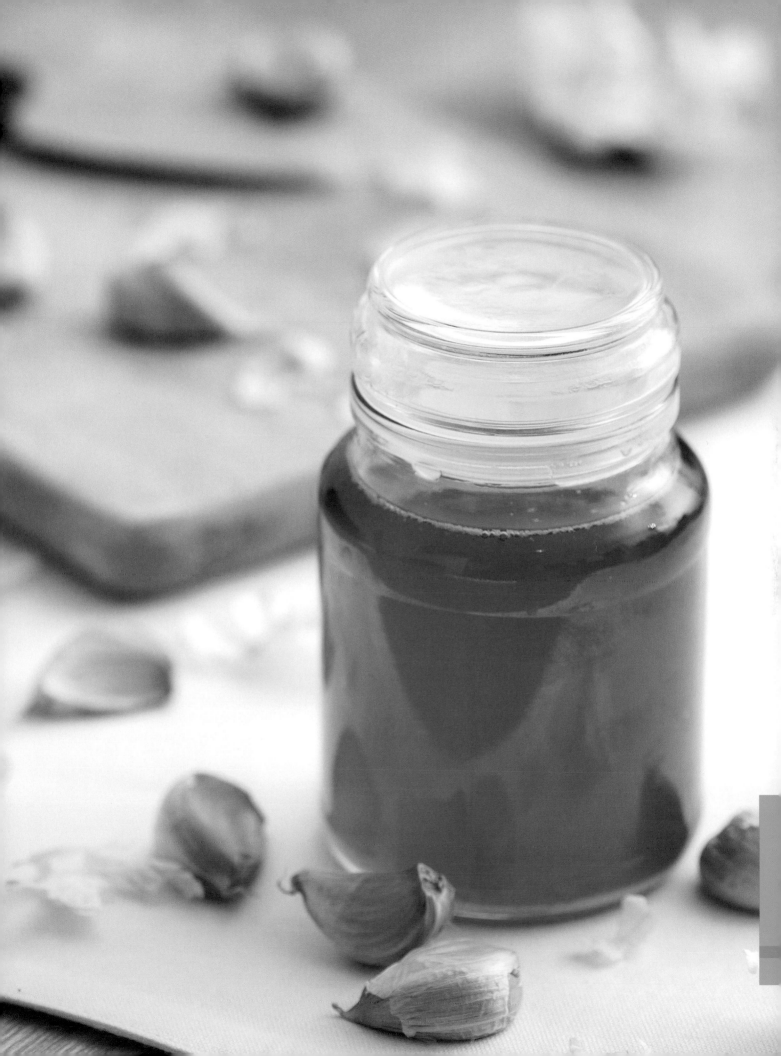

One-Size-Fits-All Stew | appropriate for the elimination phase

Pull your Crock-Pot out of your cupboard and start using it! If you don't have one, invest in a good slow cooker to make your weekly batch of homemade bone broth or prepare complete, hearty meals in a pinch. Even if you don't have a slow cooker, you can make this easy recipe in any large pot. With this simple one-size-fits-all stew recipe, you can prepare hundreds of different meals combining different meats, vegetables, and seasonings. Be creative!

INGREDIENTS

Yields at least 4-12 servings:			
Vegetables	Protein	• Beef (any big cuts, ideally on the bone) • Lamb (leg, roast, or other cuts, ideally on the bone) • Chicken (whole, drumsticks or other cuts) • Veal (osso bucco or any big cuts, ideally on the bone) • Pork (any cuts, ideally on the bone)	Fill your pot with all the protein and vegetables you can, leftovers can be used for your breakfast, lunches or snacks!
	Elimination phase	Carrots, zucchini, green beans	
	As tolerated	Onions, garlic, cabbage, turnip, butternut squash, tomato, etc.	
Seasonings	Liquid	Water or homemade bone broth	Add enough liquid to at least cover the bottom of your slow cooker.
	Elimination phase	Unrefined salt, apple cider vinegar, thyme, rosemary, basil, oregano, parsley, lemon, etc.	Add to taste.
	As tolerated	Black pepper, splash of red or white wine, red wine vinegar, balsamic vinegar, curry, coconut milk, chili powder, etc. Be creative!	
	Bonus	Add extra bones for extra nutrition (gut-healing gelatin and bone-building minerals) in your stew!	1-2 small bones are enough.

PROCESS

1. You can pan sear your meat first, but this step is optional. To pan-sear your protein, heat ghee or coconut oil in a skillet at medium-high temperature. When the fat is melted, add your protein and brown on all sides.
2. Put the raw or pan-seared meat in the slow cooker or large pot.
3. Add any combination of vegetables you like and tolerate.
4. Add enough water or bone broth to cover the protein and vegetables.
5. Add desired seasonings to taste. If unsure, start by adding a little now and wait until your stew is ready to adjust the seasoning to taste.
6. Cook at the lowest temperature possible so the stew is barely simmering for at least 6 hours to up to all day (or overnight if you want to have it for breakfast).
7. Adjust the seasoning and serve. Enjoy your meal and make sure you add enough fat, especially if the protein is lean. Drizzle ghee, olive oil or add avocado or eggs (as tolerated) to make your meal complete and satisfying.

TIPS:

A few days a week, fill your slow cooker with wholesome ingredients before leaving for work and you'll have a delicious meal at the end of the day.

Don't be afraid to make stews. You can't fail. Real food tastes good naturally. Just combine ingredients you like and you will end up with a delicious meal every time. The long cooking time will make the meat so tender and you will learn to adjust the seasonings to your personal taste. Take notes if you want to develop your own personal favorite combinations!

You can use wine in your recipes since the heat will get rid of the gut-irritating alcohol while preserving all of its wonderful flavors!

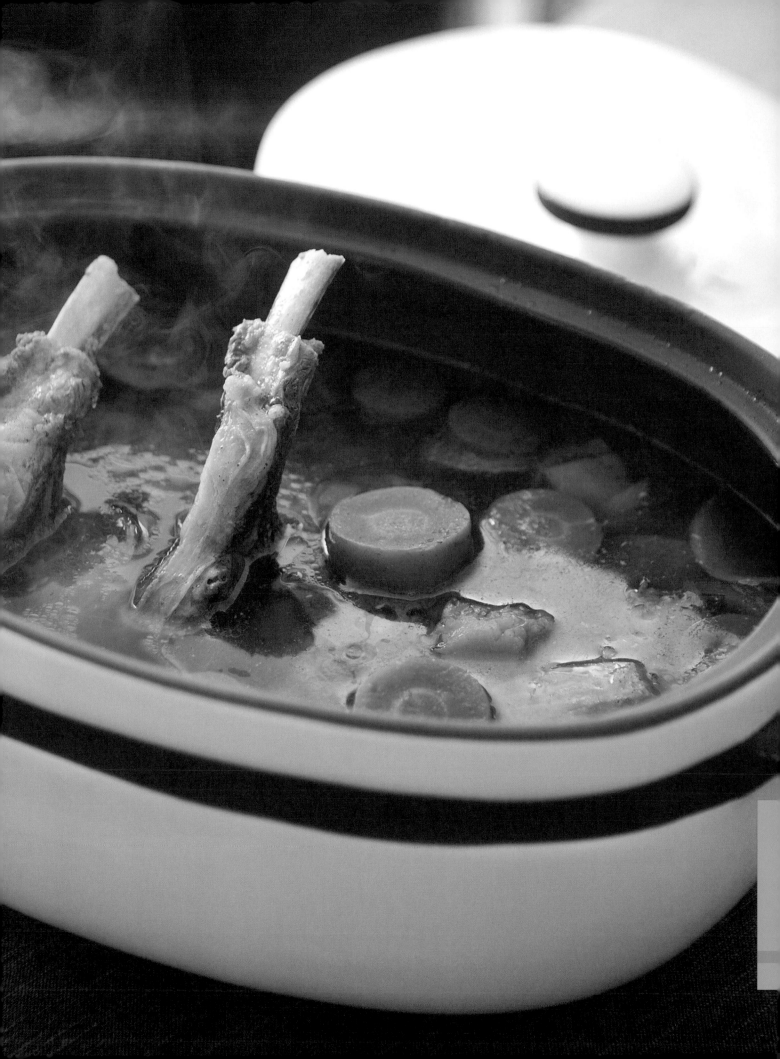

One-Size-Fits-All Soup | appropriate for the elimination phase

There's nothing more comforting than a bowl of homemade soup. Even if the only soups you've prepared came out of a can, it's easy to make a REAL food-based soup. The preparation method is very similar to making a stew, but the proportions vary depending on how liquid or thick you like it.

INGREDIENTS

Yields 4-8 servings:			
Fat	2-4 tbsp	Ghee, coconut oil or olive oil	30-60 ml
Liquid	8 cups	Homemade bone broth or water	2 L
Vegetables	2-4 cups	Any kind of tolerated vegetables, cut into bite-sized pieces (zucchini, carrots, green beans, onions, garlic, tomatoes, winter squash, asparagus, broccoli, cauliflower, etc.)	0.5-1 L
Protein (optional)	2-4 cups	Meat or poultry, raw or cooked (shredded or cut into bite-sized pieces) Or fish (without the bones) or seafood (ready-to-eat shrimp, crab, etc.)	0.5-1 L
Seasonings	To taste	Unrefined salt, pepper, herbs and spices	To taste

PROCESS

1. In a skillet or large pot, melt generous amounts of coconut oil or ghee at medium-high temperature. Add your vegetables and stir. You don't need to cook them thoroughly, but you can heat them quickly to get a bit of caramelization or browning. This step is optional, but can enhance the taste of your soup.
2. If using a large pot, add all the ingredients (liquid, protein and seasonings). If using a slow cooker, transfer all the ingredients into it. Don't worry too much about the seasonings if you're unsure how much you need. Add a little to start and you can add more before serving if needed.
3. Bring your soup to a boil.
4. Once your soup has reached the boiling point, decrease the temperature to the lowest setting allowing it to simmer gently.
5. Let simmer for at least 20 to 30 minutes to up to one to two hours.
6. Adjust the seasoning level and serve.

TIPS:

Don't be afraid to make soups. You can't fail if you use REAL food. You'll learn to adjust the seasonings to your own taste. Take notes and develop your own favorite combinations!

Try some of the following combinations to feed your inspiration. And have fun!

Asian Soup	Mediterranean Soup	Mexican Soup
Add ½-1 cup (125-250 ml) coconut milk, freshly grated ginger and either chili powder or turmeric to taste. Add chicken, fish or shrimp to make it a complete meal.	Used fresh chopped tomatoes and serve with fresh basil, oregano and thyme (or use pesto). Add chicken, fish or shrimp to make it a complete meal.	Add ½ cup (125 ml) lime juice, fresh cubed tomato, chili powder or sauce. Add chicken or beef to make it a complete meal. Garnish with cilantro before serving.

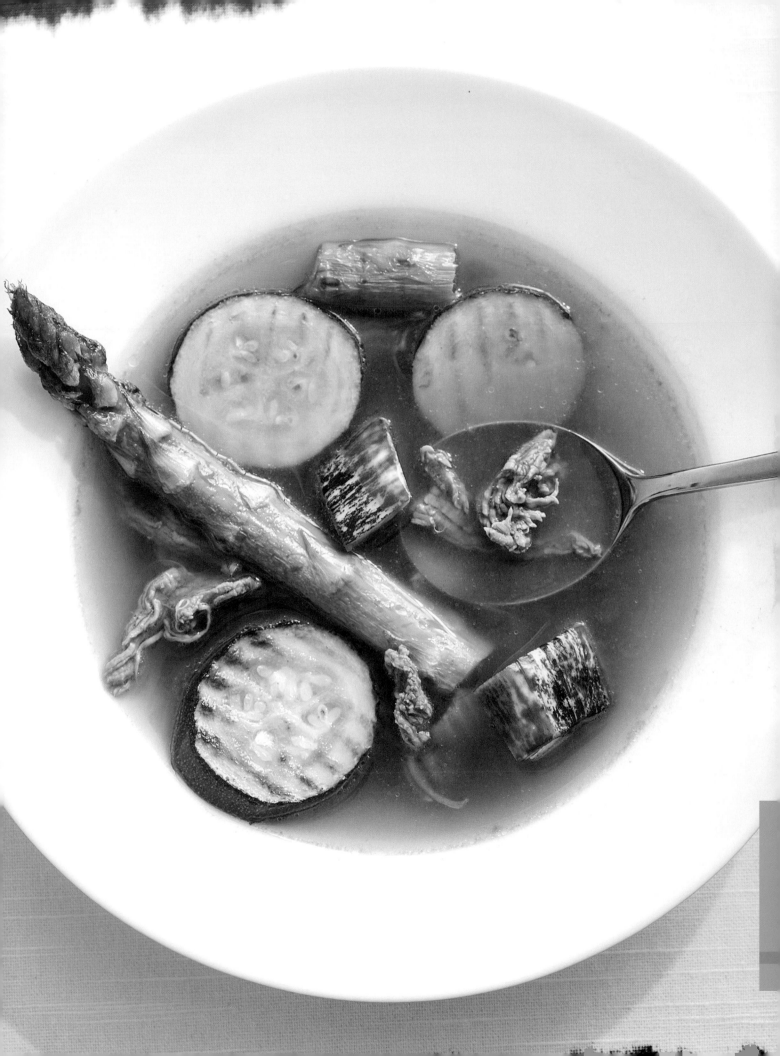

Mix-and-Match Meals | appropriate for the elimination phase

People are often afraid to switch to a REAL-food diet because they don't know how to cook or what to eat. The truth is that it couldn't be any simpler. All you have to do is mix and match the four essential components of any meal: **Protein + fat + vegetables + seasonings**.

INGREDIENTS

See Table 83: Mix-and-Match Chart p. 332

PROCESS

1. Cook your protein using your preferred cooking method. You can boil the meat, bake it in the oven, or cook it in a skillet. Use fat as needed. You can batch-cook many servings at once to have leftovers ready to use for breakfast, lunch, or snacks.
2. Cook your vegetables using your preferred cooking method. You can boil them, stir-fry them in a skillet, or bake them in the oven. Add fat if necessary. Don't forget to peel them and seed them if you have trouble digesting vegetables.
   Once your vegetables are cooked (use a fork to make sure), you can purée them using a food processor or hand blender to make them even easier to digest. You may need to add a little bit of water or homemade bone broth to give your purée the right consistency.
3. Mix and match the protein and vegetables on your plate. You can slice your protein, cube it, or leave it whole. Add fat as needed (on top, as a side, or mixed into the meal).
4. Season to taste. Season your protein and vegetables while they're cooking or season your meal at the end. Don't be afraid to try different combinations of seasonings. And don't forget the unrefined salt! Add just a little bit of seasoning at a time and taste often to make ensure you're creating a tasty dish.

TIPS:

Save time by cooking in batches. Cook many servings of protein and vegetables at once. Store extras in the fridge or freezer, so you'll have all you need on hand to create mix-and-match meals in a pinch.

Write down a list of your favorite combinations to make sure you can remember and repeat your new mix-and-match creations in the future.

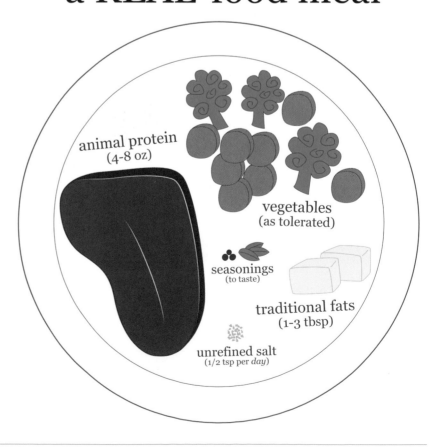

a REAL-food meal

animal protein
(4-8 oz)

vegetables
(as tolerated)

seasonings
(to taste)

traditional fats
(1-3 tbsp)

unrefined salt
(1/2 tsp per *day*)

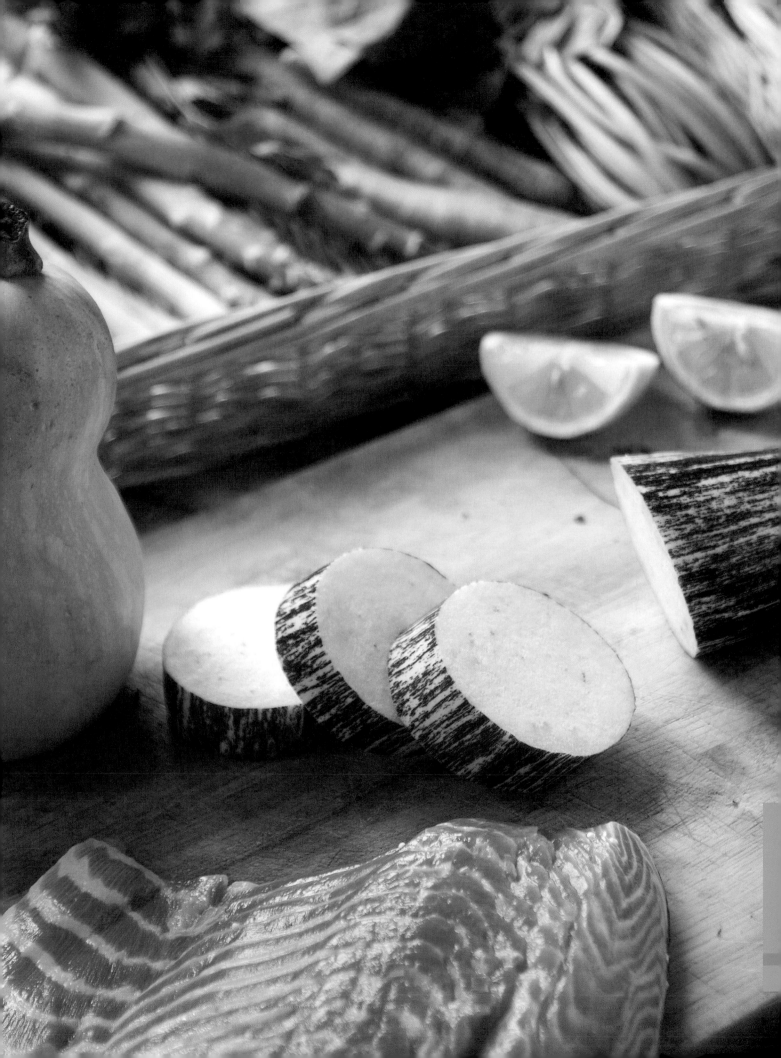

One-Skillet Meal | appropriate for the elimination phase

Even if you don't enjoy cooking and hate doing dishes, you can use this simple technique to create quick and easy meals. They take less than 30 minutes and you'll only have one skillet to wash. Use a large skillet and double the ingredients to have leftovers for tomorrow's breakfast or lunch.

INGREDIENTS:

Use Table 83: Mix-and-Match Chart p. 332 or Appendix 3

PROCESS

1. Heat your skillet under medium heat.
2. Add a cooking fat (coconut oil, ghee, duck fat, etc.).
3. Add your protein (steak, pork chops, chicken, fish, seafood, etc.). You can leave it whole, slice it, or cut it into cubes prior to cooking.
4. Add your serving of vegetables (peeled and seeded if required).
5. Add your seasonings to taste. If desired, add a bit of water or homemade bone broth (or coconut milk, balsamic vinegar, red wine, or tomato sauce) if tolerated to make your meal moister (optional). Don't forget to add unrefined salt.
6. Put a lid on your skillet and let cook.
7. Every few minutes, remove the lid and stir a little to make sure your meal isn't burning. Adjust the temperature accordingly.
8. Your meal should be ready within 10 to 15 minutes, depending on the thickness of your protein and size of your vegetables. Cut everything into smaller pieces (or use ground meat) if you want your meal to be ready more quickly.

TIPS:

Double or triple the amount to have leftovers. All you'll have to do is reheat your meal in a skillet or the microwave.

Alcohol like red or white wine can be used in cooking. The heat gets rid of the gut-irritating alcohol but leaves all the wonderful flavors.

Whether you use chicken + ghee + lemon juice + green beans or ground beef + basil + oregano + thyme + zucchini or salmon + broccoli + coconut oil + ginger, the combinations are endless. Be creative and don't be afraid to explore new combinations.

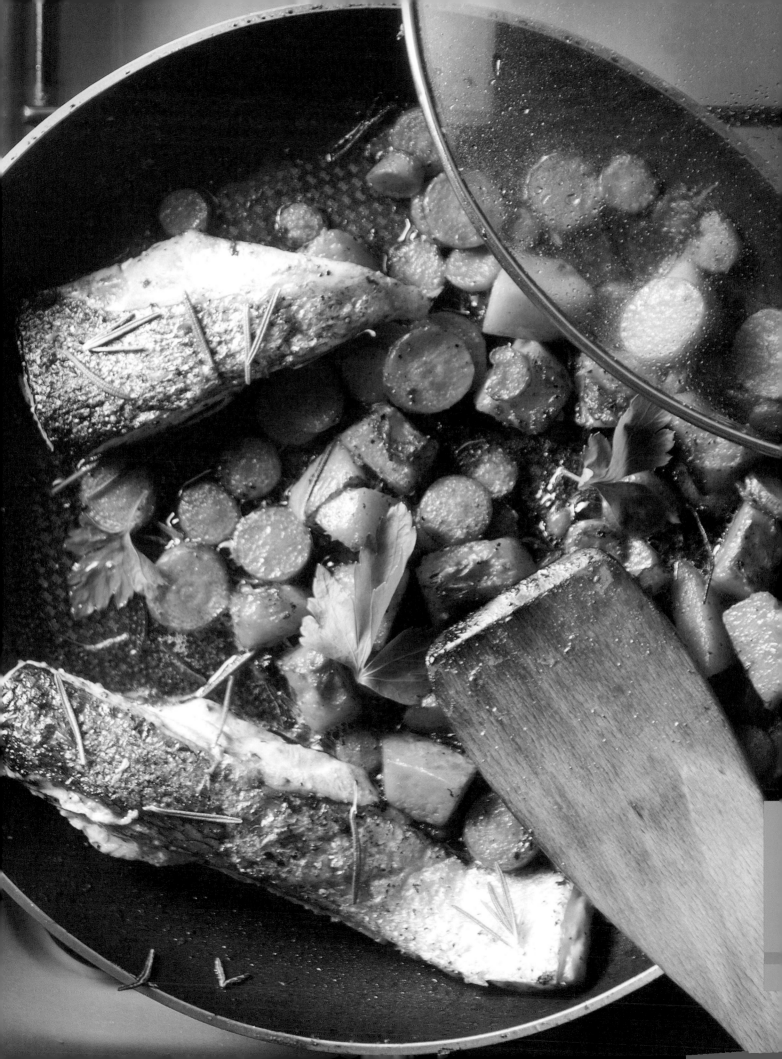

All-in-One Meal Salad | appropriate for the elimination phase

Who said eating healthy meant spending hours in the kitchen? If you keep all the ingredients you need on hand, you'll be able to prepare complete meals within minutes. Salads are not always a good option for people with digestive issues because raw vegetables can be hard to digest, but salads don't have to be made only with raw vegetables!

INGREDIENTS:

See Table 83: Mix-and-Match Chart p. 332 or Appendix 3

PROCESS

1. Cook your vegetables and protein in advance and refrigerate them in the fridge, or use leftovers.
2. Cut your cooked vegetables and cooked protein into bite-size pieces if needed and/or desired.
3. In a bowl, combine your serving of protein and vegetables. Add a serving of fat (olive oil, avocado, coconut oil, etc.) and season to taste.
4. Mix and eat!

TIPS:

You can prepare your salad in advance and refrigerate it in an airtight container to bring as a lunch to work or school the next day.

Since your all-in-one meal salad is meant to be eaten cold, it's a great meal to bring with you on the go, whether you're going on a road trip or eating out. Use ice packs to keep your salad cold until you're ready to eat it.

Your salad dressing can simply be olive oil or coconut oil mixed with your favorite seasonings.

Whether your all-in-one meal salad comprises canned tuna + cooked broccoli + lemon juice + garlic-infused olive oil or cooked chicken + spinach + zucchini + guacamole + chives or sliced stir-fried beef + cooked carrot + ghee + pesto, be creative and don't be afraid to try new combinations!

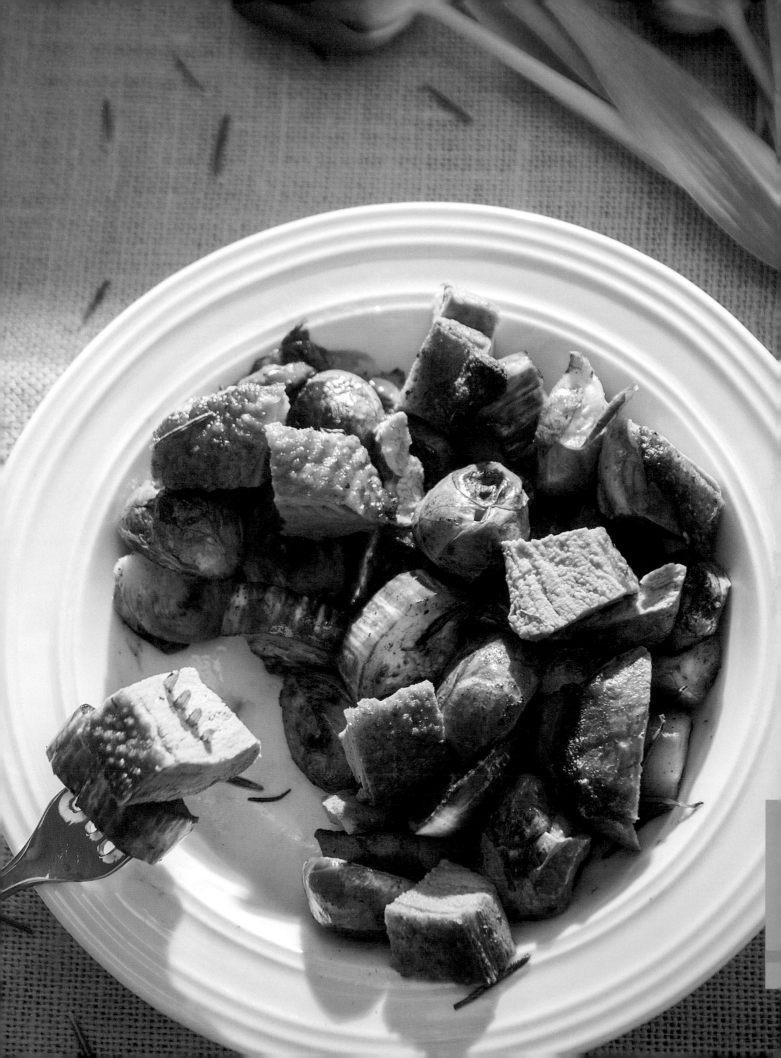

Sneaky Burgers | appropriate for the elimination phase

If you can't get yourself to eat liver, try grinding it and sneaking it into your favorite ground meat. Even kids won't even notice it! This small trick is all you need to get all the nutrients this superfood has to offer into your body.

INGREDIENTS

Yields 4-8 servings:		
1 lb	Ground meat (beef, etc.)	450 g
1 lb	Ground liver (ideally from a pastured animal)	450 g
To taste	Seasonings (any combination of unrefined salt, thyme, rosemary, basil, oregano, garlic-infused oil, pesto, vinegar, etc.)	To taste

PROCESS

1. Combine the ground meat with the ground liver.
2. Add seasonings. If you're not sure what combination you like, start with a little and add more as necessary once cooked or on your plate.
3. Shape the ground meat into burgers (or sausages or a meatloaf).
4. Cook in a skillet, bake in the oven, or grill on the barbecue until thoroughly cooked. The cooking time will vary depending on the thickness of your burgers. They will be cooked once the meat is no longer pink in the middle, which should usually take between 10 to 15 minutes in a skillet or 20 to 30 minutes at 350°F (180°C) in the oven.
5. Serve your burgers with a blended soup or any of your favorite vegetables (puréed, stir-fried, roasted, boiled, etc.) and enough fat to keep you satiated. These burgers are delicious with guacamole, salsa, or bacon.

TIPS:

You can add one cup grated carrot or zucchini to the meat mixture if you want. Once you've successfully reintroduced more vegetables, you can also add chopped onion or garlic, tomato cubes, or sun-dried tomatoes.

If you find that you can taste the liver, adjust the seasonings. You can also change the proportions slightly and use one half pound (225 grams) liver for one pound (450 grams) of ground meat.

If you use this mixture to make a meatloaf, you can add two eggs to make it stick together better. If you only tolerate egg yolks, use four of them instead of two whole eggs. If you don't tolerate eggs at all, you can experiment with replacing them with two tablespoons (30 milliliters) of flaxseed meal (ground flaxseeds) mixed with six tablespoons (90 milliliters) cold water (as long as you tolerate seeds). Let the mixture thicken before adding to the meat mixture. Bake your meatloaf in the oven at 350°F (180°C) for about an hour.

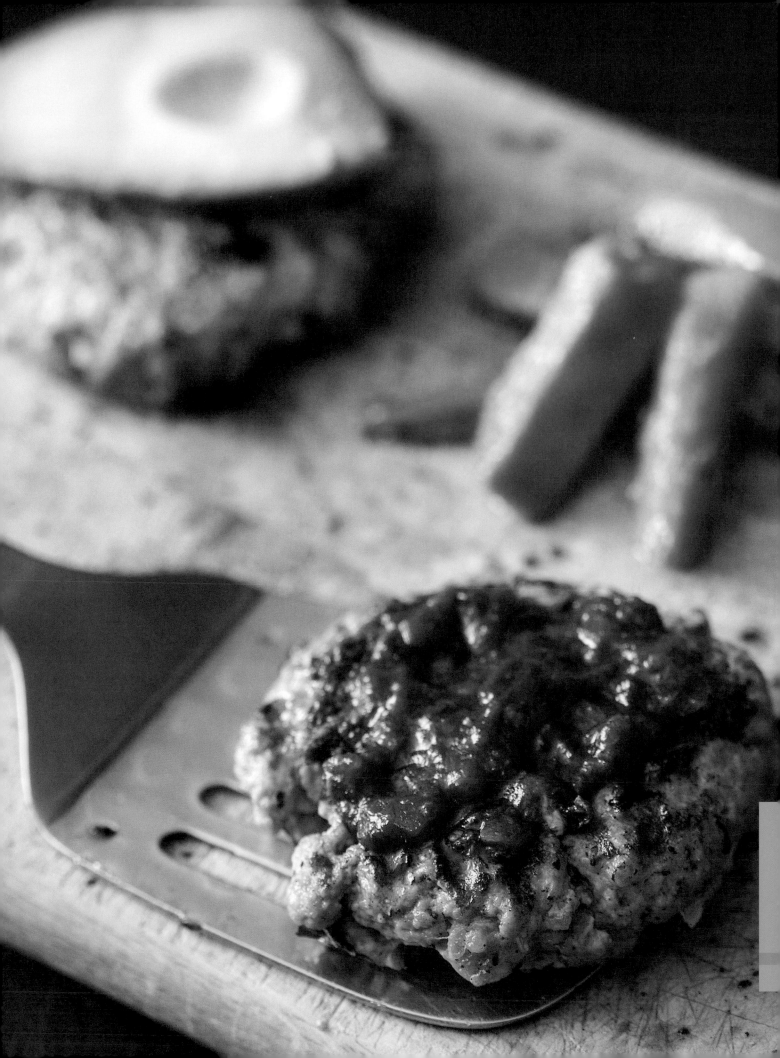

Grain-Free Chicken Pesto Pasta | appropriate for the elimination phase

You don't need wheat or any other grains to make pasta. You can make your own pasta simply by using vegetables to make your meals more fun. Zucchini works especially well, especially when trying to make an Italian-inspired pesto meal.

INGREDIENTS

For each serving:		
1-2	Medium zucchini	1-2
4-8 oz	Chicken	120-240 g
1-3 tbsp	Extra-virgin olive oil	15-45 ml
1-3 tbsp	Fresh basil leaves, finely chopped	15-45 ml
To taste	Unrefined salt	To taste

PROCESS

1. Peel the clean zucchini if needed.
2. Carefully cut the zucchini into thin slices, lengthwise. The thinner the slices, the thinner your zucchini pasta will be.
3. Put about half of the zucchini slices flat on your cutting board and slice them lengthwise again to obtain long strips similar to spaghetti.
4. Boil your zucchini pasta for five to 10 minutes or until soft.
5. Meanwhile, cook your chicken or use leftover cooked chicken.
6. Cut your cooked chicken into slices or chunks, as preferred.
7. Mix the cooked zucchini pasta with the cooked chicken.
8. Drizzle with your serving of extra-virgin olive oil and sprinkle with the freshly chopped basil leaves. Mix and enjoy!

TIPS:

If you like kitchen gadgets and enjoyed this recipe, get a spiral vegetable slicer. For less than $50, you'll be able to transform all kinds of vegetables into grain-free pastas to create many tasty and healthy gut-friendly meals.

You can also replace the zucchini pasta with spaghetti squash. Bake it whole in the microwave (pierce the skin with a fork all around your squash to prevent a squash explosion in your microwave) and bake it for about 10 to 12 minutes or until easy to pierce with a fork. You can also bake your spaghetti squash in the oven at 350°F (180°C) for about 30 minutes or until soft. Let cool down for at least 30 minutes. Cut in half. Remove the seeds. Gently scrape the flesh of the spaghetti squash to shred the pulp into long strands.

Instead of using extra-virgin olive oil and fresh basil leaves separately in this recipe, you can add pesto. Don't use commercial pesto because it often contains pine nuts, dairy ingredients, and other problematic processed ingredients. Instead, make you own simple pesto simply by blending good-quality olive oil with fresh basil leaves (see p. 280).

If you have successfully reintroduced tomatoes (nightshade), you can serve a tomato and meatball sauce (or simply a mixture of ground meat, tomato sauce, and seasonings) over your zucchini pasta.

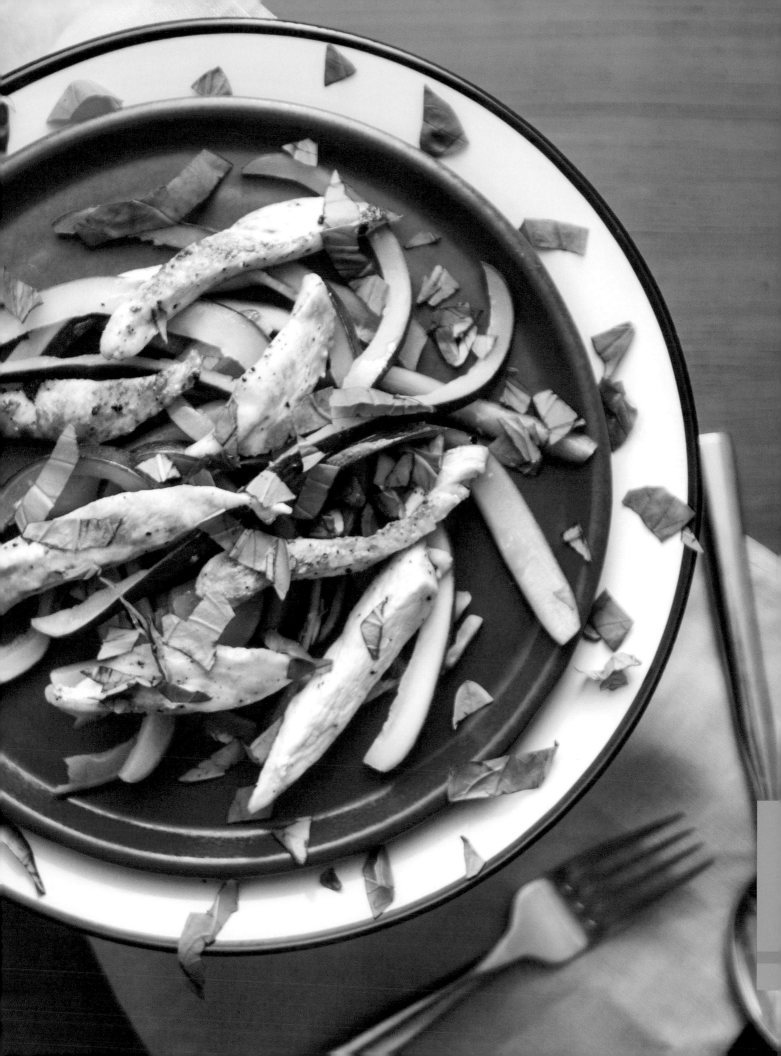

Kebabs | appropriate for the elimination phase

Changing the presentation of your meals may be all you need to get out of a food rut. Kebabs can transform ordinary foods into a special meal. If you're hosting friends for dinner or having an outdoor event, serving kebabs along with many different side dishes will allow everyone to choose what they want to eat. This recipe is also fun to make with kids. Let them assemble their own kebabs (just make sure the skewers aren't too sharp).

INGREDIENTS

For each serving:		
basic		4-8 oz (120-240 g) Chicken, pork or beef cut into cubes
	elimination phase	Zucchini slices Carrot slices (pre-cook them ahead of time to decrease cooking time)
		Marinade #1: garlic-infused olive oil (p. 284) with a bit of lemon juice, unrefined salt and a dash of rosemary or thyme (dried or fresh)
		Marinade #2: pesto (see recipe p. 280)
		Marinade #3: same as pesto recipe (p. 280), but use parsley instead
	as tolerated	Butternut squash (pre-cooked to decrease cooking time) Onion Bell pepper Asparagus Eggplant Cherry tomatoes Mushroom
		Marinade #4: equal amounts of olive oil and balsamic (or red wine) vinegar seasoned with unrefined salt, grated garlic and thyme, oregano and basil
		Marinade #5: equal amounts of coconut aminos (or gluten-free tamari sauce) with freshly grated ginger, lime juice, grated garlic and a little bit of honey

PROCESS

1. Cut the raw meat into cubes.
2. In a bowl, prepare the marinade.
3. Add the meat. Mix to coat evenly. Put a lid or plastic wrap on the bowl and refrigerate. You can also transfer the meat and marinade to a plastic bag, seal it, and put it in the fridge. Let rest for at least 30 minutes or overnight.
4. Use skewers to build your kebabs with any combination of meat and vegetable you like.
5. Grill the kebabs, turning them only once or twice, for about 10 to 15 minutes or until thoroughly cooked. Baste the marinade on the kebabs while on the grill. You can also bake them in the oven with the marinade, in a large Pyrex tray or baking sheet, at 350°F (180°C) for 30 to 45 minutes (until thoroughly cooked).

TIPS:

If you want to use the marinade as a sauce, it has to be heated (since it was in contact with the raw meat). Heat it in a skillet until hot. You can also make a fresh batch of marinade to use as a sauce instead.

Dip your kebabs in guacamole, homemade mayo (p. 288), pesto (p. 280), chimichurri, or the coconut-Asian sauce, as tolerated.

Complete your meal with extra vegetables and fat as needed.

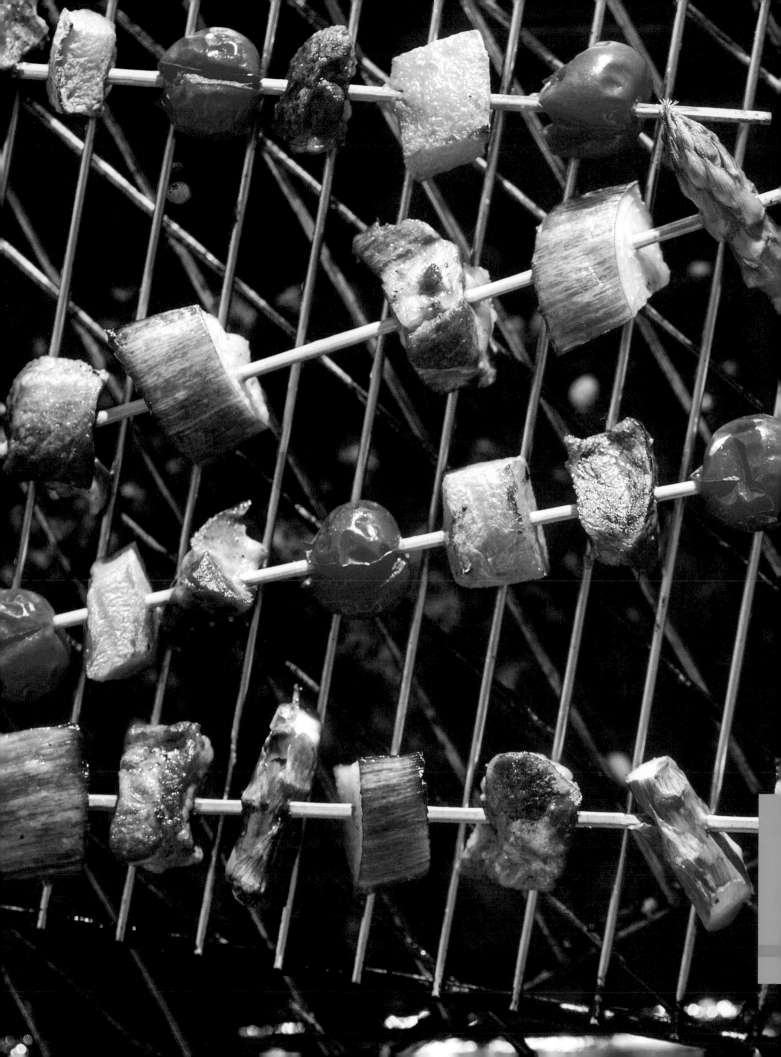

Meat Cupcakes | appropriate for the elimination phase

Even if you often eat the same foods during the elimination phase, there are thousands of ways to combine and present them to keep your meals interesting and varied. These meat cupcakes are pleasing to the eyes and taste buds and make a great potluck food. Be careful because some people could be fooled by the presentation and be surprised that your cupcakes aren't the flour- and sugar-laden kind!

INGREDIENTS

Yields 24-36 cupcakes (depending on the size):			
Meat cupcake	2 lbs	Ground meat (beef, bison, turkey, pork or any combination you like)	900 g
	½-1 cup	Grated zucchini and/or grated carrots	125-250 ml
	½ cup	Bacon, cooked and crumbled (optional)	125 ml
	½ cup	Almond meal (optional)	125 ml
	1	Egg, beaten (optional)	1
	To taste	Seasonings (unrefined salt, herbs, spices)	To taste
Icing	2-3 cups	Carrot, boiled	500-750 ml
	2-3 tbsp	Coconut oil or ghee	30-45 ml
	To taste	Unrefined salt and other seasonings	To taste

PROCESS

1. Prepare a muffin tin (or more if needed) by greasing it with coconut oil or ghee. You can also skip this step and use individual silicone muffin cups instead.
2. Put all the ingredients for the meat cupcake in a large bowl and mix. Use your (clean) hands for best results. Omit the bacon, almond meal, and egg if you're in the elimination phase or if you don't tolerate these ingredients. They can help improve the texture of the cupcakes but are not essential.
3. Fill the muffin tins with the meat mixture. Bake in the oven at 350°F (180°C) for 20 to 30 minutes or until thoroughly cooked. If you only have one muffin tin, you may have to repeat steps three and four until all your meat cupcakes are ready.
4. Meanwhile, puree the boiled carrots with a little bit of coconut oil or ghee. Add seasonings to taste.
5. Ice your cupcakes. Use a pipe for a fancier presentation. If the carrot puree is too thick, add a little water or coconut oil until you get the right consistency.
6. Eat warm or cold.

TIPS:

You can replace the carrot icing with pureed butternut squash, pureed cauliflower, or guacamole.

You can add diced onion, celery, mushroom, or any other vegetables you tolerate to the meat mixture. Sauté the vegetables in ghee or coconut oil until tender before adding them to the raw cupcake mixture.

These meat cupcakes are easy to pack in your lunch or to enjoy as a snack. They can be eaten cold, but you can also heat them for a few minutes

If you're sensitive to egg whites, you can use two egg yolks to replace the whole egg in this recipe. You can also try using one tablespoon (15 milliliters) of ground flaxseeds mixed with three tablespoons (45 milliliters) of cold water (let rest five minutes) in the mixture instead of the eggs (if you tolerate flax seeds). You can also omit the eggs completely.

You can replace the icing with tomato sauce. Spread it on each cupcake before baking in the oven for best results.

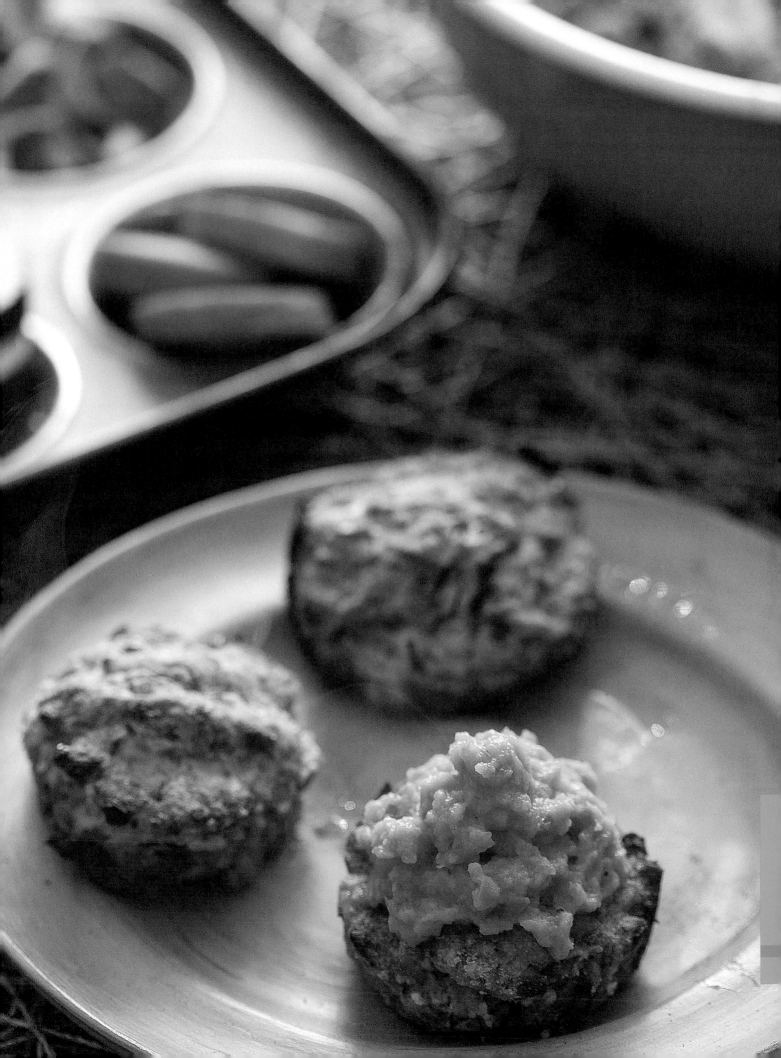

Salmon Cakes | appropriate for the elimination phase

These salmon cakes are a quick and easy way to boost your intake of anti-inflammatory omega-3 fats. Try to eat fish two to three times a week to get all the omega-3s you need. Make extra salmon cakes to bring for lunch the next day.

INGREDIENTS

For each serving:		
4-8 oz	Canned salmon	120-240 g
2-4 tbsp	Unsweetened dried coconut (optional)	30-60 ml
1	Egg, beaten (optional)	1
To taste	Unrefined salt	To taste
To taste	Seasonings (cilantro, lime juice, grated ginger, dill)	To taste

PROCESS

1. Drain the canned salmon and put it in a large bowl. Remove the skin, but keep the bones. Use a fork to mash the bones and salmon meat until homogenous.
2. Add all the other ingredients. If you're on the elimination phase, skip the unsweetened dried coconut and egg. The salmon cakes won't hold as well without the egg, but it will still work.
3. Shape the salmon mixture into patties and set aside.
4. Heat coconut oil or ghee in a skillet. Once melted, add your salmon cakes and cook for about five minutes or until lightly browned.
5. Flip each salmon cake and grill the other side until browned.
6. Serve warm or cold.

TIPS:

Serve your salmon cakes with lemon juice and fresh cilantro. You can also use homemade mayo, guacamole, coconut milk, or a mango salsa as a dip for your salmon cakes.

You can substitute the whole egg with two egg yolks or omit it completely if you don't tolerate eggs.

You can add diced onions, grated garlic, and diced celery to the salmon mixture before cooking.

Turmeric or curry powder are good ways to season your salmon cakes and enhance their anti-inflammatory properties.

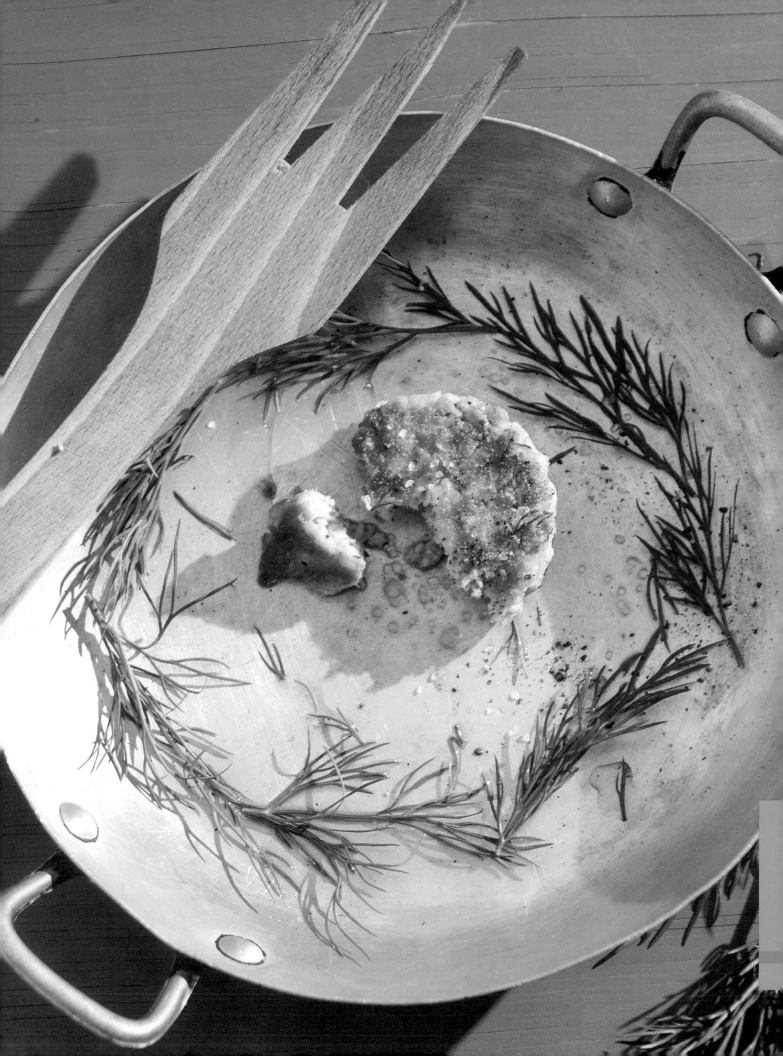

More Easy REAL-Food Inspiration!

Preparing and eating REAL food doesn't have to be complicated. You don't need complex recipes. Simply assemble a variety of ingredients you tolerate and you'll create delicious new meals every time. If you miss your old grain-free meals, experiment with some of the ideas below to get the taste you like without the problematic flours, sugars, and refined oils.

Table 84: Substitutions for Your (Old) Favorite Foods

Meals	Substitutions	How?	Toppings
Burgers	• Bun-less burgers • Portobello mushrooms caps • Eggplant slices	Drizzle mushroom caps or eggplant slices with olive oil and sprinkle with salt. Bake or grill in oven until soft and use as a bun for your burger.	Serve your grain-free burger with guacamole, bacon, a fried egg, tomato sauce, pesto or homemade mayo.
Pizza	• Eggplant • Zucchini	Slice eggplant or zucchini lengthwise. Place on lined baking sheet and drizzle with olive oil. Season to taste and grill until soft. Rearrange slices on baking sheet to form a "crust." Prepare pizza as usual.	A pizza doesn't need cheese—just use ingredients you tolerate. For example: • Pesto, chicken, and extra olive oil • Tomato sauce, ground meat, thyme and basil Also make good toppings: Smoked salmon, bacon, prosciutto, eggs, avocado, garlic-infused oil, all the vegetables you enjoy and can eat safely.
Pizza	• Portobello mushroom caps	Bake mushroom caps in oven until soft. Use each cap to prepare individual mini-pizzas.	
Pizza	• Cauliflower dough	Layer cauliflower dough at bottom of lined baking sheet and prepare pizza as usual.	
Pizza	• Ground meat	Layer raw ground meat (plain or seasoned) at bottom of lined baking sheet. Cook in oven 25-30 minutes, until cooked thoroughly. Use this ground meat "crust" to prepare your pizza (or "meatza!").	
Sandwiches and Wraps	• Lettuce leaves • Nori sheets	Put your favorite sandwich toppings on lettuce leaves or nori sheets (algae) and wrap!	Protein: Leftover protein (ground meat, chicken, fish, seafood), deli meat (ham, prosciutto, bacon), eggs Fats: Pesto, homemade mayo, tomato salsa, guacamole, nut butter
Sandwiches and Wraps	• Thin omelet	Pour a thin layer of beaten eggs in a skillet (with coconut oil or ghee) and cook on both sides. Use as you would use a tortilla.	
Pasta	• Spaghetti squash	Pierce the skin of your butternut squash and bake it in the oven at 350°F (180°C) for about 30 minutes or until soft. Let cool for at least 30 minutes. Cut in half. Remove the seeds. Gently scrape the flesh of the spaghetti squash to shred the pulp into long strands.	Sauces: • Pesto • Tomato sauce • Garlic-infused olive oil • Puréed avocado Protein: • Ground meat • Chicken • Salmon • Tuna • Shrimp • Prosciutto • Ham Seasonings: • Fresh or dried herbs Vegetables: • As tolerated (spinach, onions, mushroom, squash, etc.)
Pasta	• Zucchini noodles	Cut your zucchini lengthwise then lengthwise again on the other side to obtain zucchini noodles. Or use a spiral vegetable slicer.	
Pasta	• Bell pepper boat	Halve your bell pepper. Pour your pasta topping and bake in the oven until ready.	
Pasta	• Zucchini boat	Halve your zucchini. Scoop out some of the flesh and fill with your pasta topping. Bake in the oven until ready.	
Pasta	• Kelp noodles	Follow the instructions on the package.	
Lasagna	• Zucchini slices • Eggplant slices	Grill zucchini and/or eggplant slices in the oven (drizzled with olive oil and sprinkled with salt) until soft. Use instead of wheat pasta to layer your lasagna with ingredients you tolerate.	See the pasta category. Remember that lasagna doesn't need to have cheese. Use only ingredients you tolerate well.

Table 84: Substitutions for Your (Old) Favorite Foods (cont.)

Meals	Substitutions	How?	Toppings
Sushi	• Cauli-rice • Coconut aminos or gluten-free tamari sauce	Use cauli-rice instead of rice to prepare your sushi. Replace soy sauce with coconut aminos or gluten-free tamari sauce and replace tempura with the breading options below. Avoid imitation crab (contains gluten/grains) and use the real thing instead. Or just make sashimi (fresh raw-fish slices).	• Smoked salmon • Fresh fish • Shrimp and crab • Homemade mayo • Ginger • Wasabi • Cucumber and carrot julienne • Avocado
Stir-Fry	• Cauli-rice • Zucchini noodles • Kelp noodles	Use cauli-rice, zucchini noodles, or kelp noodles as a base for your stir-fry. Mix with vegetables, protein, fat and seasonings to taste.	• Chicken, fish, pork, beef, shrimp • Mushroom, carrot, bok choy, broccoli, cabbage as tolerated • Ginger, coconut aminos, coconut milk, nut butter
Breading	• Coconut flour • Almond meal • Unsweetened dried coconut	Dip your protein in beaten eggs then dip in coconut flour, almond meal or unsweetened dried coconut (plain or mixed with seasonings). Repeat these steps as needed. Bake in the oven on a lined baking sheet until cooked. (If you don't tolerate eggs, coat your protein with one of these options. It won't stick as well but will still work.)	• Chicken (whole breast, slices or chicken cut into chicken nuggets) • Fish • Shrimp
Chili	• No beans and corn • More meat	This one is easy. Remove the beans and corn from your favorite chili recipe and use more meat instead. You can even sneak in some minced liver for extra nutrition. Avoid this recipe if you're sensitive to nightshades (tomatoes, chili powder, etc.).	Serve over cauli-rice, baked butternut squash, zucchini noodles, or sweet potatoes, as tolerated.
Chips or Crackers	• Kale chips	See recipe (p. 298)	Sprinkle with different dried herbs (basil, oregano, thyme, parsley, rosemary) and spices (cinnamon, turmeric, chili powder) to create interesting varieties!
	• Coconut chips	See recipe (p. 296)	
	• Chicken skin	Put pieces of chicken skin on lined baking sheet. Season to taste and grill in oven until crispy.	
Appetizers	• Cucumber slices	Peel the cucumber if its high fiber content is problematic for your intestines.	• Smoked salmon and guacamole • Shrimp and homemade mayo
	• Endives	Wash fresh endives and pat them dry.	• Tuna salad with homemade mayo
	• Bacon slices	Cook them until crispy	• Spread with guacamole
	• Bacon-wrapped anything	Wrap raw or cooked bacon around one of the options on the right. Bake in the oven until cooked if desired.	• Asparagus • Baked sweet potato bites • Dates • Figs • Apricots • Sausages • Shrimp • Scallop • Chicken

Nutritious Vegetables | appropriate for the elimination phase

Roasted carrots look and taste quite different from puréed or stir-fried carrots. Use this to your advantage and keep things interesting by varying the way you prepare the vegetables you tolerate. Combine them with different fats and seasonings and you won't feel like you are eating the same foods over and over, even if your diet is limited.

INGREDIENTS

See Table 86: Vegetable and Seasoning Options p. 333

PROCESS

1. Wash your vegetables.
2. Peel and de-seed them if needed to make them easier to digest.
3. Cut the vegetables into cubes or slices or julienne them. You can also use a mandoline to make thin slices, cut them into fries, or use a spiral vegetable slicer for pasta-like vegetable strips.
4. Choose one of the following cooking methods:

Table 85: Cooking Methods for Vegetables

Boiling	Steaming	Stir-Frying	Roasting	Puréeing
Put water or bone broth in a saucepan. Add the prepared vegetables and seasoning as desired. Boil for at least 5-10 minutes to up to one hour, or until the vegetables are tender when pierced with a fork (the smaller the vegetable pieces, the shorter the cooking time). Add water if necessary if it evaporates.	Place a steaming basket or metal colander in a saucepan. Add water to the bottom (the water shouldn't be in direct contact with the vegetables). Add your vegetables and bring the water to a boil. Steam, with a lid on, for at least 5-10 minutes or as long as needed for your vegetables to be cooked thoroughly. Add water if necessary.	Heat fat (coconut oil, ghee, olive oil, or duck fat) in a skillet under medium to high temperature. Once the skillet is hot, add the vegetables and stir-fry as long as needed to get your vegetables cooked thoroughly or al dente. Adjust the heat to prevent burning. You can also add more fat or some bone broth to keep the vegetables from sticking.	Put your cut vegetables in a Pyrex dish. Add generous amounts of fat (coconut oil, ghee, olive oil, or duck fat). Add seasonings to taste and mix. Roast in the oven at 400°F (200°C) for about 45-60 minutes or until the vegetables are cooked thoroughly and slightly golden. This works especially well with root vegetables such as winter squashes and beets, but it also works very well with cauliflower, Brussels sprouts, onion, zucchini, bell pepper, and eggplant.	Cook your vegetables any way you like. Add to a blender or food processor. Add a little bit of water, bone broth, and seasonings if desired. Purée until smooth. Add more liquid if needed to get just the right consistency. Or add even more liquid to transform your purée into a blended soup.

TIPS:

Always make large batches of vegetables and reheat leftovers as needed.

Use Table 86 (p. 333) to remember all the vegetable and seasoning options you have during the elimination and reintroduction phases, as tolerated.

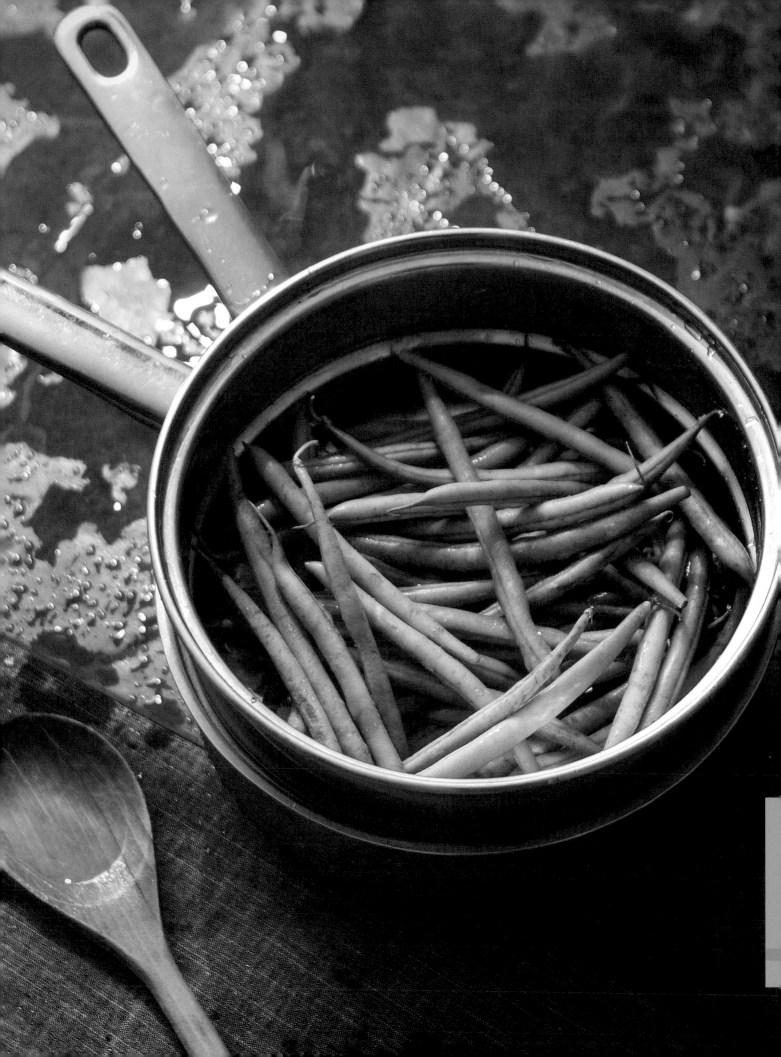

Vegetable Fries | appropriate for the elimination phase

Even though some people don't tolerate potatoes because of their high starch content or because they belong to the nightshade family, you can still enjoy fries as a tasty side dish. Not only are vegetable-based fries more nutrient dense, but their lower carbohydrate content won't feed a gut dysbiosis and is better for your blood-sugar levels.

INGREDIENTS

Yields as many fries as you prepare:	
As much as you want!	Carrots, turnips, beets, butternut squash, jicama, sweet potatoes Olive oil or coconut oil Seasonings (unrefined salt, dried herbs or spices)

PROCESS

1. Choose a vegetable you tolerate.
2. Peel it if necessary and cut it into fries.
3. Put the vegetable fries on a lined baking sheet.
4. Drizzle with generous amounts of olive or coconut oil and season to taste.
5. Bake in the oven at 350°F (180°C) for 15 to 45 minutes or until your fries are crispy (it can take more or less time depending on the vegetable you choose and the thickness of your fries).

TIPS:

Serve your vegetable fries with tomato sauce (add seasonings to make it a salsa or blend it for a sugar-free ketchup), with homemade mayonnaise (seasoned to taste) or guacamole.

Add a splash of balsamic vinegar or drizzle a little honey over your fries before baking to enhance their natural sweetness.

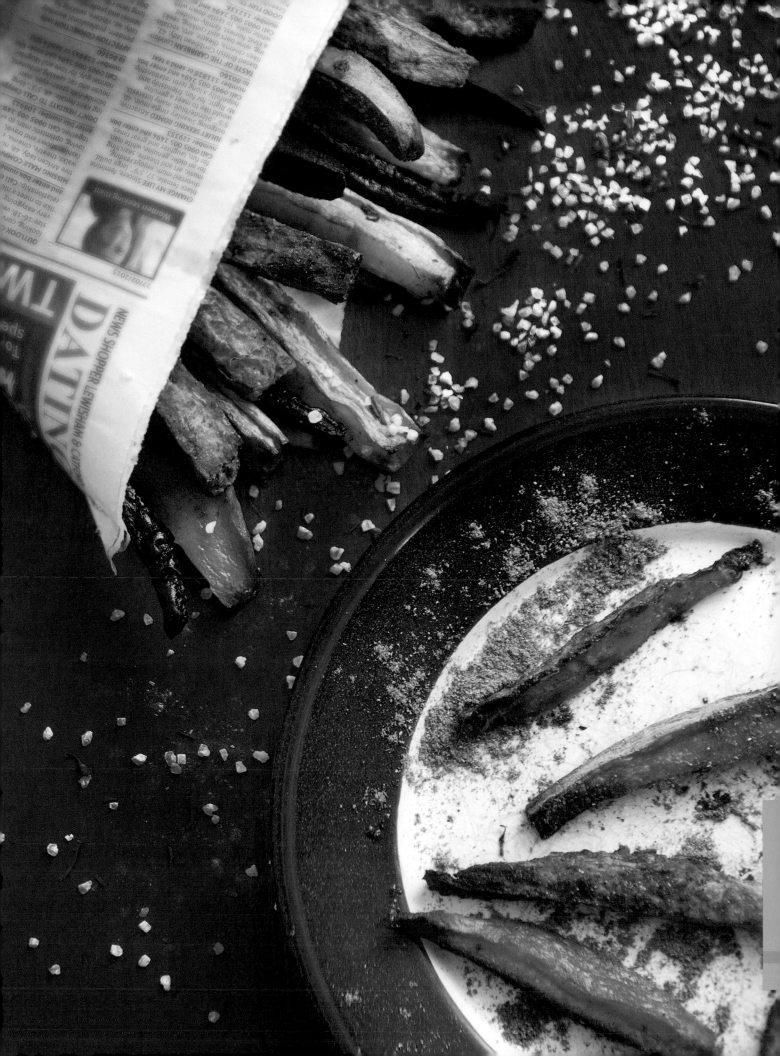

Mashed Cauliflower | contains cauliflower

Once you can reintroduce cauliflower into your diet, you will be able to use this versatile vegetable to imitate a variety of high-carb side dishes made with starchy potatoes or grains. If you miss comfort foods like mashed potatoes, cauliflower makes a tasty and more nutrient-dense substitute.

INGREDIENTS

About 3-4 cups (0.75-1L):		
1 head	Cauliflower	1 head
6 tbsp	Ghee, coconut oil, or butter	90 ml
To taste	Unrefined salt	To taste
To taste	Seasonings	To taste

PROCESS

1. Remove the leaves from your cauliflower head and break it into florets.
2. Put in a large saucepan, cover with water, and bring to a boil.
3. Boil for about 10 to 15 minutes or until the cauliflower is soft when pierced with a fork.
4. Drain the water from the saucepan.
5. Add the fats and seasonings to the boiled cauliflower.
6. Mash the cauliflower with a potato masher or hand blender, or transfer to a food processor and blend until you obtain the right consistency. Add more fat or a bit of water or bone broth if too thick.

TIPS:

Use garlic-infused oil, or herbed butter if desired.

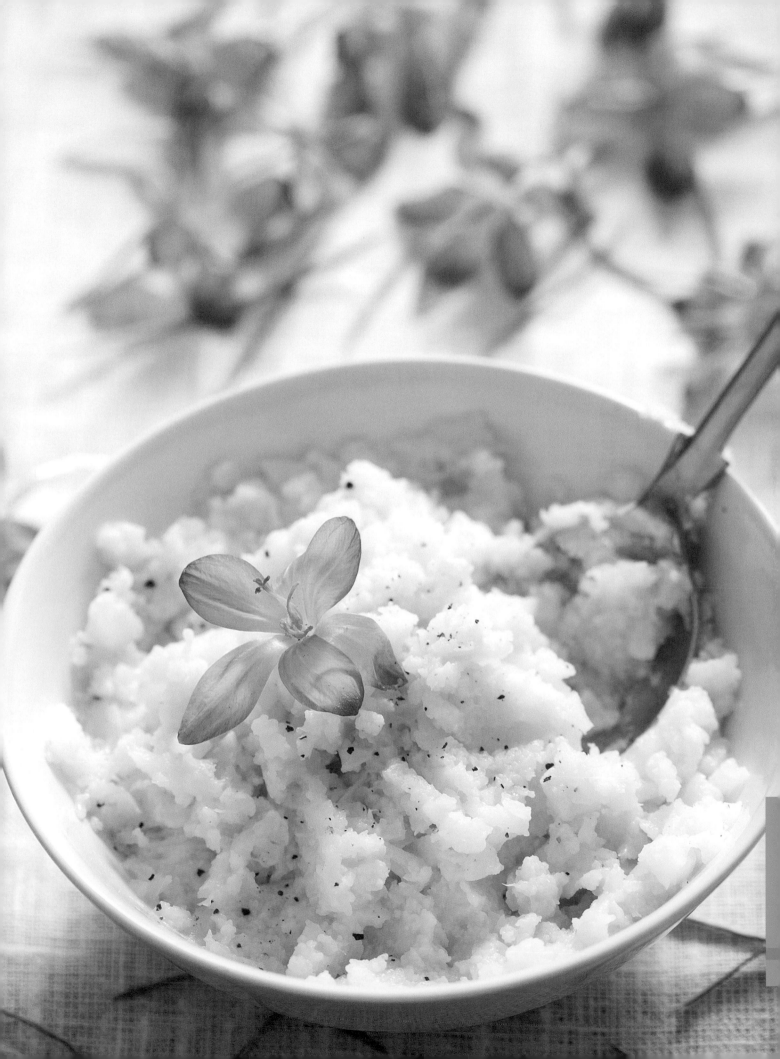

Cauli-rice | contains cauliflower

What the heck is cauli-rice? Cauli-rice is a grain-free rice imitation made from one of the most versatile of all vegetables: cauliflower. Serve your cauli-rice as you would serve rice. It works great as a side dish, in stir-fries, or even in sushis.

INGREDIENTS

Yields 3-4 cups (0.75-1L):		
1 head	Cauliflower	1 head
3-4 tbsp	Ghee, coconut oil, duck fat, or olive oil	45-60 ml
To taste	Seasonings (unrefined salt, herbs and spices)	To taste

PROCESS

1. Remove the leaves around the cauliflower.
2. Grate the raw cauliflower by hand using a cheese grater or a food processor. The grated cauliflower will resemble rice grains.
3. Put aside in a large bowl.
4. In a skillet, heat your fat under medium temperature.
5. Add the cauli-rice to the skillet and cook for five to 10 minutes until soft. You may need to do more than one batch and add more fat as needed. Season to taste.

TIPS:

Keep your cauli-rice raw or cooked in the fridge for three to four days.

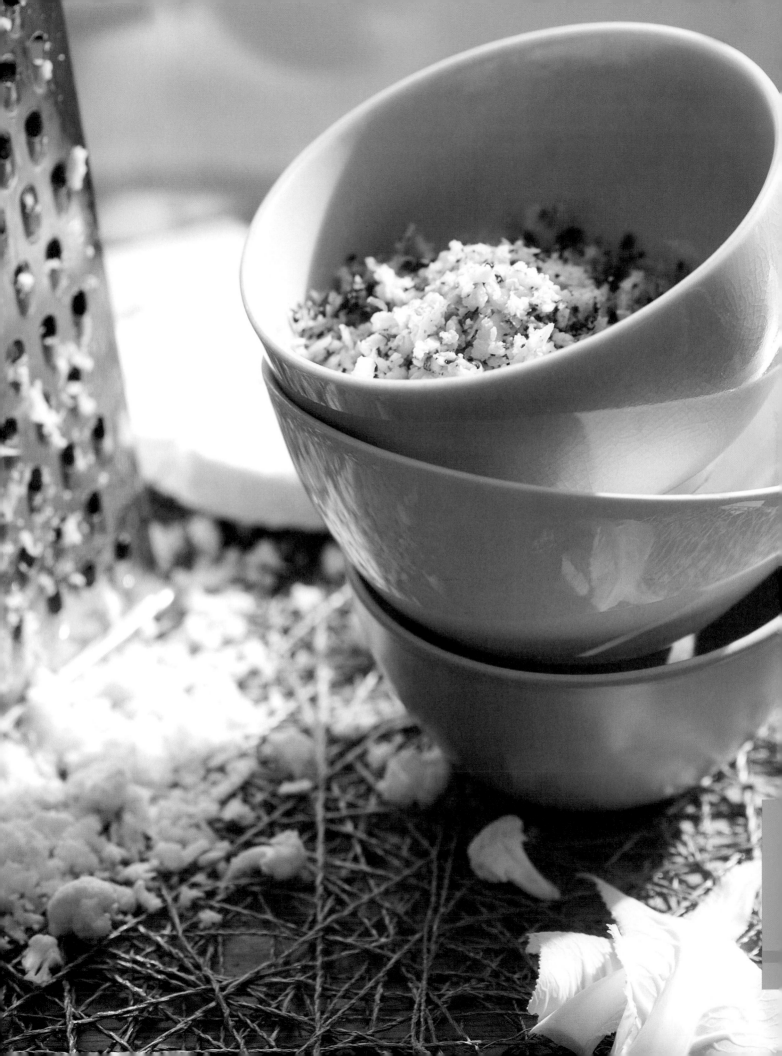

Lemon Butter Sauce | appropriate for the elimination phase

This lemon butter sauce only uses two ingredients and goes wonderfully with fish, seafood, chicken, and green vegetables. Beware of commercial varieties containing sugar as the first ingredient, followed by wheat glucose syrup, preservatives and vegetable gums.

INGREDIENTS

Yields just over 1 cup (250 ml):		
1 cup	Ghee	250 ml
4 tbsp	Lemon juice (2 lemons)	60 ml

PROCESS

1. Combine the ghee and lemon juice.
2. Refrigerate for a firmer consistency or melt in a small saucepan for a liquid sauce.

TIPS:

Add dried or fresh herbs (such as sage, rosemary, oregano, parsley, or thyme) if desired.

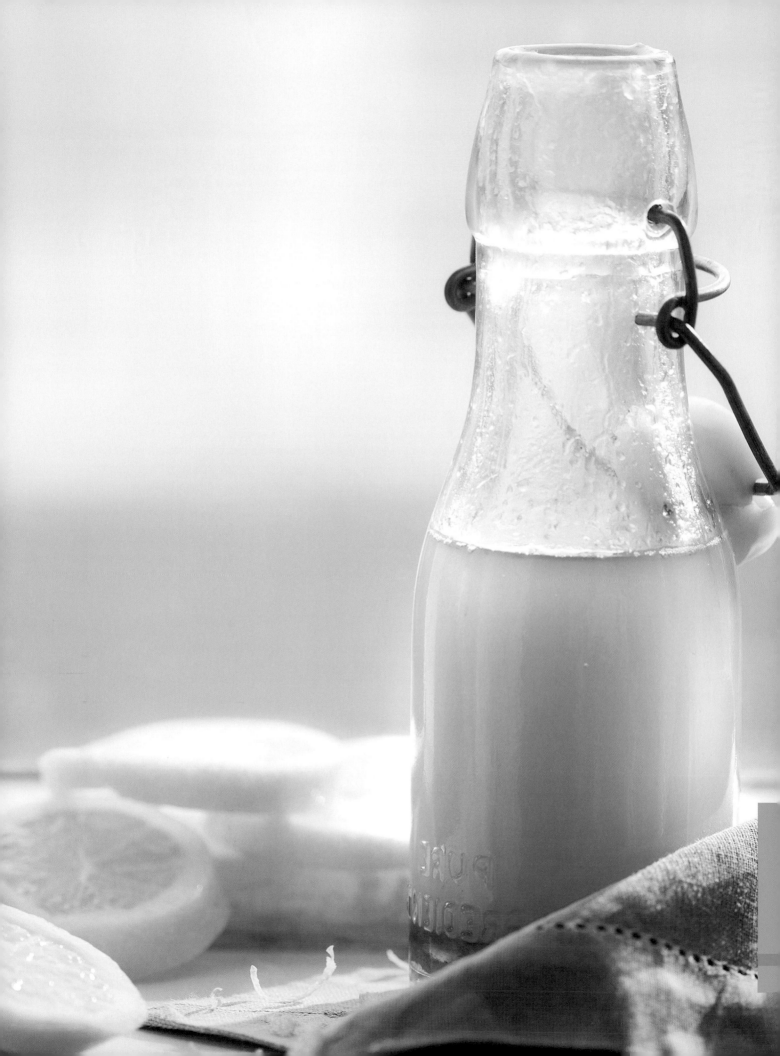

Pesto | appropriate for the elimination phase

Commercial pesto often contains nuts (pine nuts), dairy (Parmesan cheese), and other ingredients that could be problematic for your digestion. These ingredients play a small role in enhancing the taste of pesto, but most of the flavors actually come from the basil leaves and olive oil. You can make pesto using only the most basic ingredients to craft a delicious sauce for your steak, chicken, or vegetables. You can even use it as a marinade.

INGREDIENTS

Yields 1 cup (250 ml):		
2 cups	Fresh basil leaves	500 ml
¼ - ½ cup	Extra-virgin olive oil	60-125 ml
½ tsp	Unrefined salt	2 ml

PROCESS

1. Put all the ingredients in a blender. Start with the smallest amount of olive oil.
2. Process until smooth, adding more olive oil as necessary to get the consistency just right.
3. Transfer to a glass container and keep in the fridge for five to six days, or freeze your pesto in an ice-cube tray for easy-to-use single servings.

TIPS:

You can use garlic-infused oil (see recipe p. 284) if you like.

Add homemade bone broth (one half to one cup or 125 to 250 milliliters) to your pesto to turn it into a sauce. Heat and serve over your meat or vegetables.

Replace the basil leaves with other herbs (cilantro, parsley, or other) to create new pesto varieties.

You can also replace part or all of the herbs with sun-dried tomatoes if desired. Use dried ones (not soaked in oil since the oil used is often refined). Pour boiling water over your sun-dried tomatoes, let rest about five to 10 minutes, and drain. Use these hydrated sun-dried tomatoes for this homemade pesto or in any of your favorite recipes (if you tolerate nightshades).

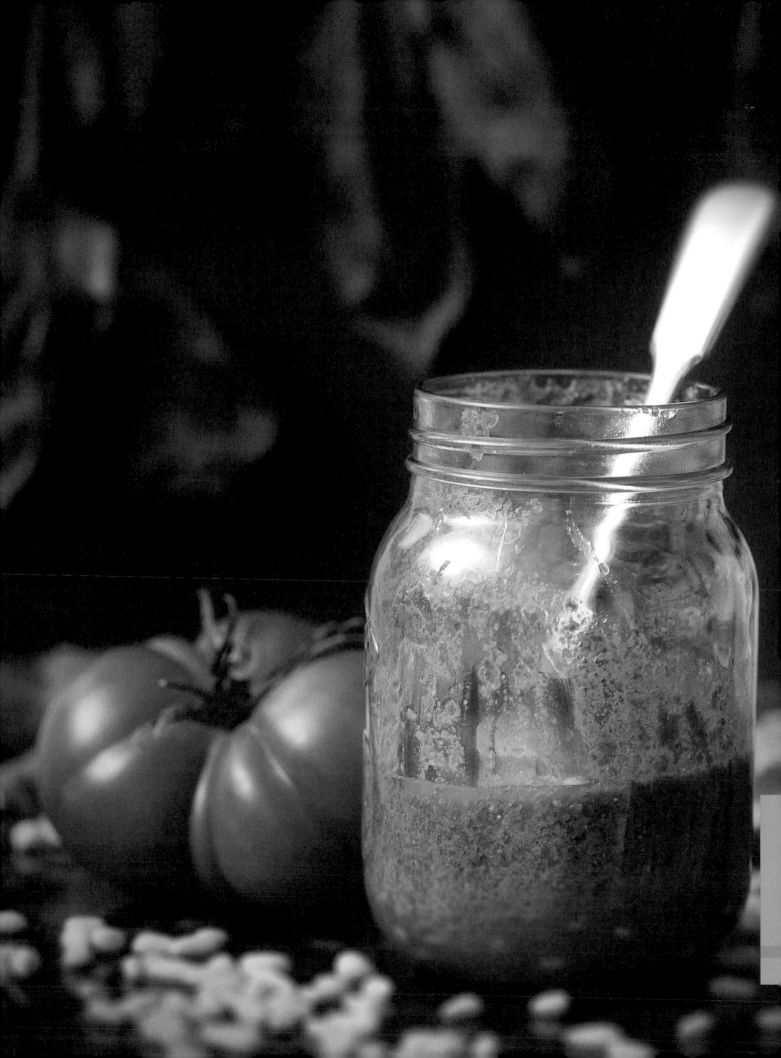

Herbed Ghee (or Herbed Butter) | appropriate for the elimination phase

A higher-fat diet doesn't have to be boring and smothered with unappetizing oils. Be creative with your fats and aromatize them to keep your diet varied and interesting. This herbed ghee is delicious served with any kinds of protein or vegetables.

INGREDIENTS

Yields 1 cup (250 ml):		
1 cup	Ghee	250 ml
2-3 tbsp	Fresh herbs, finely chopped	30-45 ml

PROCESS

1. In a bowl, mix your ghee (room temperature) with the fresh herbs. Season to taste with unrefined salt (if your ghee is unsalted).
2. Keep at room temperature or in the refrigerator.

TIPS:

Replace the ghee with butter (if tolerated).

Try different combinations of fresh herbs like tarragon, thyme, parsley, oregano, or rosemary leaves.

Pipe the herbed ghee/butter into small serving dishes for a festive look.

You can also simply mix equal amounts of ghee or butter with equal amounts of pesto for a delicious and antioxidant-rich spread (this spread will be softer than pure ghee or butter even if kept in the refrigerator).

Freeze your herbed ghee/butter in an ice-cube tray. When you need it, simply take a cube or two and use it to prepare your meal.

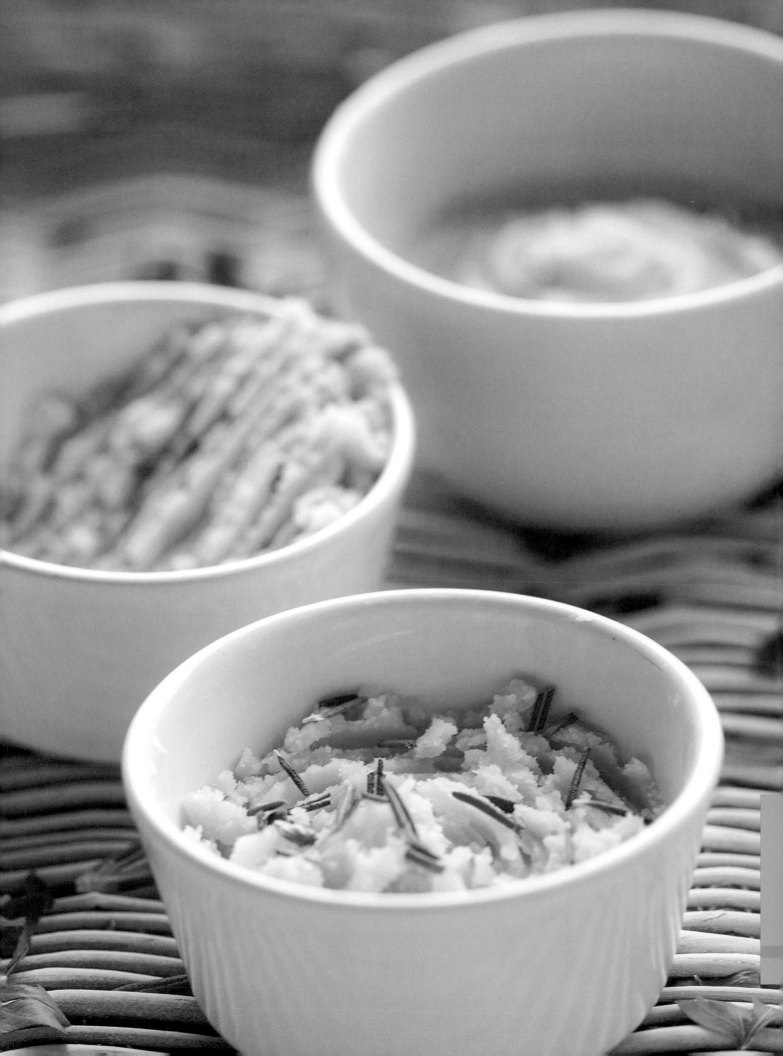

Garlic-Infused Oil | appropriate for the elimination phase

You can extract the aroma of garlic without its FODMAPs by using olive oil. Use this oil for cooking your food, preparing your salad dressing, vinaigrettes, or homemade mayonnaise. Or simply drizzle it over your grain-free zucchini-noodle dishes.

INGREDIENTS

Yields 1 cup (250 ml):		
1 cup	Olive oil (or macadamia or avocado oil)	250 ml
5-6	Garlic cloves	5-6

PROCESS

1. Peel the garlic cloves and cut each one in half.
2. Put the garlic cloves in a small skillet with the olive oil.
3. Heat at a low temperature until the oil is hot. Keep the temperature as low as possible to allow the garlic to infuse without damaging the fats of olive oil (a temperature of 110°F or 45°C is best; use a thermometer if you have one).
4. Let the garlic infuse for about 10 minutes or until the garlic is soft and slightly golden.
5. Let cool down, strain the oil, and discard the garlic.

TIPS:

Make a garlic puree with the caramelized garlic cloves and give it to someone who can handle FODMAPs. This garlic purée is delicious spread on a steak or added to homemade sauces and mayonnaises.

Freeze your garlic-infused oil in an ice-cube tray. When you need it, simply take a cube or two and use it to prepare your meal.

Add herbs (a branch of rosemary or a few leaves of thyme, for instance) while infusing your oil with garlic to add extra flavors to your oil.

While there is nothing wrong with using extra-virgin olive oil, it can be a waste of money since the heat is likely to destroy its vitamin E and antioxidants. You'll get better value for your money using regular olive oil for this recipe.

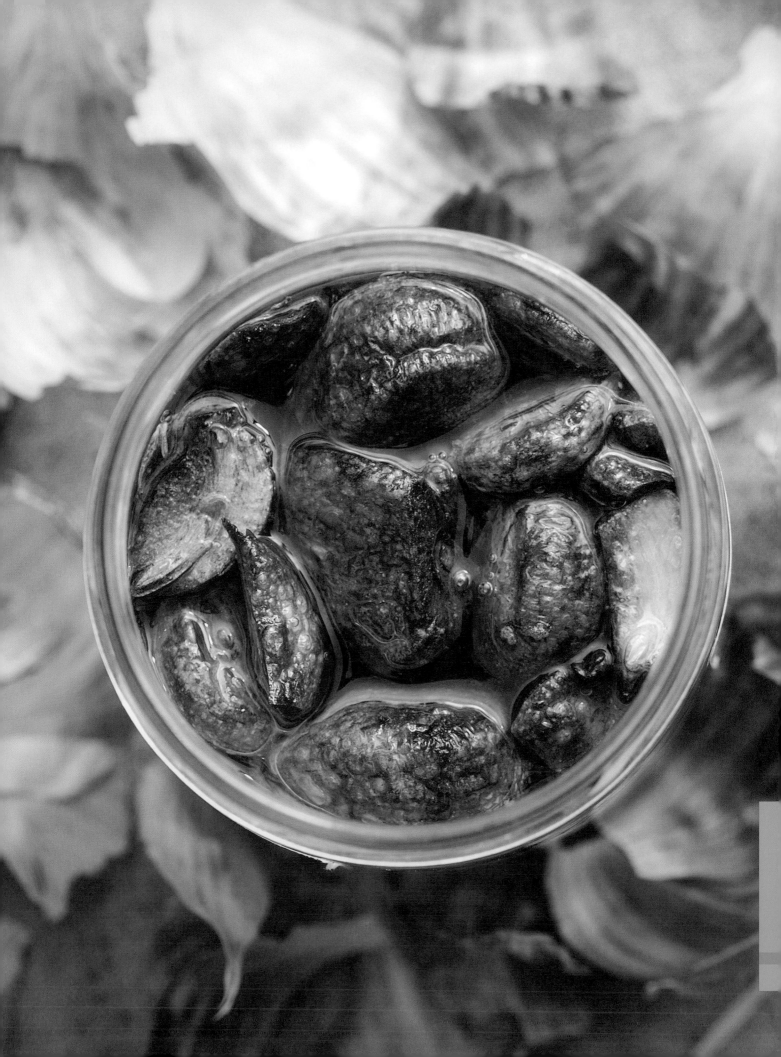

Reduction Sauce | appropriate for the elimination phase

A reduction sauce is an application of French cooking techniques to concentrate the flavors of the meat and bones you use to make your homemade bone broth. Use this reduction to serve as a sauce for your meat or use it to stir-fry or purée your vegetables.

INGREDIENTS

Yields about 1-2 cups (250-500 ml):		
3-4 cups	Homemade bone broth	0.75-1 L
To taste	Seasonings	To taste

PROCESS

1. Pour your bone broth in a large skillet.
2. Bring to a boil.
3. Let simmer at high intensity for as long as it takes to let most of the water evaporate and concentrate the flavors in the reduction.

TIPS:

You can make your reduction in the same skillet you used to cook your protein. Once the protein is ready, remove it and deglaze the skillet with one half to one cup (125 to 250 milliliters) of wine. Heating the wine will get rid of the alcohol while preserving its flavors. If you don't want to use wine, use some bone broth. Then add the remaining bone broth and follow steps two and three.

Add one to two teaspoons (five to 10 milliliters) of gelatin to thicken your reduction if desired.

You can make this reduction into a gravy by adding coconut flour. Mix one to two teaspoon (five to 10 milliliters) of coconut flour with some water before adding it to the skillet. Use a whisk to mix it and get rid of any lumps.

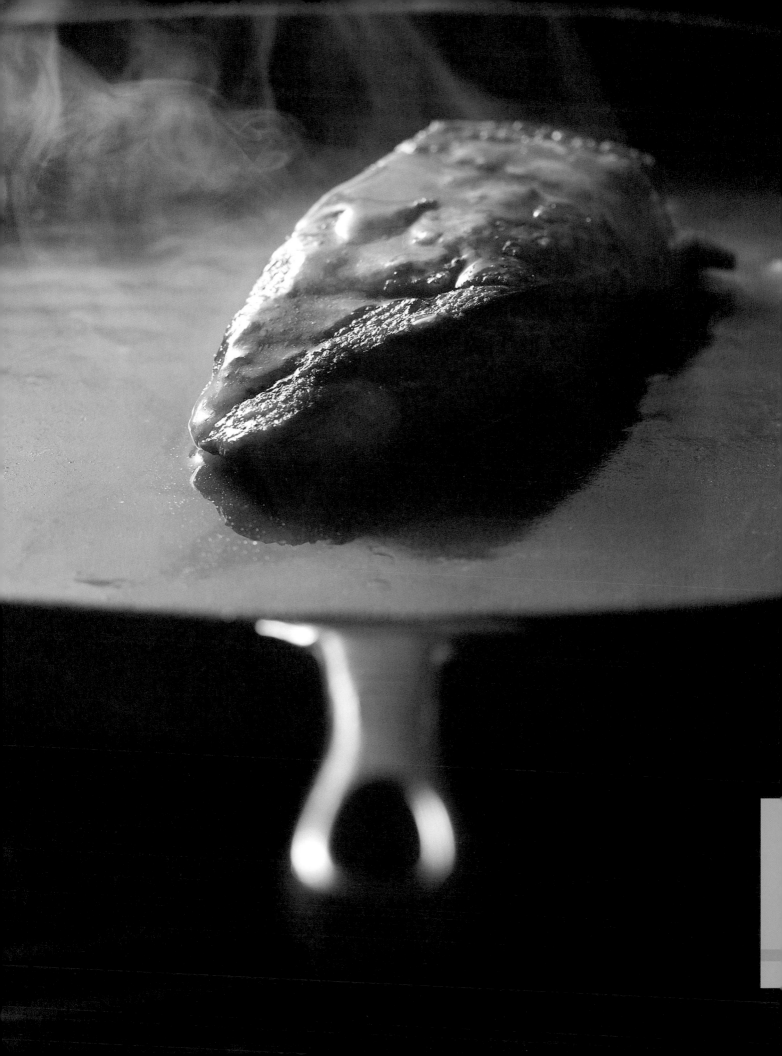

Homemade Mayonnaise | contains eggs

Commercial mayonnaise is filled with refined inflammatory omega-6 fats (vegetable oil, especially soybean oil) and other processed ingredients. But mayonnaise is not necessarily bad for you. If made with the right oils, it's an excellent vessel to add more healthy fats to your diet. Use your healthy mayo to dip veggies, meat, fish, or seafood or to prepare creamy salad dressings or deviled eggs.

Don't use extra-virgin olive oil for this recipe; its taste is too strong. Although light-tasting olive oil is more processed, it's a better option for making mayonnaise. If you don't want to use olive oil, try avocado oil or macadamia oil.

INGREDIENTS

Yields about 1 cup (250 ml):		
1 cup	Oil (olive oil, avocado oil, or macadamia oil)	250 ml
2	Egg yolks (or 1 whole egg)	2
1 tbsp	Lemon juice or apple cider vinegar	15 ml
To taste	Unrefined salt and seasonings	To taste

PROCESS

1. Put the egg yolk (or whole egg), lemon juice (or apple cider vinegar), and seasonings in a blender. Mix.
2. Keep the blender on and pour the oil into the blender *very slowly*. The oil should emulsify (thicken) with the egg yolk as you pour the oil. You can also use a hand blender or do this by hand with a whisk, but you will need the help of someone else to pour the oil while you emulsify the mayonnaise with one hand and hold the bowl with the other.
3. Store your mayo in the fridge for up to five to seven days.

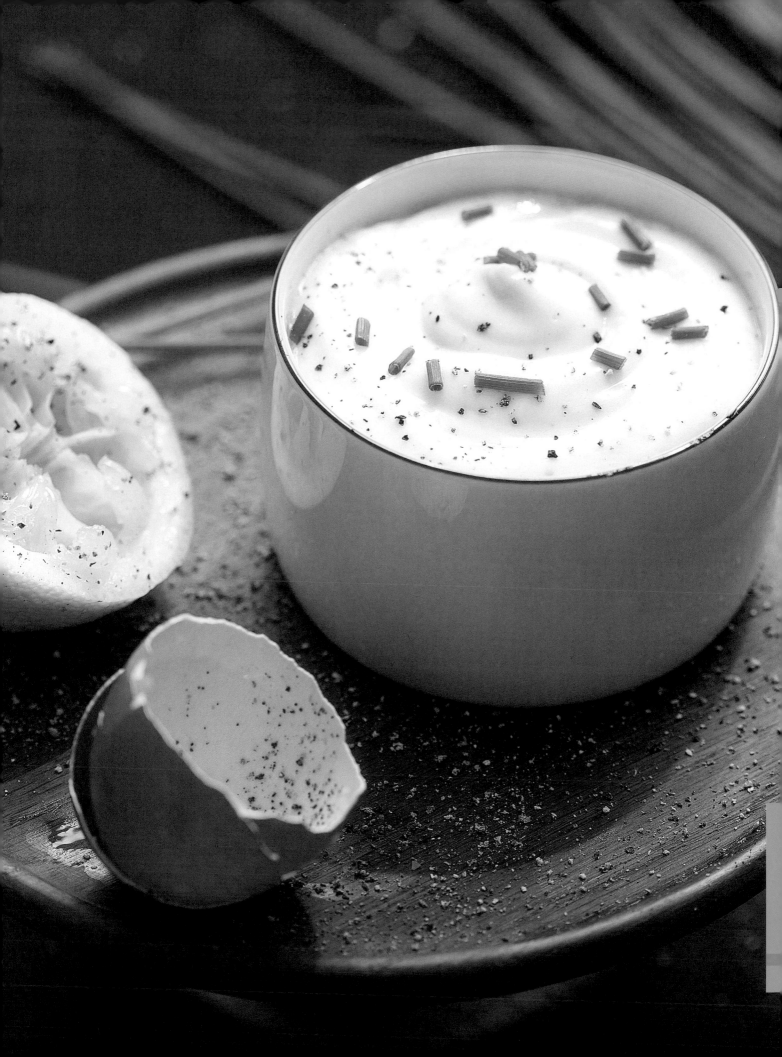

Basic Vinaigrette | contains vinegar

This simple and versatile vinaigrette is great not only for salads, but also as a marinade for your steaks or kebabs. You can also drizzle it over your cooked vegetables or use it as a dip for raw vegetables.

INGREDIENTS

Yields 1 cup (250 ml):		
½ cup	Olive oil, macadamia oil or avocado oil	125 ml
¼ cup	Vinegar (balsamic, red wine, tomato, etc.)	60 ml
To taste	Unrefined salt and other seasonings	To taste

PROCESS

1. Mix all ingredients and season to taste.
2. Shake well before serving.

TIPS:

If using balsamic vinegar, always go for quality. Cheap balsamic vinegar is not prepared according to the Italian tradition and may contain a lot of added sugar. Choose "aged" balsamic vinegar to make sure you have the real, sugar-free kind.

Keep your vinaigrette at room temperature. Don't put it in the fridge or it will turn solid and will be difficult to use.

Combine all ingredients in a glass bottle, shake, and your vinaigrette is ready!

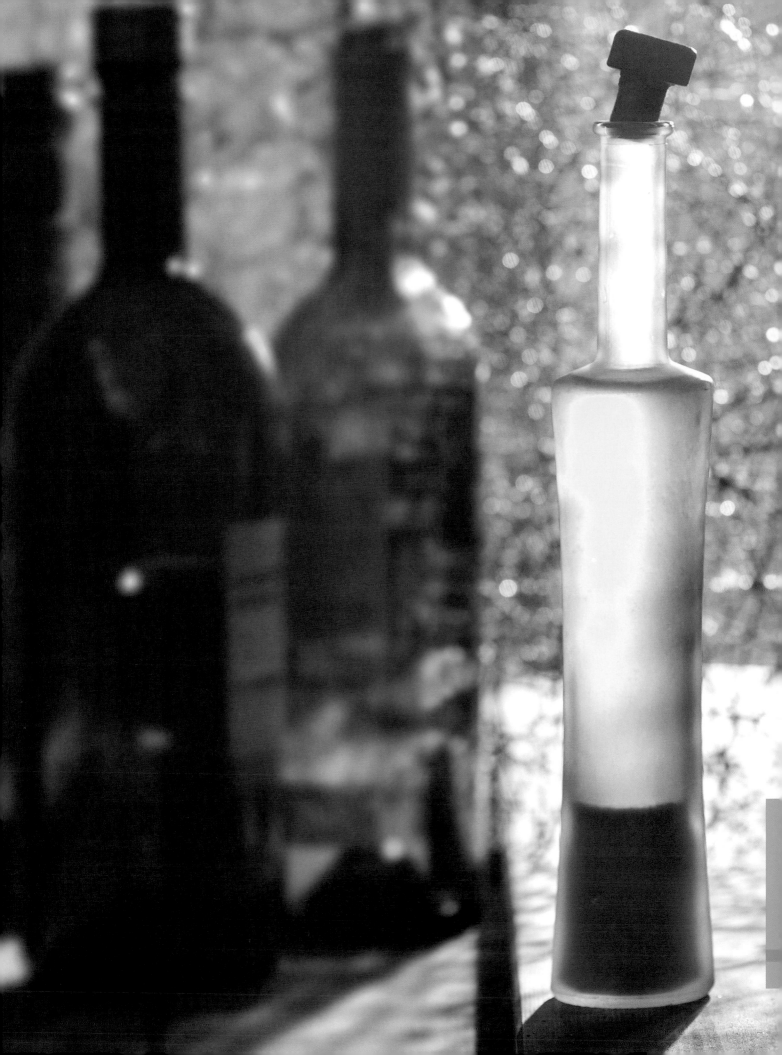

Green Tea and Raspberry Gelatin Squares | appropriate for the elimination phase

Gelatin is one of the beneficial ingredients naturally found in homemade bone broth. You can get a bit more of the gut-healing amino acids gelatin contains by using powdered gelatin to make sugar-free jelly treats. If you can, use gelatin from grass-fed or pastured cows, such as Great Lakes Gelatin—but any gelatin is definitely better than none! These gelatin squares are an excellent way to get your gut-healing gelatin when the weather is too hot to make bone broth.

INGREDIENTS

Yields 3 cups (750 ml):		
4-6 tsp	Dry powdered gelatin (or 6 gelatin sheets)	20-30 ml
3 tbsp	Cold water	45 ml
3 cups	Warm water	750 ml
1 tbsp	Green tea leaves	15 ml
10	Frozen raspberries	10

PROCESS

1. Mix the dry powdered gelatin with the cold water. Let rest for about five minutes to allow the gelatin to absorb the water.
2. Meanwhile, prepare your green tea by infusing about three cups of hot water. For best results, don't use boiling water to prepare green tea. To prevent your green tea from being bitter, use hot water with a temperature around 175°F or 80°C.
3. Add the green tea leaves and the frozen raspberries. Let infuse about five minutes. You can also mash the frozen raspberries once they thaw so they release more of their natural flavors and colors.
4. Filter your tea and discard the green tea leaves and raspberries.
5. Add the tea to the gelatin and mix well.
6. Pour the liquid in a Pyrex container or individual silicone muffin cups.
7. Refrigerate for at least two to three hours or until the mixture gels.
8. Cut into squares and keep in the fridge for up to four to five days.
9. Enjoy these delicious sugar-free, gut-healing treats whenever you like (as a snack or dessert).

TIPS:

Use frozen blueberries instead of raspberries. Avoid blackberries if you are sensitive to FODMAPs.

Rooibos tea or other herbal teas can also be used to make different flavors.

Instead of tea leaves and frozen berries, try using lemon or lime juice.

Add one to two tablespoons (15 to 30 milliliters) of honey or other tolerated sweeteners if desired.

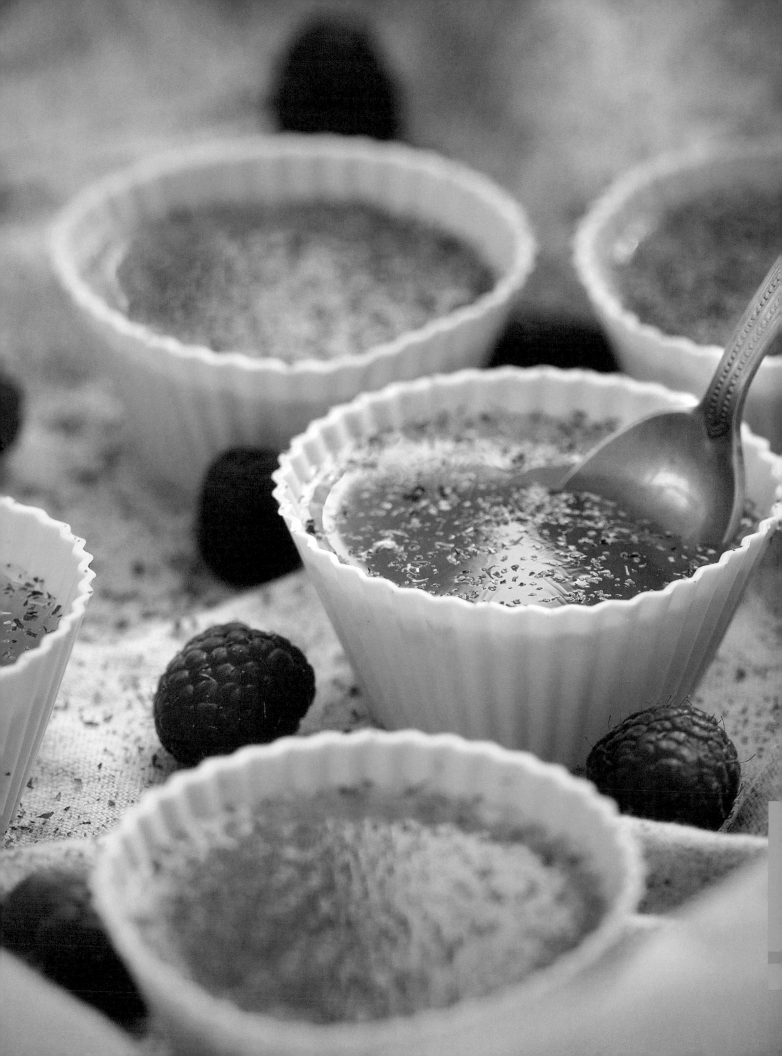

Chicken Liver Pâté | contains onion, garlic and vinegar

Liver truly is a superfood; It's Mother Nature's multivitamin. Chicken liver pâté is a delicious and easy way to introduce liver into your diet to get all the benefits it has to offer, including a good dose of vitamins A, D, and K_2, and many B vitamins, as well as a variety of essential minerals. Wait until you tolerate red wine vinegar and eliminate any ingredients you don't tolerate (especially garlic and onion). Ghee can be used instead of butter.

INGREDIENTS

Yield about 2 cups (500 ml):		
1 lb	Organic chicken liver	450 g
½	Large onion (optional)	½
2	Cloves of garlic (optional)	2
To taste	Salt, pepper, thyme and rosemary	To taste
½ cup	Red wine vinegar	125 ml
¼ cup	Butter (or ghee)	60 ml

PROCESS

1. In a skillet, cook the onions, garlic, and chicken livers in ghee.
2. Once the onions are transparent and the chicken livers are cooked, add the red wine vinegar and seasonings. Let cook at medium heat for 10 to 15 minutes. Once most of the vinegar has evaporated, turn off the heat and let cool.
3. Once cooled, put the mixture in a food processor, add the butter, and process until smooth.
4. Serve on cucumber slices or eggplant crackers, or use as a dip for carrot sticks.

TIPS:

When choosing chicken livers, choose the reddest ones you can find, ideally from pastured chickens allowed to eat their natural diet, including insects and worms. Red livers are more likely to come from healthy animals than are those with a gray or brown color.

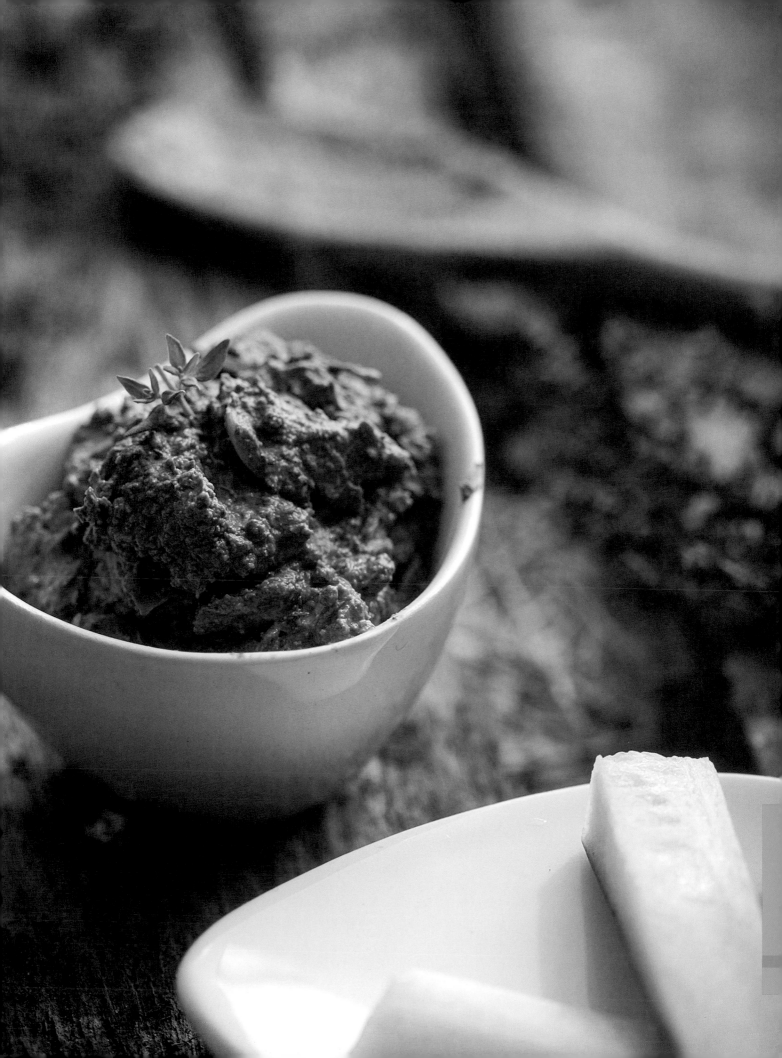

Coconut Chips | contains coconut

If you want a snack food for occasional nibbling, coconut chips are a great option. Coconut is low in carbohydrates and high in helpful MCTs (medium-chain triglycerides). Toasting the unsweetened coconut flakes enhances their natural sweetness.

INGREDIENTS

Yields 2 cups (500 ml):		
2 cups	Large flakes of unsweetened dried coconut	500 ml

PROCESS

1. Heat a non-stick skillet under medium to high temperature.
2. Add the large flakes of unsweetened coconut to form a thin layer.
3. Stir often, with a wooden spoon, to allow the coconut flakes to caramelize evenly without burning. Lower the temperature if your coconut chips start to burn. Stay close as the coconut flakes will caramelize within a few minutes.
4. Once the coconut chips have reached the desired color, turn off the heat and transfer the coconut chips to a plate to let them cool. Resist the temptation of tasting them right away if you don't want to burn your tongue!

TIPS:

Sprinkle your coconut chips with salt, cinnamon, or other seasonings once ready and still hot, if desired.

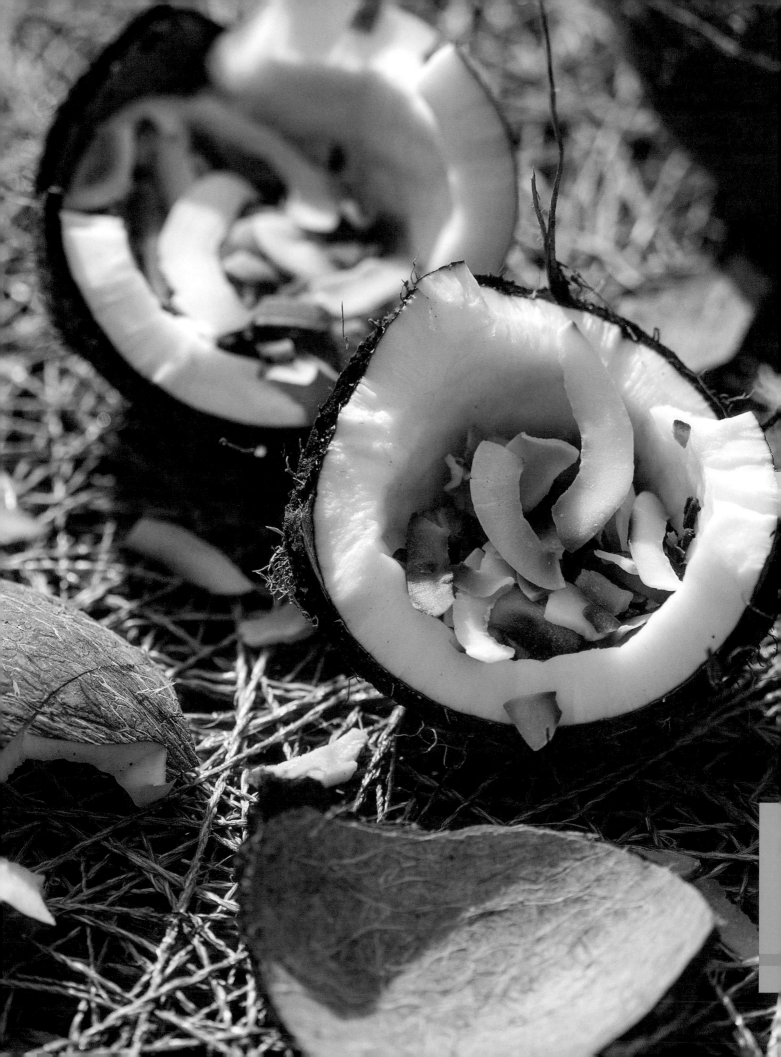

Kale Chips | contains kale

Kale is one of the most-nutrient dense vegetables, and it can be dehydrated and enjoyed in chip form. Choose organic kale if possible because conventionally grown kale tends to contain more pesticide residues than most vegetables.

INGREDIENTS

Yields 4-6 cups (1-1.5L):		
1 bunch	Kale, fresh (ideally organic)	1 bunch
1-2 tbsp	Olive oil	15-30 ml
To taste	Unrefined salt and seasonings	To taste

PROCESS

1. Wash the kale and pat it dry with a towel.
2. Remove the stems.
3. In a bowl, mix the kale with the olive oil and seasonings.
4. Put a single layer of the kale leaves on a lined baking sheet.
   Use two baking sheets if possible or simply do multiple batches.
5. Bake in the oven at 325°F (160°C), turning once or twice to prevent burning, for 15 to 20 minutes or until dried and crispy.
6. Let cool and enjoy.

TIPS:

Mix the olive oil with balsamic vinegar before drizzling on the kale for a different flavor.

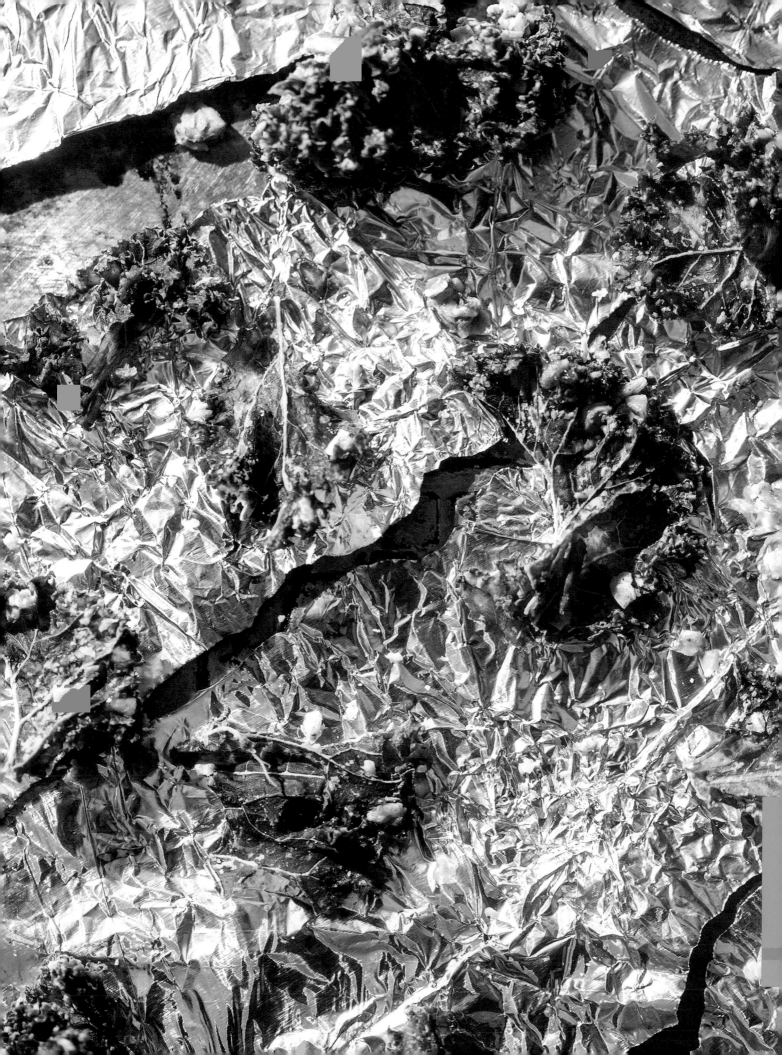

Nut Bars | contains nuts, dates and coconut

Commercially prepared bars are likely to contain ingredients you don't tolerate. Some bars may only contain nuts and fruits, but they can be quite expensive. Making your own allows you to choose only the ingredients you want without spending a fortune.

INGREDIENTS

Yields 4 servings:		
6	Large dates, pitted	6
½ cup	Nuts	125 ml
½ cup	Unsweetened dried coconut	125 ml
1 tbsp	Coconut oil	15 ml
Dash	Salt	Dash

PROCESS

1. Combine all the ingredients in a food processor and blend until smooth.
2. Spread the bar mixture into a small Pyrex dish and refrigerate for two to three hours (or until firm).
3. Cut into four bars. Wrap individually with plastic wrap if desired.
4. Keep your bars for a few days in the refrigerator or freeze them.

TIPS:

Experiment with different combinations of nuts, including macadamia, almonds, walnuts, pecans, and hazelnuts.

Replace the nuts with nut butter if desired.

Replace the dates with figs if desired.

If you don't tolerate nuts, use coconut butter. If you don't tolerate coconut, use only nuts.

Add lemon or lime zest, cocoa powder, spices (cinnamon, nutmeg, cardamom), whole nuts, and whole dried fruits (as tolerated) if desired.

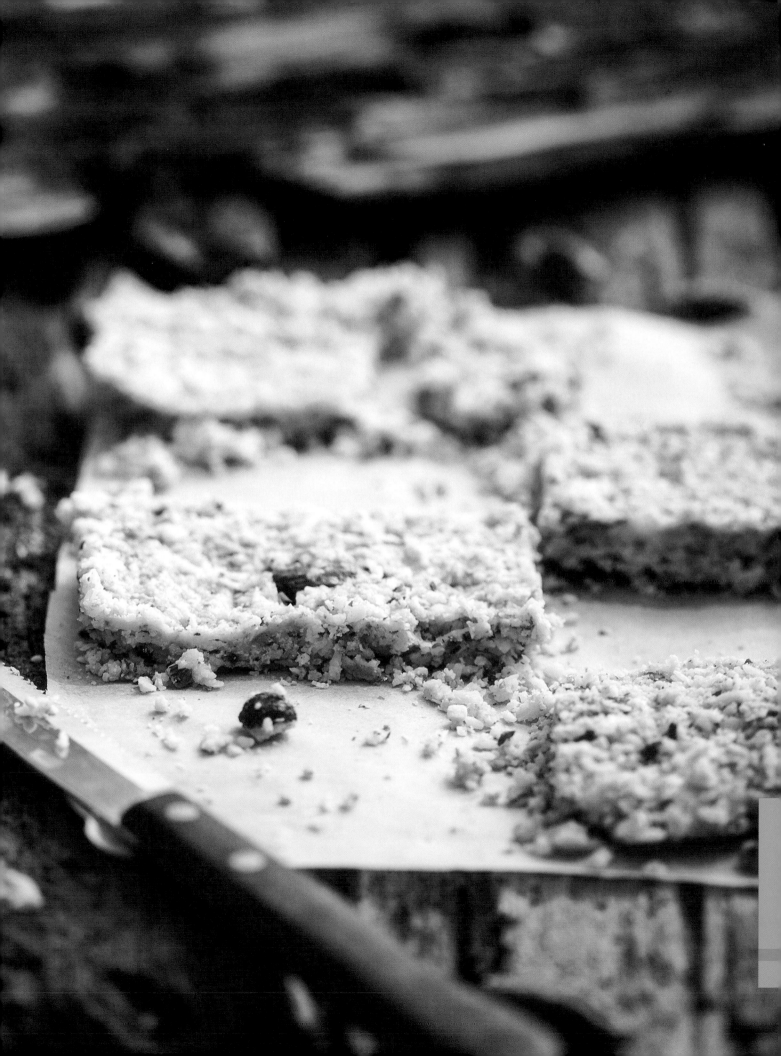

Sauerkraut | contains cabbage

Making your own sauerkraut is the cheapest and most effective way to get gut-friendly bacteria into your diet without having to worry about dairy, FOS, or any other ingredients often found in probiotic supplements. All you need is some cabbage, unrefined salt, and a bit of elbow grease and Mother Nature will do the rest. It may be intimidating to make your own sauerkraut for the first time, but it's easier than it looks. And a single batch can last you for weeks!

INGREDIENTS

Yields 4-6 cups (1-1.5 L):		
Basic ingredients	1 1-2 tbsp	Medium cabbage Sea salt	1 15-30 ml
Optional	Shredded carrots, shredded red cabbage, 1 tbsp. (15 ml) caraway seeds, garlic	

PROCESS

1. Remove a few outer leaves of the cabbage and keep them for later.
2. Cut the rest of your cabbage into smaller pieces of two to three inches (five to seven centimeters).
3. Shred the cabbage. You can core it if you like, but this is not necessary. It is easier to use a food processor to shred the cabbage. If you don't have one, do it manually with a cheese grater or slice it as thinly as you can with a chef's knife.
4. In a large bowl, mix the shredded cabbage evenly with the sea salt and optional ingredients.
5. Fill about one third of a glass jar or Mason jar with the cabbage mixture. Use a wooden spoon (or ideally a wooden pounder designed for making sauerkraut) and pound the cabbage until it starts to release its juice.
6. Add a bit more cabbage and continue pounding until the jar is almost full. Make sure to leave about one to two inches (two to five centimeters) empty at the top of the jar to allow for expansion during fermentation.
7. Press the pounded cabbage as much as you can until it's covered with its released juice. If there isn't enough juice, you probably haven't pounded the cabbage enough. You can add a brine made with one tablespoon (15 milliliters) of unrefined salt for every two cups (500 milliliters) of water (bottled or non-chlorinated, since the chlorine in tap water can hinder fermentation) if needed. Make sure all the cabbage is covered and not exposed to air.
8. Fold or roll one of the whole cabbage leaves you put aside and fit it on top of the pounded cabbage before replacing the lid. The cabbage leaf will maintain enough pressure to prevent the sauerkraut from floating and being exposed to oxygen.
9. Use more than one jar if needed, following the same steps.
10. Put the lids on your jars and place them on a baking sheet or shallow container. The fermentation process can result in spillover.
11. Leave at room temperature for at least 10 to 14 days.
12. Check your sauerkraut daily to make sure it's always covered with liquid and not in contact with the air. If you see mold forming, simply remove it.
13. After one week, start tasting your sauerkraut each day to see how the taste changes as the fermentation progresses. Once you like its taste, stop the fermentation by transferring your sauerkraut to the refrigerator.
14. Your sauerkraut can be kept in the fridge for months.
15. Add sauerkraut to your soups, stews, meats, eggs, and vegetables.

TIPS:

The time it takes for your sauerkraut to ferment and reach its optimal taste can vary depending on the ambient temperature.

Even if you don't tolerate cabbage because of its FODMAPs, you should be able to tolerate sauerkraut because the fermentation process allows them to break down.

Start gradually with very small amounts of sauerkraut juice and sauerkraut solids to allow time for your gut flora to adjust and minimize unpleasant side effects.

Avoid heating or cooking your sauerkraut to prevent killing its beneficial probiotics (you can place it on warm foods if their temperature is close to your body temperature).

Don't reduce the salt content of the recipe. The salt is necessary to prevent the growth of harmful bacteria and allow only the good probiotic bacteria present in the cabbage to ferment your cabbage safely.

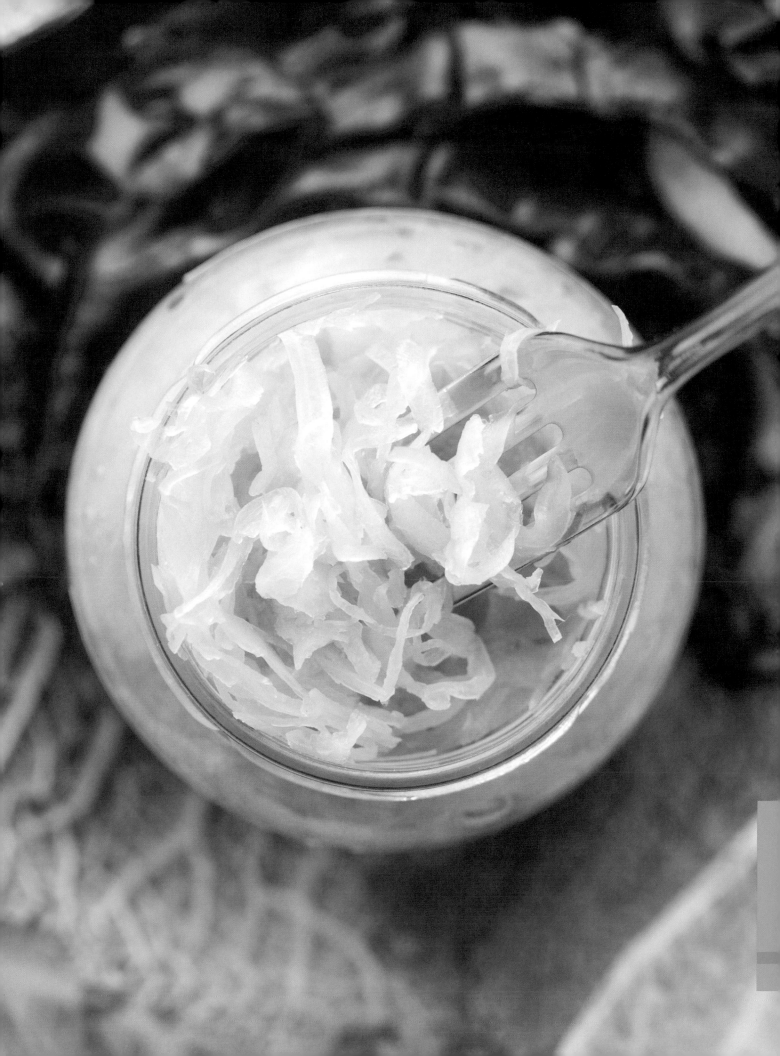

Fermented Carrots | appropriate for the elimination phase

This ferment is probably the easiest to do and the most likely to please unaccustomed taste buds and deliver a wide range of gut-friendly probiotics. The natural sweetness of carrots masks the natural acidity produced by the fermentation process.

INGREDIENTS

Yields 4 cups (1 L):			
Basic ingredients	4 cups	Grated carrots	1 L
	1 tbsp	Sea salt	15 ml
Optional	1 tbsp	Ginger, freshly grated	15 ml

PROCESS

1. Grate the raw carrots with a food processor or cheese grater until you have about four cups grated. You should need about one pound (450 grams) of carrots.
2. In a large bowl, mix the grated carrots evenly with the sea salt (and ginger, if desired).
3. Fill about one third of a glass jar or Mason jar with the carrot mixture. Use a wooden spoon (or a wooden pounder for making sauerkraut) to pound your carrots. Pound the carrots until they start to release their juice.
4. Add more carrots and continue pounding until the jar is almost full. Make sure to leave about one to two inches (two to five centimeters) empty at the top of the jar to allow for expansion during fermentation.
5. Press the pounded carrots as much as you can so they are covered with their released juice. If there isn't enough natural carrot juice, you probably haven't pounded them enough. You can add a brine made with one tablespoon (15 milliliters) of unrefined salt for every two cups (500 milliliters) of water (bottled or non-chlorinated, since the chlorine in tap water can hinder fermentation) if needed. Make sure all the carrots are covered and not exposed to air.
6. Use more than one jar if needed, following the same steps.
7. Put the lids on your jars and place them on a baking sheet or shallow container. The fermentation process can result in spillover.
8. Leave at room temperature for at least three to five days.
9. Check on your fermented carrots daily to make sure they are always covered with liquid and not in contact with the air. If you see mold, simply remove it.
10. After three days, start tasting your fermented carrots each day to see how the taste changes as the fermentation progresses. Once you like the taste, stop the fermentation by transferring them to the refrigerator.
11. Your fermented carrots can be kept in the fridge for months.
12. Eat a little bit before your meals or add it to your soups, stews, meat, eggs, or vegetables.

TIPS:

You can follow the same steps to ferment almost any vegetables, such as cauliflower, onions, cucumbers, etc.

Avoid heating or cooking your carrots to prevent killing their beneficial probiotics (you can put them on warm foods if their temperature is close to your body temperature).

Do not reduce the salt content of this recipe. The salt is necessary to prevent the growth of harmful bacteria and allow only the good probiotic bacteria present in the carrots to ferment them safely.

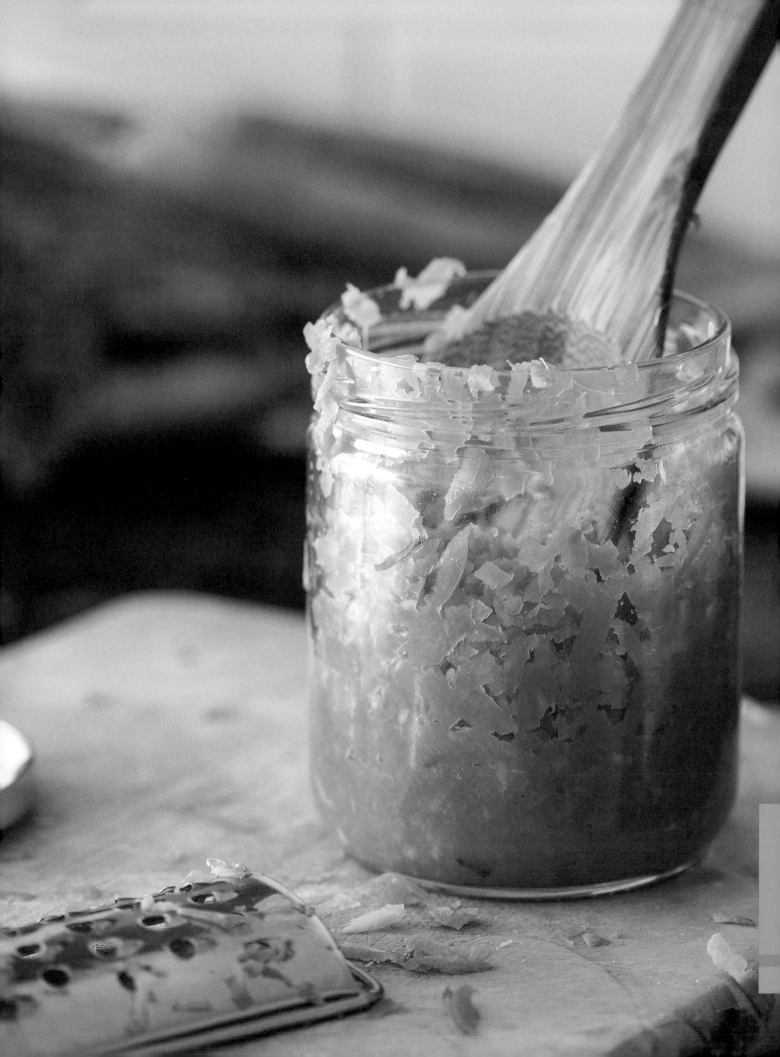

Homemade Yogurt | contains dairy

If you tolerate dairy, or want to give it a try, making your own yogurt is a great food experiment. By fermenting your yogurt for 24 hours, you'll be able to get rid of almost all the natural lactose in the milk. You can experiment with different types of milk: regular cow's milk, Jersey cow's milk, or goat milk. Keep in mind that raw milk and the milk from grass-fed cows and goats is usually better tolerated. Each serving (one half cup or 125 ml) of homemade yogurt will provide you with 350 billion CFU of probiotics, making it a very cheap and effective way to replenish your gut flora. You will need a yogurt maker for this recipe, which you can find online or at your local kitchen store for $30 to $50.

INGREDIENTS

	Yields the same amount of yogurt as the amount of milk used:		
Basic ingredients	4-8 cups	Milk	1-2 L
Fresh batch	1	Yogurt starter kit	1
Ongoing batch	½ cup	Previous batch	125 ml

PROCESS

1. In a large pot, heat the milk. Stir regularly to keep it from burning at the bottom.
2. Use a thermometer and heat until the milk reaches 180°F (80°C). Stir the milk to ensure the temperature is even. This step helps kill any harmful bacteria to prevent them from growing in your yogurt.
3. Turn off the heat and remove the milk from the stove. Let it cool down until it reaches room temperature (67 to 77°F or 20 to 25°C). Don't move on to the next step before the milk has cooled down enough or you risk killing the beneficial probiotic bacteria you'll add in the following steps.
4. Pour the milk through a fine sieve to remove the film that forms on top (optional).
5. In a smaller bowl, mix your yogurt starter kit (one eighth of a teaspoon for four cups or one quarter teaspoon for eight cups; one half milliliter for one liter or 2 milliliters for two liters) with a little bit of the cooled down milk. Alternatively, you can use active yogurt from a previous batch of yogurt. Once dissolved, add the beneficial bacteria to the whole batch of milk and whisk until homogenous.
6. Pour in a yogurt maker, following the instructions provided by your specific model.
7. Put the lid on and plug it in. Your yogurt maker will keep the temperature just right for the fermentation process.
8. Put your yogurt maker in a safe and temperature-stable area of your home. Let ferment for 24 hours.
9. After 24 hours of fermentation, unplug the yogurt maker and transfer your batch of yogurt to the refrigerator.
10. Let it rest for eight hours to allow it to cool fully and set before eating.

TIPS:

The probiotic bacteria will stay alive for two weeks in your yogurt. Your homemade yogurt will be safe to eat for up to three weeks, but the probiotic content will be significantly decreased by the third week.

If you want to use a small amount of a previous batch of yogurt as your starter kit, make sure it's younger than two weeks. If your yogurt seems to be getting weaker with every batch, start fresh with a new yogurt starter kit next time.

You can mix your yogurt with fruit, honey, or maple syrup as desired.

If you want your yogurt to be thicker (similar to Greek yogurt), use a cheese cloth and a sieve to drip it overnight in the fridge.

Introduce your homemade yogurt very gradually to allow your gut flora to adjust.

If you react to 24-hour fermented yogurt, it's likely due to a casein (milk protein) sensitivity.

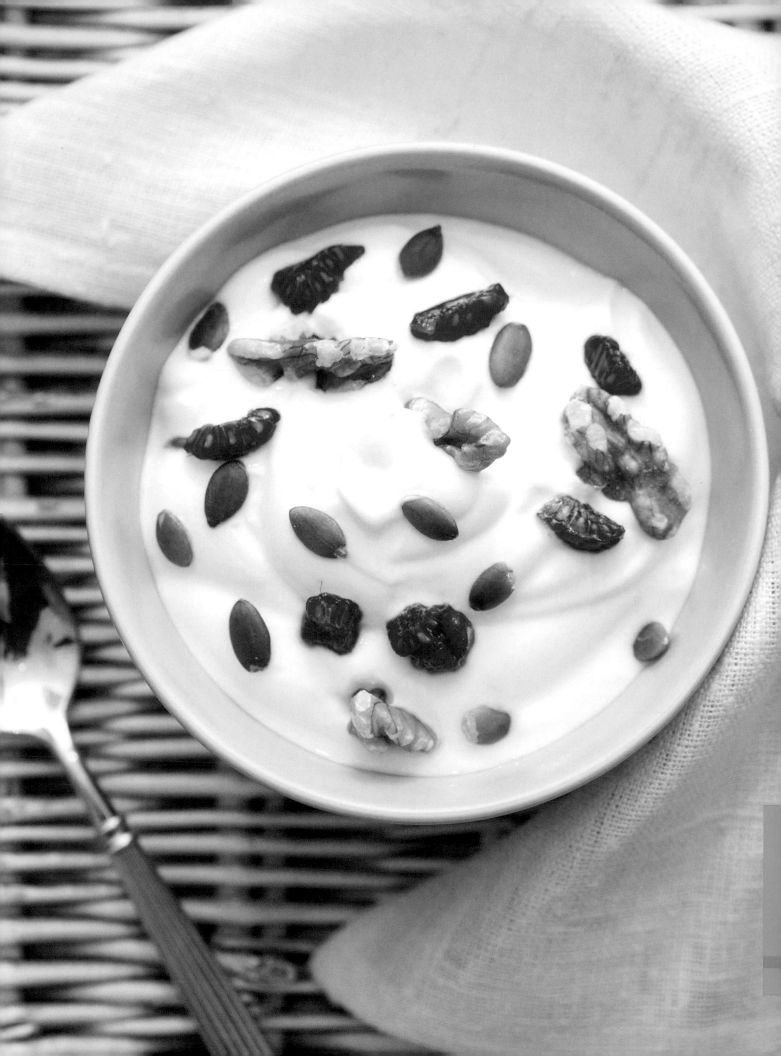

Breakfast Sausages | appropriate for the elimination phase

Breakfast can be the most difficult meal to get used to for many people on this elimination diet protocol. These breakfast sausages are a great option if you don't like to cook in the morning or don't have a lot of time. Prepare a batch on the weekend and you'll have your breakfast ready for one to two weeks (depending on your protein serving size)!

INGREDIENTS

Yields 12 servings of 4 oz (120 g) or 6 servings of 8 oz (240 g):		
3 lb	Ground turkey (or ground beef, bison, pork, etc.)	1.35 kg
2 tsp	Unrefined salt	10 ml
To taste	Seasonings (any combination of thyme, rosemary, basil, oregano, garlic-infused oil, pesto, vinegar, etc.)	To taste

PROCESS

1. Combine the ground meat with the seasonings.
2. Line a baking sheet with a double layer of foil.
3. Spread the ground meat on the lined baking sheet to form a flat loaf.
4. Sprinkle with more seasonings if desired.
5. Wrap the extra foil around your meat.
6. Bake in the oven for 1.5 to two hours at 300°F (150°C). Check the temperature to make sure the sausages are cooked thoroughly (or cut them in the center to ensure they're no longer pink).
7. Cut your block of cooked sausages into equal squares (or other shapes if you prefer). This recipes yield 12 four-ounce (120-gram) servings, eight six-ounce (180-gram) servings, or six eight-ounce (240-gram) servings.
8. Reheat your breakfast sausages in a skillet, with generous amounts of ghee or coconut oil, until browned before serving.

TIPS:

Your breakfast sausages will keep in the fridge for a few days. Freeze your sausages individually so you have an easy breakfast option on hand whenever you need one.

Try to sneak in a little minced organ meat (liver or other) for extra nutrition.

Don't forget to combine your breakfast sausages with plenty of traditional fats (olive oil, coconut oil, ghee, duck fat) and vegetables as tolerated for a complete, nutritious meal.

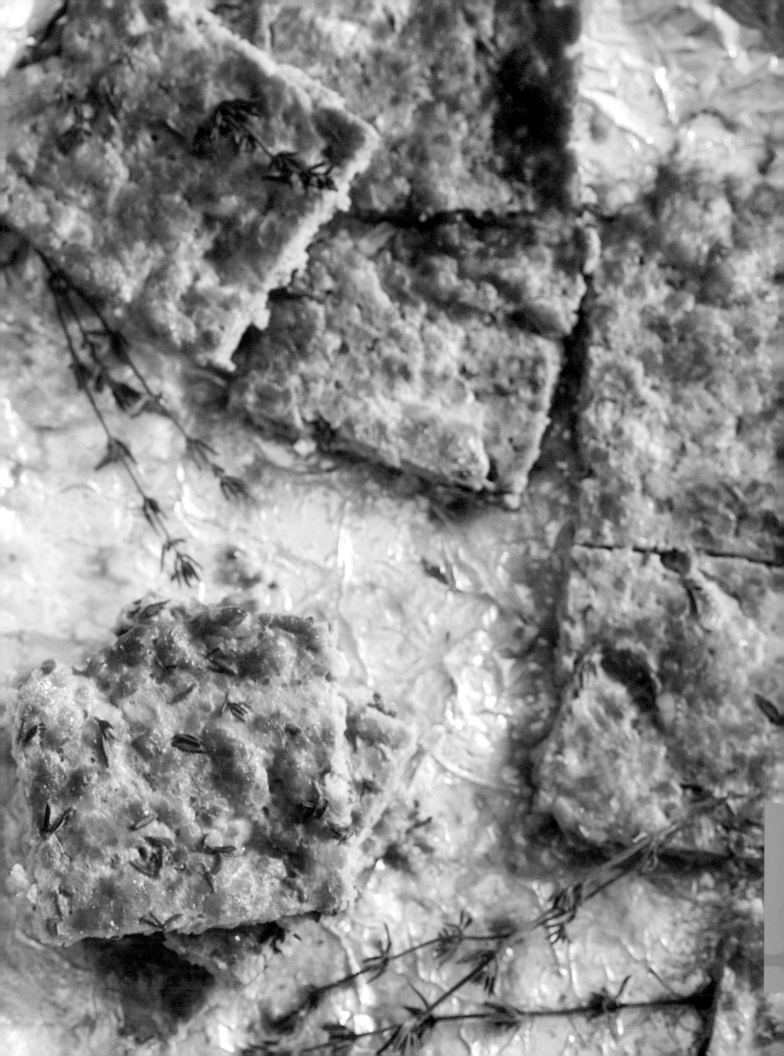

Coconut "Oatmeal" | contains coconut

Do you miss your morning bowl of oatmeal? Grains, even gluten-free oats, can be hard to digest and trigger food-sensitivity reactions. Instead, try this grain-free version using only easy-to-digest REAL food ingredients.

INGREDIENTS

Yields 1 serving:		
¼ cup	Unsweetened dried coconut	60 ml
½-¾ cup	Coconut milk (without guar gum)	125-175 ml
Dash	Unrefined salt	Dash
To taste	Vanilla, cinnamon, banana, mashed pumpkin, berries or nuts (optional)	To taste

PROCESS

1. Put the dried coconut and coconut milk in a small saucepan.
2. Heat under medium heat until it thickens slightly.
3. Combine with the different seasonings and enjoy warm.

TIPS:

Add one to two tablespoons (15 to 30 milliliters) of almond meal or one half tablespoon (seven milliliters) of coconut flour at the first step to thicken your coconut "oatmeal" if desired.

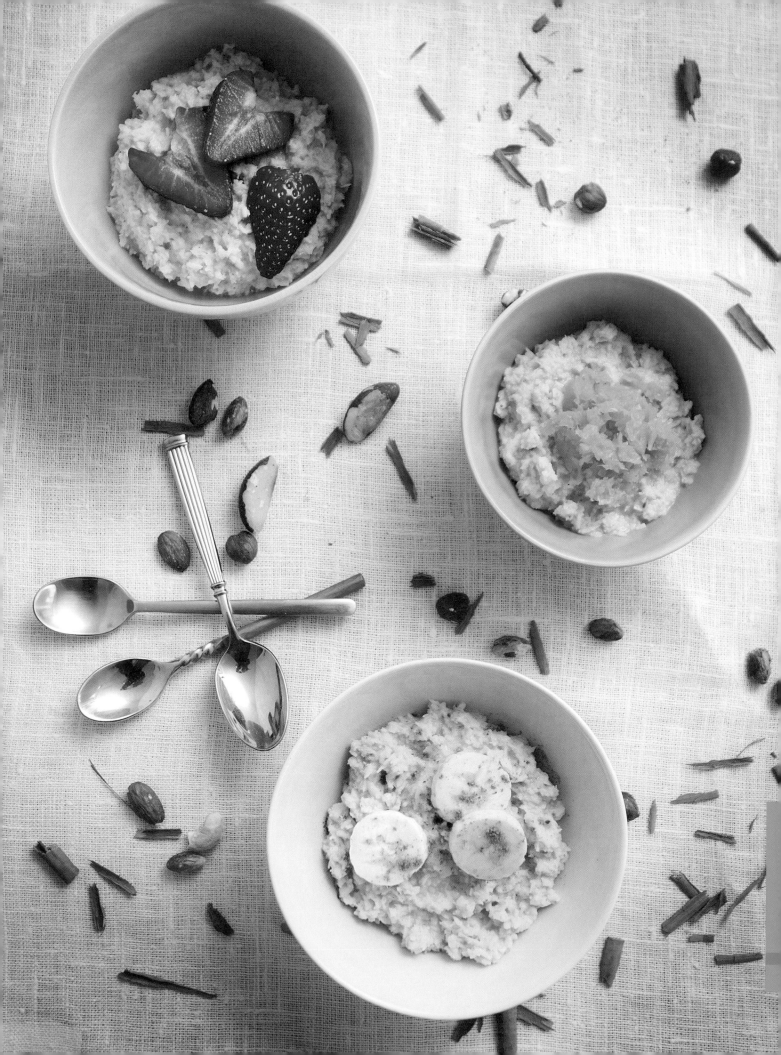

Deviled Eggs | contains eggs

Deviled eggs are a healthy Paleo snack (or breakfast) option if you tolerate eggs. Make your own mayonnaise to get healthy fats since most commercial mayonnaises are made from processed vegetable oils and seed oils (soybean oil, canola oil, etc.). If you don't want to make mayonnaise, use mashed avocado or guacamole with a bit of lemon juice to mix with the cooked egg yolks. Yummy!

INGREDIENTS

Yields 6 deviled eggs (12 halves):		
6	Eggs	6
¼-½ cup	Homemade mayonnaise or guacamole	60-125 ml
To taste	Unrefined salt and seasonings	To taste

PROCESS

1. Put your eggs in a small saucepan.
2. Add just enough water to barely cover them.
3. Bring to a boil. Once the water boils, turn off the heat to keep the water just simmering (the eggs can break if the water boils too long).
4. Cook for about six minutes.
5. After six minutes, drain the hot water from the eggs and cool down under cold water (to prevent a dark circle from appearing around the edge of the yolk).
6. You can also prepare your hard-boiled eggs in advance and refrigerate them until you're ready to make your deviled eggs.
7. Peel the eggs, cut them in half and scoop the yolks out.
8. Put the yolks in a bowl. Add homemade mayonnaise or guacamole and seasonings. Mash everything together until you obtain a smooth consistency.
9. Spoon the yolk mixture back into the egg whites and serve.

TIPS:

Deviled eggs can keep a few days in the fridge, but they don't freeze well.

Pipe the yolk mixture for a fancier presentation.

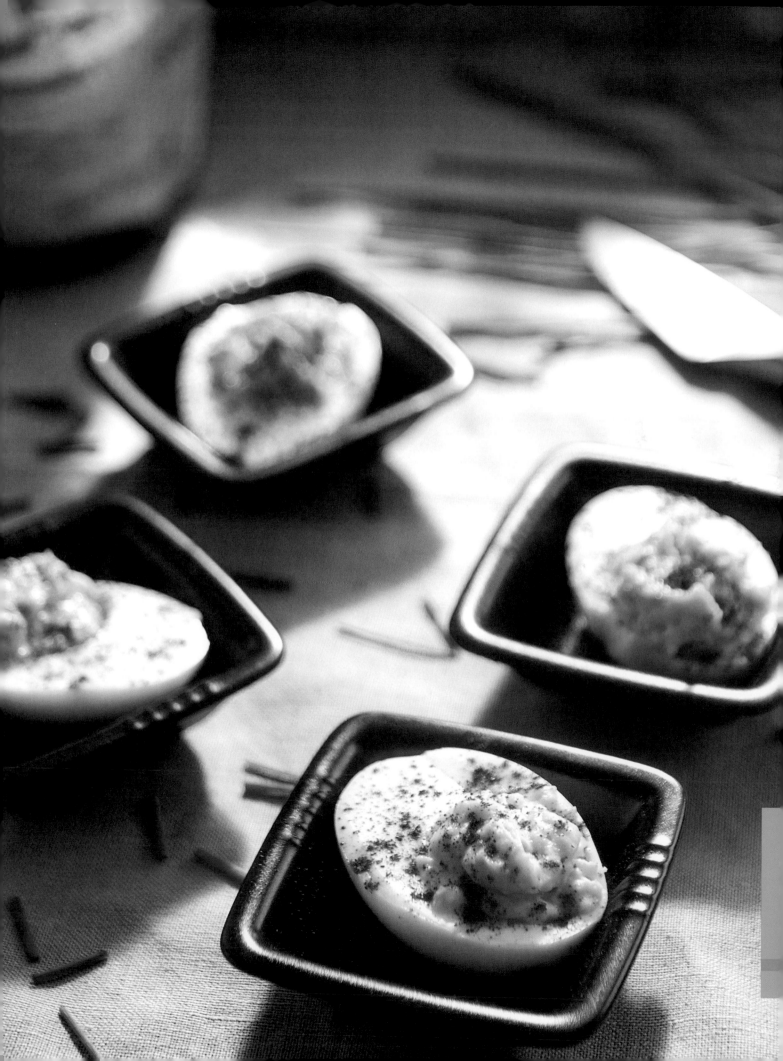

Frittata | contains eggs

This frittata recipe can be used to make hundreds of different frittatas simply by varying the vegetables and seasonings. Try spinach, tomatoes and pesto; mushrooms, broccoli and ginger; or zucchini and lemon.

INGREDIENTS

Yields 1 serving:		
1-2 tbsp	Ghee or coconut oil	15-30 ml
2-4	Eggs, beaten	2-4
½-1 cup	Vegetables	125-250 ml
1-2 oz	Ground meat or chicken, cooked (optional)	30-60 g
To taste	Unrefined salt and other seasonings	To taste

PROCESS

1. Prepare your chosen vegetables by washing them and cutting them as you prefer (diced, sliced, or grated).
2. Heat the fat in a skillet under medium temperature.
3. Add the vegetables. Cook for five to 10 minutes until tender.
4. In a bowl, beat the eggs and add the seasonings to taste (unrefined salt, herbs and spices). Add the cooked ground meat or chicken if desired (optional).
5. Pour the eggs over the vegetables. Cook for about five minutes or until the bottom of the frittata is well cooked.
6. Use a plate to flip your frittata and cook it on the other side. You can also put your skillet (if it is oven proof) in the oven under the grill for about five minutes, or until the top is cooked, instead. If both of these techniques are too complicated, scramble your frittata by breaking it into pieces and turning them to cook the eggs evenly.
7. Serve hot or warm.

TIPS:

Add pieces of bacon, cooked sausages or cheese (as tolerated).

Make a larger batch of frittata and keep leftovers in the fridge to have a quick breakfast or snack the next day.

Make a basic frittata (with eggs only) and once it is cooked, use it as a base for a grain-free pizza!

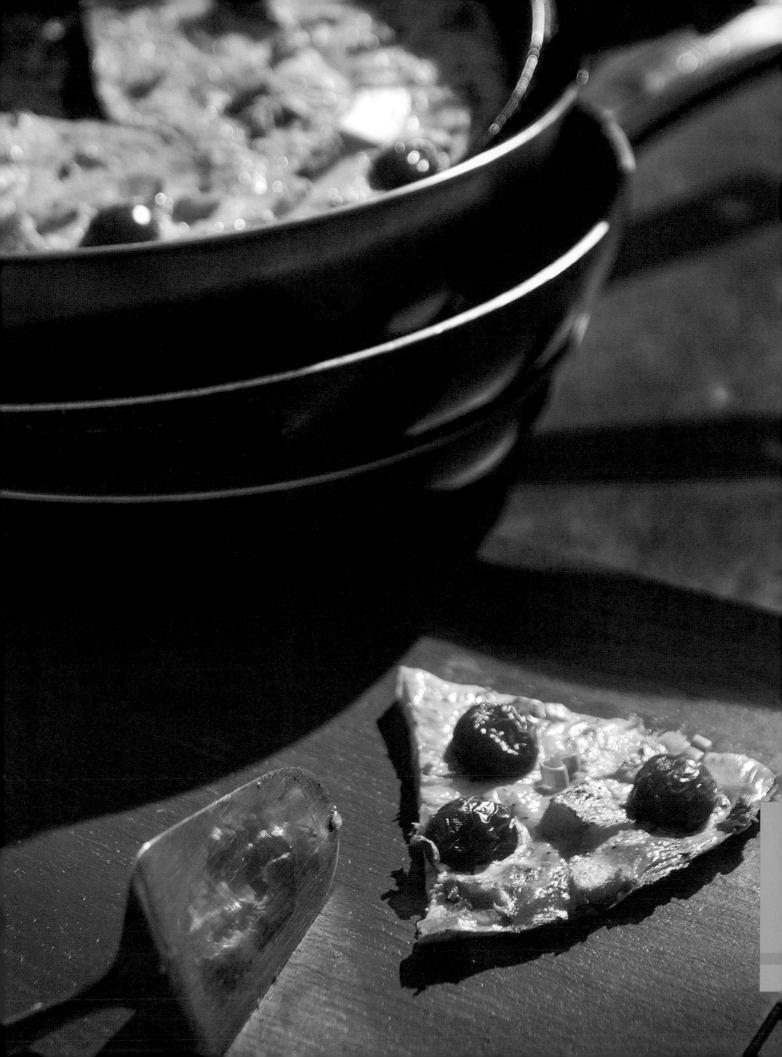

Egg Drop Soup | contains eggs

This recipe makes a simple but quick breakfast or snack combining nutritious protein-rich eggs and gut-healing bone broth. It's a nice way to serve your eggs differently.

INGREDIENTS

Yields 1 serving:		
1-1.5 cup	Bone broth	250-375 ml
2-3	Eggs	2-3
To taste	Unrefined salt and seasonings (chives)	To taste

PROCESS

1. Add your homemade bone broth to a saucepan and bring to a boil.
2. Meanwhile, beat the eggs in a bowl.
3. Once the broth boils, slowly pour the beaten eggs in the boiling broth and whisk constantly to form long strands of cooked eggs.
4. Season to taste with unrefined salt and other seasonings. Fresh chive works great with this soup.
5. Enjoy immediately.

TIPS:

Add Asian flavors by using a bit of freshly grated ginger and coconut aminos (or gluten-free tamari sauce) to your broth.

If desired, you can start your soup by cooking onions and other vegetables in ghee or coconut oil in the saucepan before adding the broth and following the next steps.

If you prefer, you can cook the beaten eggs in a separate skillet to form a crêpe. Once cook, cut into long strings and add to the bone broth.

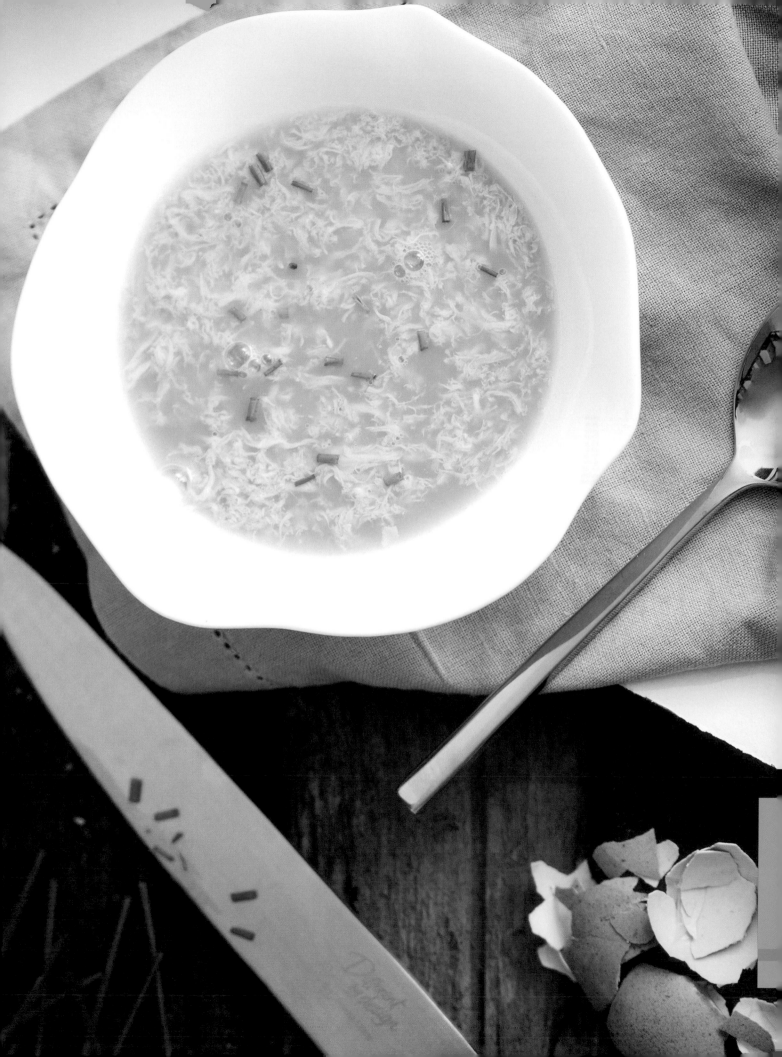

Carrot Treat | appropriate for the elimination phase

If you want to satisfy your sweet tooth without flours, sugars, or fruits, try this coconut treat. The cinnamon and coconut oil bring out the natural sweetness of carrots. Use as much cinnamon as you like. This spice has antibacterial properties and can even help with blood-sugar regulation.

INGREDIENTS

Yields 1 serving:		
½-1 cup	Carrots, puréed	125-250 ml
1-2 tsp	Cinnamon	5-10 ml
1-2 tbsp	Coconut oil	15-30 ml

PROCESS

1. Mix the puréed carrots with the coconut oil and cinnamon. Start with a small amount of cinnamon and increase to taste. You can also omit the coconut oil and use it to top your carrot treat instead.
2. Enjoy warm or cold.

TIPS:

Add one or two raw egg yolks (if they come from free-range eggs and if you trust your source) for extra creaminess.

Prepare your carrot treat with a little extra fat and one or two raw egg yolks and refrigerate overnight, then enjoy it for breakfast. You can have it warm or cold (the coconut oil will harden and give it an interesting texture).

Make a large batch. Carrot purée will keep in the fridge for at least four to five days.

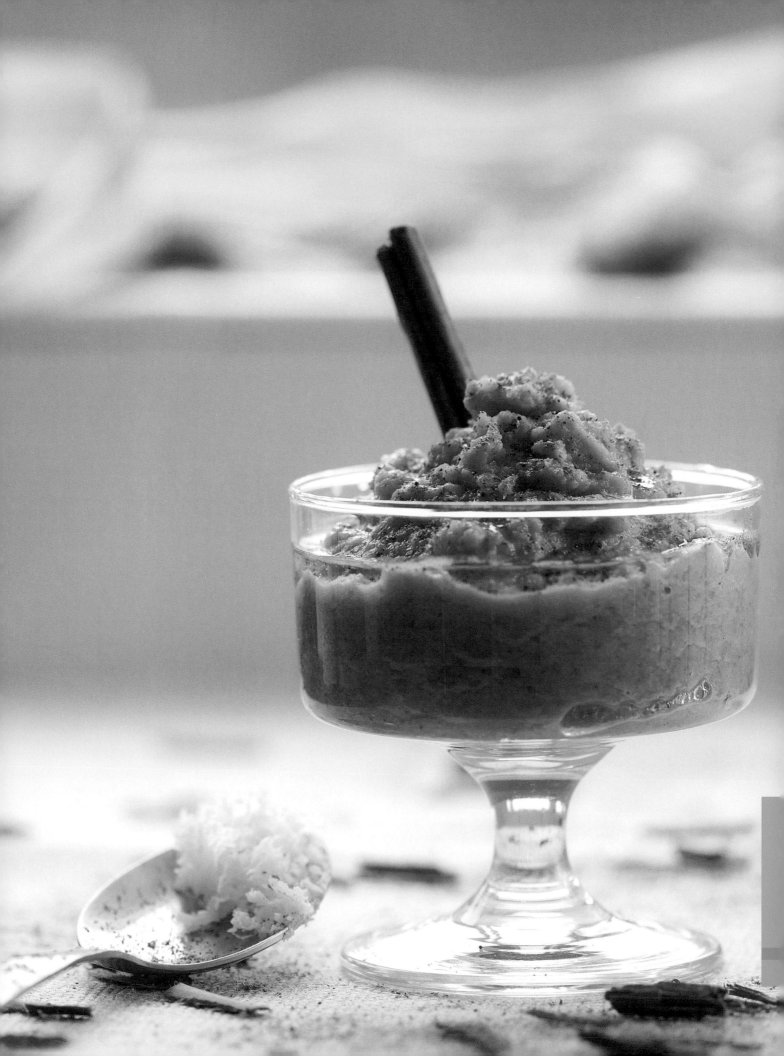

Grain-Free, Sugar-Free Carrot Cupcakes | contains eggs

These carrot cupcakes are a great treat to add to your diet as soon as you can successfully reintroduce eggs. If you're eating out, bring a few of these grain-free and sugar-free cupcakes with you to have a safe dessert to enjoy with everyone else.

INGREDIENTS

Yields 12 cupcakes:		
4-5	Eggs	4-5
1.5-2 cups	Carrot purée	375-500 ml
2 tsp	Cinnamon (more if desired)	10 ml
¼-½ cup	Coconut oil (optional)	60-125 ml

PROCESS

1. Beat the eggs.
2. Add the carrot purée and cinnamon. Mix well.
3. Add the melted coconut oil if desired.
4. Pour the batter in a greased muffin tin (or used silicone muffin cups).
5. Bake at 350°F (180°C) for about 20 minutes or until golden.
6. Let cool and serve spread with coconut oil or butter.
7. The cupcakes can be kept in the fridge for a few days.

TIPS:

Replace the carrot with grated zucchini or puréed butternut squash.

You can ice your cooled cupcakes with creamy ghee (plain or seasoned to taste with unsweetened dried coconut, vanilla extract, honey, or maple syrup).

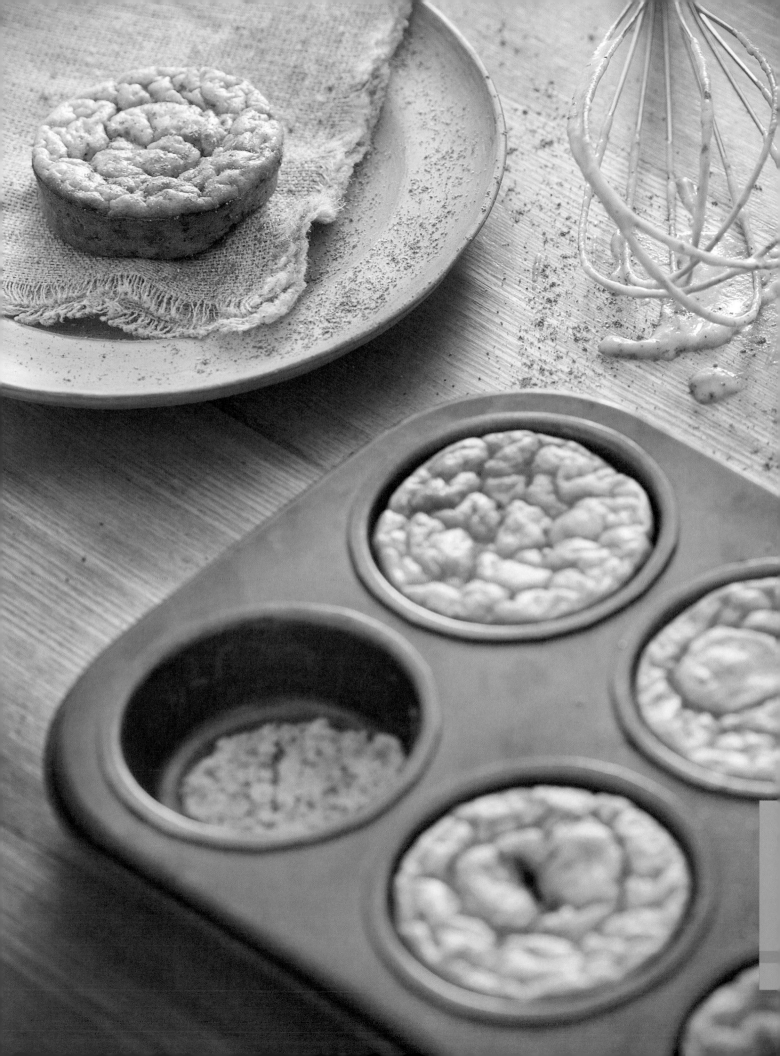

Baked Apple Pudding | contains coconut and apple

This pudding is so rich and unctuous, you won't miss the dairy-based kind. It's perfect for dessert or anytime you need a little pick-me-up energy boost between meals.

INGREDIENTS

Yields about 2-3 cups (500-750 ml):		
1 can	Coconut milk	1 can
2	Apples, grated or cut into cubes	2
To taste	Vanilla extract, cinnamon and nutmeg (optional)	To taste

PROCESS

1. Put the apple in a baking dish.
2. Cover with the coconut milk.
3. Bake in the oven at 350°F (180°C) for about 30 to 45 minutes, or until the apples are cooked (it will take less time if the apples are grated and more time with large apple cubes).
4. Let cool, season to taste, and enjoy warm or cold.

TIPS:

Make a large batch and enjoy this baked apple pudding for breakfast or snack.

You can also make your apple pudding on the stove. Bring the coconut milk to a boil and let the apple simmer for about 25 to 30 minutes or until tender.

Add almond butter or roasted walnuts if desired for extra protein.

The tangy taste of green apples combines nicely with the natural sweetness of coconut milk, but red apples work just as well.

Blend your pudding in a blender or food processor for a smoother consistency.

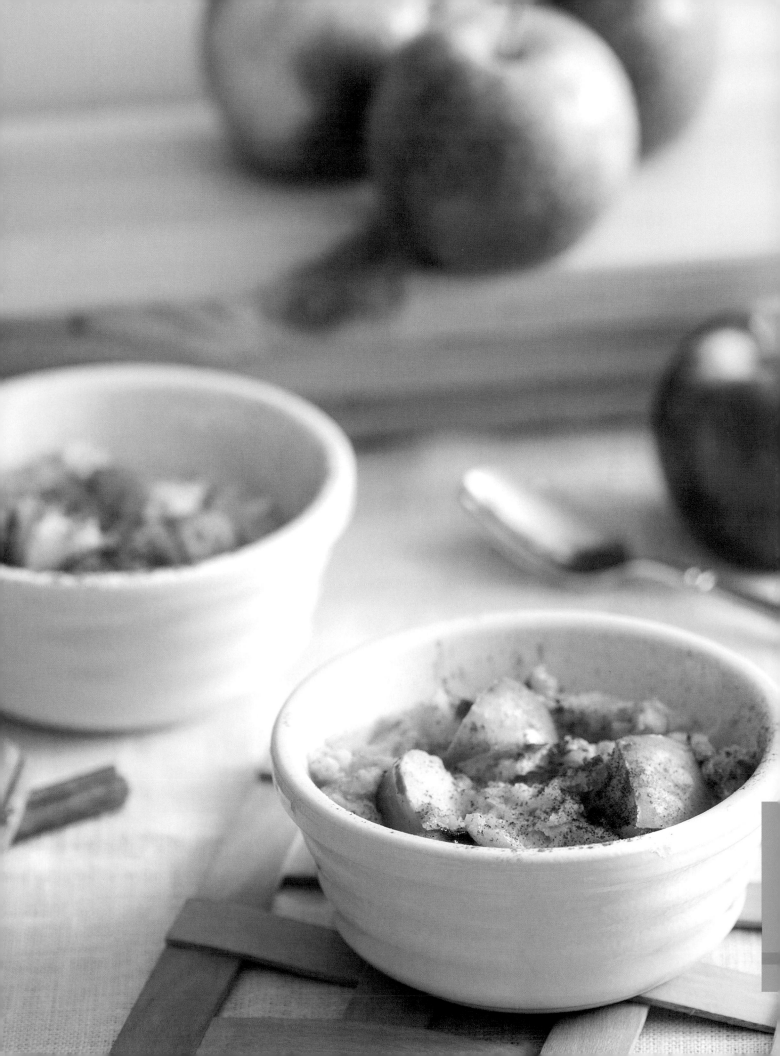

Avocado Mousse | contains avocado, coconut, and/or nuts

You don't need dairy to enjoy a delicious mousse for dessert. Don't let the green color of this mousse put you off: Its delicate taste and creaminess are divine. Serve with a dollop of coconut whipped cream if desired.

INGREDIENTS

Yields 1 serving:		
½-1	Avocado	½-1
1-2 tbsp	Nut butter or coconut butter	15-30 ml
2 tbsp	Unsweetened dried coconut (optional)	30 ml

PROCESS

1. Put all the ingredients in a food processor and blend until smooth, adding just enough nut butter or coconut butter to obtain a smooth texture.
2. Enjoy!

TIPS:

Add one to two tablespoons (15 to 30 milliliters) unsweetened cocoa powder and a bit of vanilla for a chocolate version of this avocado mousse.

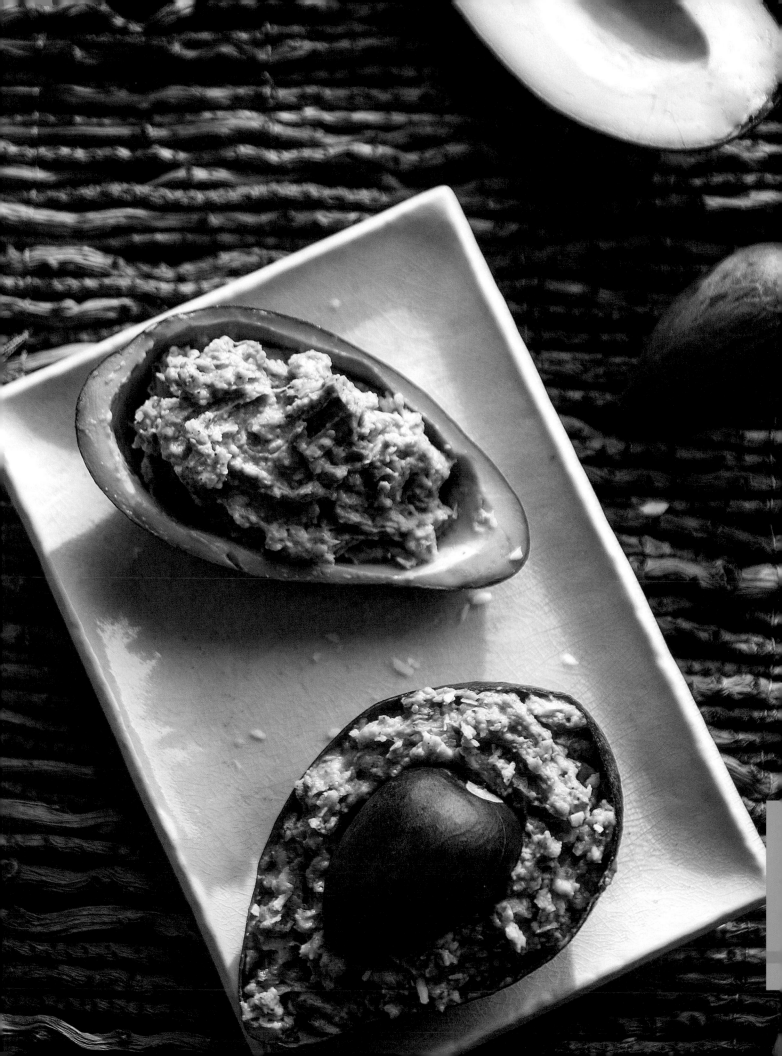

Coconut Macaroons | contains eggs and coconut

Coconut macaroons don't contain any flour or grain: only egg whites and coconut flakes. French macaroons are similar, but contain almond meal instead of coconut, in addition to dairy in the icing and some added colorings and sugars.

INGREDIENTS

Yields about 12 macaroons:		
2	Egg whites	2
2 ½ cups	Unsweetened coconut flakes	625 ml
Dash	Unrefined salt	Dash

PROCESS

1. Whisk the egg whites in a clean bowl until thick.
2. Gently fold in the coconut flakes and the salt.
3. Drop the macaroon mixture on a lined baking sheet.
4. Bake in the oven at 350°F (180°C) for about 10 to 12 minutes or until the coconut macaroons are lightly golden.
5. Let cool and serve.

TIPS:

Add one quarter cup of honey, unsweetened cocoa powder, or nuts if desired.

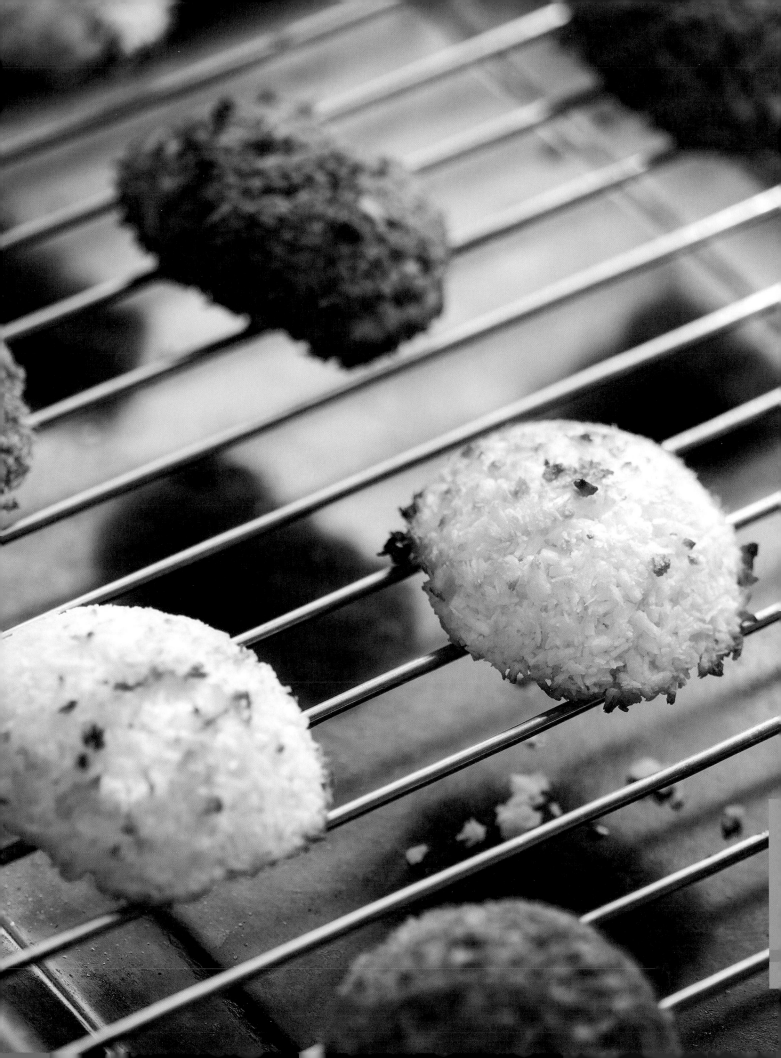

No-Bake Frozen Cookies | contains coconut and nuts

If you don't enjoy baking, try these no-bake frozen cookies. They're a cinch to make and are a refreshing and crunchy treat to enjoy year-round.

INGREDIENTS

Yields about 12 cookies:		
1/3 cup	Coconut oil	80 ml
1/3 cup	Nut butter	80 ml
2 cups	Unsweetened dried coconut	500 ml

PROCESS

1. Drop the cookies on a lined baking sheet.
2. Freeze for two to three hours or until firm.
3. Place the frozen cookies in a hermetic container and keep in the freezer.
4. Enjoy cold or let warm up a few minutes at room temperature before eating.

TIPS:

Add one third cup (80 milliliters) honey or maple syrup and two tablespoons (30 milliliters) of unsweetened cocoa powder if tolerated.

Add dried fruits and nuts if desired.

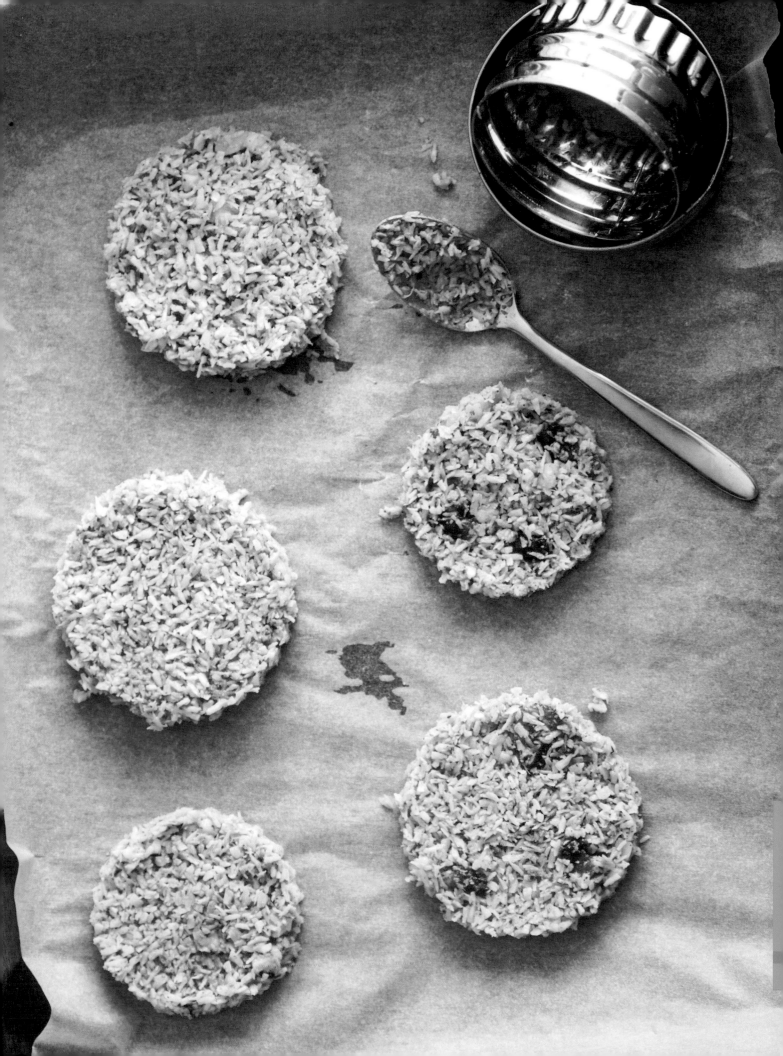

Infused Water | appropriate for the elimination phase

If you don't like drinking plain water, try infusing water with the natural flavors of fresh herbs, tea leaves, and fruits.

INGREDIENTS

Fresh herbs	Tea	Vegetables	Fruits
elimination phase as tolerated			
Mint	Green tea	Cucumber	Watermelon
Rosemary	Rooibos tea		Berries
Sage	Herbal tea		Pineapple
Thyme			Oranges
Lavender			Lemon
Tarragon			Lime
Basil			Kiwi

PROCESS

1. Add a combination of herbs, tea leaves, vegetables, and fruits in a pitcher or large glass jar.
2. Fill with water and leave in the fridge overnight.
3. Strain your infused water and enjoy cold!

TIPS:

If you use tea, brew a large pot of tea. Add fruits if desired. Let cool, then transfer to a glass pitcher or jar and refrigerate overnight.

Raspberry and mint, lemon and mint, and orange and lavender are great combinations, but don't be afraid to experiment with different infusions to come up with your own creations!

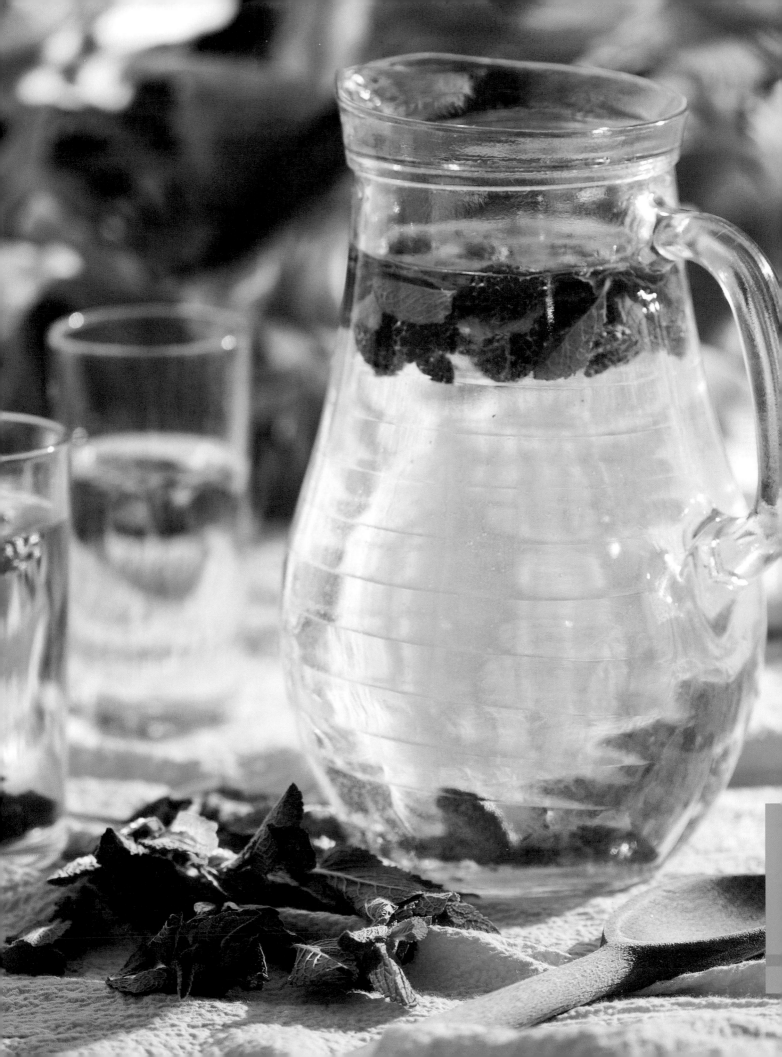

(Find this recipe on pg. 252)

Table 83: Mix-and-Match Chart

	Protein	Fats	Vegetables	Seasonings
Serving	4-8 oz (120-240 g) per person per meal, adjusted as needed to stay full until next meal	1-3 tbsp (15-45 ml) per person per meal, adjusted as needed to stay full until next meal	¼-¾ cup (60-175 ml) per person per meal at first, increased as tolerated	☑ ½-1 tsp (2-5 ml) of unrefined salt per day ☑ Other seasonings can be used to taste
Elimination Phase	☑ Beef ☑ Chicken ☑ Duck ☑ Turkey ☑ Lamb ☑ Pork ☑ Venison ☑ Wild boar ☑ Bison ☑ Fish ☑ Seafood	☑ Ghee ☑ Coconut oil ☑ Olive oil ☑ Avocado oil ☑ Macadamia oil ☑ Duck fat ☑ Lard ☑ Tallow	☑ Carrots ☑ Zucchini ☑ Spinach ☑ Green beans ★ Boiled, steamed, stir-fried, roasted, puréed or vegetable fries Always cooked thoroughly and ideally peeled, de-seeded, and puréed	☑ Unrefined salt ☑ Apple cider vinegar ☑ Fresh herbs ☑ Dried herbs ☑ Lemon ☑ Lime ☑ Cinnamon ☑ Garlic-infused oil ☑ Homemade pesto ☑ Ginger ☑ Chives ☑ Green onions (green part) ☑ Asafoetida powder ☑ Lemon butter sauce ☑ Herbed ghee ☑ Reduction sauce
As Tolerated	☑ Eggs ☑ Shrimps ☑ Sausages (gluten-free) ☑ Ham, prosciutto and deli meat (gluten-free and sugar-free) ☑ Smoked fish	☑ Avocado ☑ Butter ☑ Homemade mayo ☑ Hollandaise sauce ☑ Cream ☑ Coconut milk and coconut cream (without guar gum) ☑ Unsweetened dried coconut ☑ Uncured bacon ☑ Nuts ☑ Nut butters ☑ Basic vinaigrette ☑ Guacamole ☑ Avocado dressing	☑ Cauliflower ☑ Broccoli ☑ Cabbage ☑ Tomato ☑ Onion ☑ Garlic ☑ Asparagus ☑ Bok choy ☑ Beets ☑ Butternut squash ☑ Spaghetti squash ☑ Turnip ☑ Eggplant ☑ Brussels sprouts ☑ Bell pepper ☑ Mushroom	☑ Balsamic vinegar ☑ Red wine vinegar ☑ Black pepper ☑ Chili powder ☑ Chili sauce ☑ Turmeric and other spices ☑ Coconut aminos ☑ Tamari sauce (gluten free) ☑ Sea vegetables ☑ Sundried tomato ☑ Mustard powder ☑ Tomato sauce ☑ Fermented foods

(Find this recipe on pg. 270)

Table 86: Vegetable and Seasoning Options

	Elimination Phase	As Tolerated				
		High-FOD-MAPs	Cruciferous	Nightshades	Medium carb vegetables	Starchy vegetables*
Vegetables	Carrots	Asparagus	Cauliflower	Tomato	Pumpkin	Sweet potato
	Zucchini	Onion	Broccoli	Cherries	Butternut squash	White potato**
	Spinach	Artichoke	Brussels sprouts	Eggplant	Acorn squash	Taro root
	Green beans	Mushrooms	Bok choy	Bell pepper	Beet	Yucca/cassava
		Snow peas	Cabbage		Turnip	Parsnip
		Fennel	Kale		Rutabaga	
		Celery	Swiss chards		Jicama	

	Vary your vegetables and spice things up!	Elimination Phase	As Tolerated
Seasonings	Add during or after cooking	Rosemary, basil, oregano, parsley, thyme, chives, green part of green onions, ginger, lemon/lime zest or juice, asafoetida powder, garlic-infused oil	Balsamic or red wine vinegar, tomato sauce, coconut milk, coconut-Asian sauce, honey
	Add after cooking	Pesto, lemon-butter sauce, reduction sauce	Avocado dressing, hollandaise sauce, butter, basic vinaigrette, caramelized onion jam, caramelized garlic, cream
	Extra fats for your purées or to dip your vegetables	Ghee, coconut oil, creamy ghee, garlic-infused oil, herbed ghee/butter, pesto, lemon-butter sauce, fresh and dried herbs, cinnamon, nutmeg, cardamom	Avocado dressing, creamy salad dressing, guacamole, homemade mayonnaise, egg yolks, cream, coconut-Asian sauce, caramelized garlic, caramelized onion jam

*Avoid starchy vegetables for a while if you have SIBO; **White potatoes are also a nightshade

Want More Recipes?

There are also plenty of great recipe resources online or in cookbooks—just make sure to look for recipes in line with the principles of the Paleo diet, GAPS plan, or SCD. Keep in mind that you'll always need to make a few adjustments according to your personal tolerances, but at least you'll have grain-free, dairy-free, legume-free, and sugar-free recipes that can be modified easily for your personal BYO diet. Here's a quick list to get you started!

PALEO PRINCIPLES:

- The Healthy Gluten-free Life: 200 Delicious Gluten-Free, Dairy-Free, Soy-Free and Egg-Free Recipes! By Tammy Credicott (2012)
- Make it Paleo: Over 200 Grain Free Recipes For Any Occasion by Bill Staley, Hayley Mason and Mark Sisson (2011)
- Everyday Paleo Family Cookbook: Real Food for Real Life by Sarah Fragoso (2012)
- Practical Paleo: A Customized Approach to Health and a Whole-Foods Lifestyle by Diane Sanfilippo, Bill Staley and Robb Wolf (2012)
- Paleo Slow Cooking: Gluten Free Recipes Made Simple by Chrissy Gower and Robb Wolf (2012)
- Paleo Comfort Foods: Homestyle Cooking for a Gluten-Free Kitchen by Julie Sullivan Mayfield, Charles Mayfield, Mark Adams and Robb Wolf (2011)
- Well Fed: Paleo Recipes for People Who Love to Eat by Melissa Joulwan, David Humphreys and Kathleen Shannon (2011)
- Eat Like a Dinosaur: Recipe & Guidebook for Gluten-free Kids by Paleo Parents and Elana Amsterdam (2012)

WESTON A. PRICE PRINCIPLES:

- Nourishing Traditions: The Cookbook that Challenges Politically Correct Nutrition and the Diet Dictocrats by Sally Fallon and Mary Enig (1999)

GAPS DIET:

- Internal Bliss – GAPS Cookbook (Recipes designed for those following the Gut and Psychology Syndrome Diet) by GAPSdiet.com (2010)

SPECIFIC CARBOHYDRATE DIET (SDC):

- Breaking the Vicious Cycle: Intestinal Health Through Diet by Elaine G. Gottschall (1994)
- Recipes for the Specific Carbohydrate Diet: The Grain-Free, Lactose-Free, Sugar-Free Solution to IBD, Celiac Disease, Autism, Cystic Fibrosis, and Other Health Conditions by Raman Prasad (2008)

Other Resources:

FIND GOOD-QUALITY FOODS:

- Eatwild.com (meat, eggs, and dairy)
- Localharvest.org (produce)
- U.S. Wellness Meats (meat and dairy)
- Tropical Traditions (coconut products and soy-free eggs)

You can also contact your local chapter of the Weston A. Price Foundation for help finding quality foods in your area of the world.

Chapter 11: Meal Plans

In this chapter, you'll find two weekly meal plans: one for the elimination phase (p. 339) and one for a more varied BYO diet following the reintroduction phase that includes eggs and more vegetables (p. 340). You'll also find a table with many snack and treat ideas (p. 341) for all phases of this nutrition protocol as well as a section detailing portion sizes (Table 87 below) to help you get enough calories.

You don't have to follow these meal plans to the letter, but let them inspire you to get started on a REAL-food-based diet. All the meals are interchangeable. You can also cook a larger batch of any one meal and eat it multiple days in a row to save time in the kitchen.

The Numbers

To be successful with your elimination diet, it's important to eat *enough* to satisfy your body's energy requirements. If you don't, you'll be more likely to suffer cravings and end up eating something your digestive system doesn't like.

Most women need around 2,000 calories per day to *maintain* a healthy weight, while most men need around 2,500 calories. You can go a little lower if you're trying to lose weight or a bit higher if trying to gain weight. In either case, make sure you eat enough. Eat at least 1,600 calories per day to ensure you provide your body with all the nutrients and energy it needs to heal.

Table 87 tells you how many serving of protein and fat you need each day and at each meal to get enough calories and Table 88 shows you what each serving of protein and fat corresponds to.

Table 87: How Much to Eat to Get Your Calories

Recommended Intake			1,600 calories	2,000 calories	2,500 calories	3,000 calories
Daily Total		Protein	15 oz (450 g)	18 oz (540 g)	24 oz (720 g)	27 oz (810 g)
		Fat	6 tbsp (90 ml)	8 tbsp (120 ml)	10 tbsp (150 ml)	12 tbsp (180 ml)
		Vegetables	As tolerated	As tolerated	As tolerated	As tolerated
Intake Per Meal	3 meals per day	Protein	5 oz (150 g)	6 oz (180 g)	8 oz (240 g)	9 oz (270 g)
		Fat	2 tbsp (30 ml)	2-3 tbsp (20-45 ml)	3-4 tbsp (45-60 ml)	4 tbsp (60 ml)
		Vegetables	As tolerated	As tolerated	As tolerated	As tolerated
	4 meals per day	Protein	3.5-4 oz (100-120 g)	4.5 oz (135 g)	6 oz (180 g)	6.5-7 oz (195-210 g)
		Fat	1.5 tbsp (22 ml)	2 tbsp (30 ml)	2.5 tbsp (38 ml)	3 tbsp (45 ml)
		Vegetables	As tolerated	As tolerated	As tolerated	As tolerated

*One calorie is equivalent to 4.18 kilojoules; don't forget to add seasonings to taste!

Table 88: Serving Equivalents

Food Groups	Serving Size	Foods
1 oz Protein	1 oz (30 g)	Poultry, meat, fish, liver, seafood, etc.
	1 large	Egg
1 Tbsp Fat	1 tbsp (15 ml)	Ghee, coconut oil, olive oil, homemade mayonnaise, butter, etc.
	½ oz (15 g) of nuts	Nuts (10 walnut halves, 5-8 macadamia kernels, or 12 almonds)
	1 tbsp (15 ml)	Nut butter
	¼ large or ½ small	Avocado
	½ cup (125 ml)	Guacamole
	3 tbsp (45 ml)	Dried, unsweetened coconut
	1.5 tbsp (22 ml)	Coconut butter
	¼ cup (60 ml)	Coconut milk
1 Serving Carbs	½-1 cup (125-250 m)	Fruits, winter squashes, starchy vegetables, roots, and tubers

If you're worried about your weight, eliminate one tablespoon of fat or two ounces of protein for each serving of carbs you reintroduce into your diet.

Now that you know how much to eat to get the calories you need in the elimination phase, see Table 89 below for an example of what a week of eating might look like in this phase.

Table 89: Weekly Meal Plan: Elimination Phase

Days	Meal #1	Meal #2	Meal #3
Mon	Breakfast sausages (p. 308) with puréed carrots and coconut oil	Chicken pesto zucchini pasta (p. 260)	Lamb and carrot stew (p. 248)
Tue	Leftovers from last night: lamb and carrot stew	Chicken with lemon butter sauce (p. 278) and green beans	Steak seasoned with rosemary, with roasted zucchini and drizzled with garlic-infused oil (p. 284)
Wed	Breakfast sausages (p. 308) with puréed carrots and coconut oil	Monday-lunch leftovers: chicken pesto zucchini pasta	Beef or bison patties mixed with basil and oregano, with carrot fries (p. 272)
Thu	Leftovers from last night: beef patties with pesto (p. 280) and leftover veggies	Canned tuna mixed with olive oil, lemon juice and cooked spinach	Chicken, carrot, and zucchini soup (p. 250) with green onions (green part only)
Fri	Salmon cakes with cooked spinach drizzled with lemon juice and olive oil (freeze leftovers)	Pork chops with green beans and ghee	Chicken cooked in olive oil and ginger with carrot fries (p. 272)
Sat	Thursday-dinner leftovers: chicken, carrot, and zucchini soup with green onions (green part only)	Chicken kebabs (p. 262) dipped in pesto (p. 280) served with roasted zucchini and carrots and drizzled with olive oil	Zucchini noodles with steak and reduction sauce (p. 286)
Sun	Meat cupcakes (p. 264) with carrot purée (freeze extra cupcakes without icing for next week)	Breakfast sausages (p. 308) with puréed carrots and coconut oil	Salmon filet and green beans cooked in ghee and seasoned to taste

Once you hit the reintroduction stage, you'll be able to start trialing new foods. Table 90 gives you a snapshot of a week on this branching-out phase.

Table 90: Weekly Meal Plan: Reintroduction Phase (Includes eggs, more vegetables, and seasonings)

Days	Meal #1	Meal #2	Meal #3
Mon	Breakfast sausages (p. 308) with broccoli and coconut oil	Salad of avocado and hard boiled eggs, drizzled with olive oil and lemon juice	Stew (p. 248): lamb, rosemary, carrots, onions, and turnips
Tue	Omelet baked in a muffin tin (based on the frittata recipe on p. 314) with fermented carrots (p. 304) (freeze leftover for snacks or breakfasts next week)	Leftover stew from last night	Salad (p. 256) with leafy greens, tomatoes, chicken, avocado, and basic vinaigrette (make a double batch to have extra for lunch tomorrow)
Wed	Leftover salad from last night	Leftover stew with sauerkraut (p. 302) or fermented carrots (p. 304)	Steak served with guacamole, sauerkraut (p. 302), and cauliflower mashed (p. 274) with herbs and butter and roasted vegetables (p. 270)
Thu	Leftover stew from Tuesday night with a bit of sauerkraut (p. 302)	Frittata (p. 314) with mushroom, spinach, ginger, and coconut aminos (or gluten-free tamari sauce)	Salmon cakes (p. 266) served with curry mayonnaise (p. 288) and roasted Brussels sprouts (p. 270)
Fri	Fried eggs served with leftover vegetables and bacon	Zucchini noodles with tomato sauce and ground beef	Chicken with coconut aminos or gluten-free tamari sauce and bok choy cooked in coconut oil
Sat	Omelet muffins (based on the frittata recipe on p. 314)	Leftovers from last night	Bison burger with portobello mushroom caps (p. 268), sauerkraut (p. 302), and butternut squash fries (p. 272)
Sun	Eggs Benedict made with portobello mushroom caps, poached eggs and home hollandaise	Leftover bison burger served over leafy greens with basic vinaigrette (p. 290)	Shrimp dipped in garlic-infused oil (p. 284) with cauli-rice (p. 276), stir-fried in olive oil with onions and bell pepper

If you need a little extra something to complete a meal or a pick-me-up to sustain your energy until your next meal, Table 91 gives you some more ideas to try.

Table 91: Snack and Treat Ideas

	Savory	Sweet
Elimination Phase	• Leftovers • Canned tuna • Tea with coconut oil • Homemade bone broth (p. 244) • Cooked vegetables with ghee (p. 246) or coconut oil • Soups (regular or blended, p. 250)	• Carrot treat (p. 318) • Spoonful of ghee (p. 246) or coconut oil • Green tea and raspberry gelatin squares (p. 292) • Infused water (p. 330)
Reintroduction Phase (As Tolerated)	• Roasted vegetables (p. 270) with ghee, butter, or coconut oil • Vegetable fries (p. 272) with avocado dressing, homemade mayonnaise (p. 288), or guacamole • Omelet "muffins" • Salad (leftover vegetables + meat + olive oil + seasonings) • Olives • Avocado and tomato slices drizzled with olive oil and balsamic vinegar • Avocado slices drizzled with coconut milk • Frittata (p. 314) • Jerky • Bacon, prosciutto, or deli meat • Prosciutto- or bacon-wrapped asparagus • Shrimp dipped in garlic-infused oil (p. 284) (or garlic butter) or tomato sauce • Guacamole rolled in smoked salmon slices • Pickles • Chicken liver pâté (p. 294) on cucumber slices • Eggplant crackers • Vegetables dipped in homemade mayonnaise (p. 288) or guacamole • Kale chips (p. 298) • Deviled eggs (p. 312) • Avocado & egg salad with mayonnaise (p. 288) • Egg-drop soup (p. 316) • Chicken kebabs (p. 262)	• Fresh fruit (plain or drizzled with coconut milk) • Puréed pumpkin or squash mixed with coconut butter, coconut milk, cinnamon, and/or butter • Butternut squash fries (p. 272) • Butternut purée with cinnamon and coconut oil or butter • Coconut butter • Coconut chips (p. 296) • Nuts and nut butter • Avocado mousse (p. 324) • Dairy-free ice cream • Nut bars (p. 300) • Scrambled coconut eggs • Carrot "cupcakes" (p. 320) • Baked apple pudding (p. 322) • Baked pear • Grilled fruit kebabs • Dairy-free smoothie • Coconut macaroons (p. 326) • No-bake frozen cookies (p. 328)

Appendices, References

Appendix 1: Track Your Progress

Monitor your symptoms before starting on the elimination diet and a few months down the road to track your progress.

Before								
Symptoms	Frequency					Severity		
Date: _____	Daily	Almost Daily	3-4 Times Per Week	1-2 Times Per Week	Rarely	Mild	Moderate	Severe
Bloating								
Abdominal pain								
Flatulence								
Belching								
Feeling of urgency								
Acid reflux								
Fatigue								
Depression								
Brain fog								
Bowel movements	Average frequency: Appearance on the poop chart (circle): 1 2 3 4 5 6 7 a b							

After								
Symptoms	Frequency					Severity		
Date: _____	Daily	Almost Daily	3-4 Times Per Week	1-2 Times Per Week	Rarely	Mild	Moderate	Severe
Bloating								
Abdominal pain								
Flatulence								
Belching								
Feeling of urgency								
Acid reflux								
Fatigue								
Depression								
Brain fog								
Bowel movements	Average frequency: Appearance on the poop chart (circle): 1 2 3 4 5 6 7 a b							

Appendix 2: Your Weekly Health Journal

Date	Time	Food and Supplements	My Health
Monday _____			Symptoms: Bowel movements: _____ Type: 1 2 3 4 5 6 7 a b Sleep: ___ hrs Stress: ___ /10
Tuesday _____			Symptoms: Bowel movements: _____ Type: 1 2 3 4 5 6 7 a b Sleep: ___ hrs Stress: ___ /10
Wednesday _____			Symptoms: Bowel movements: _____ Type: 1 2 3 4 5 6 7 a b Sleep: ___ hrs Stress: ___ /10
Thursday _____			Symptoms: Bowel movements: _____ Type: 1 2 3 4 5 6 7 a b Sleep: ___ hrs Stress: ___ /10
Friday _____			Symptoms: Bowel movements: _____ Type: 1 2 3 4 5 6 7 a b Sleep: ___ hrs Stress: ___ /10
Saturday _____			Symptoms: Bowel movements: _____ Type: 1 2 3 4 5 6 7 a b Sleep: ___ hrs Stress: ___ /10
Sunday _____			Symptoms: Bowel movements: _____ Type: 1 2 3 4 5 6 7 a b Sleep: ___ hrs Stress: ___ /10

Appendix 3: Mix-and-Match Chart

What to eat? Use the mix-and-match chart and make sure you get enough of each food group at every meal.

	Protein	Fats	Vegetables	Seasonings
Serving*	4-8 oz (120-240 g)	1-3 tbsp (15-45 ml)	¼-¾ cup (60-175 ml) as tolerated	½-1 tsp (2-5 ml) of unrefined salt per day and other seasonings to taste
Elimination Phase	☑ Beef ☑ Chicken ☑ Duck ☑ Turkey ☑ Lamb ☑ Pork ☑ Venison ☑ Wild boar ☑ Bison ☑ Fish ☑ Seafood	☑ Ghee ☑ Coconut oil ☑ Olive oil ☑ Avocado oil ☑ Macadamia oil ☑ Duck fat ☑ Lard ☑ Tallow	☑ Carrots ☑ Zucchini ☑ Spinach ☑ Green beans ★ Boiled, steamed, stir-fried, roasted, puréed, or vegetable fries Always cooked thoroughly and ideally peeled, de-seeded, and puréed	☑ Unrefined salt ☑ Apple cider vinegar ☑ Fresh herbs ☑ Dried herbs ☑ Lemon ☑ Limes ☑ Cinnamon ☑ Garlic-infused oil (p. 284) ☑ Homemade pesto ☑ Ginger ☑ Chives ☑ Green onions (green part only) ☑ Asafoetida powder ☑ Lemon butter sauce (p. 278) ☑ Herbed ghee (p. 282) ☑ Reduction sauce (p. 286)
As Tolerated	☑ Eggs ☑ Shrimps ☑ Sausages (gluten-free) ☑ Ham, prosciutto, and deli meats (gluten free and sugar free) ☑ Smoked fish	☑ Avocado ☑ Butter ☑ Homemade mayo (p. 288) ☑ Hollandaise sauce ☑ Cream ☑ Coconut milk and coconut cream (guar gum-free) ☑ Unsweetened dried coconut ☑ Uncured bacon ☑ Nuts ☑ Nut butters ☑ Basic vinaigrette (p. 290) ☑ Guacamole ☑ Garlic-infused oil (p. 284)	☑ Cauliflower ☑ Broccoli ☑ Cabbage ☑ Tomato ☑ Onion ☑ Garlic ☑ Asparagus ☑ Bok choy ☑ Beets ☑ Butternut squash ☑ Spaghetti squash ☑ Turnip ☑ Eggplant ☑ Brussels sprouts ☑ Bell pepper ☑ Mushroom	☑ Balsamic vinegar ☑ Red wine vinegar ☑ Black pepper ☑ Chili powder ☑ Chili sauce ☑ Turmeric and other spices ☑ Coconut aminos ☑ Tamari sauce (gluten-free) ☑ Sea vegetables ☑ Sundried tomatoes ☑ Mustard powder ☑ Tomato sauce ☑ Fermented foods (p. 302-307)

*Per person per meal, adjusted as needed to stay full until next meal;

a REAL-food meal

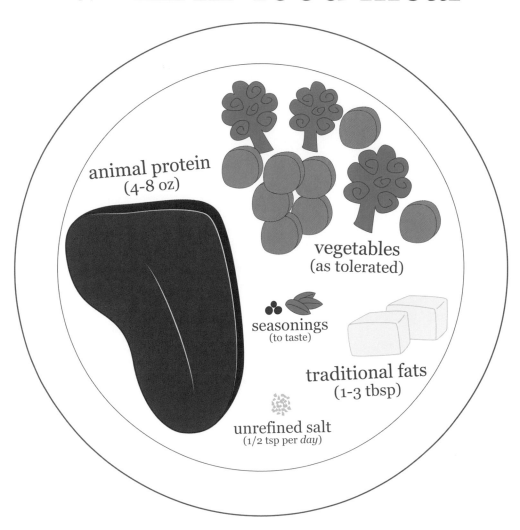

animal protein
(4-8 oz)

vegetables
(as tolerated)

seasonings
(to taste)

traditional fats
(1-3 tbsp)

unrefined salt
(1/2 tsp per *day*)

macronutrient balance for digestive health

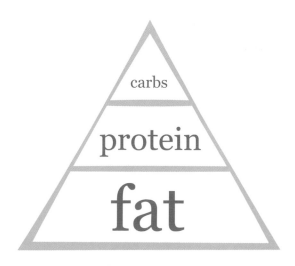

carbs

protein

fat

Appendix 4: Shopping List

Food Groups	Shopping List for the First 2-4 weeks	Amount for One
Animal Protein**,***	☑ Meat (beef, bison, venison, lamb, wild boar, pork) ☑ Organ meat and offal (liver, tongue, kidneys) ☑ Poultry (chicken, turkey, duck) ☑ Fish (salmon, sardines, herring, mackerel, sole) ☑ Seafood (scallops, oysters, crab, lobster, mussels)	Around 4-8 oz (120-240 g) per meal (and possibly some at snack time) = 5-10 lbs (2.5-5 kg) per week
Traditional Fats	☑ Extra-virgin coconut oil ☑ Ghee ☑ Butter (to make your own ghee) ☑ Extra-virgin olive oil (or macadamia oil or avocado oil) ☑ Duck fat, tallow, or lard	At least 1-3 tbsp (15-45 ml) per meal (and possibly some at snack time) = 1.5-4 cups (300 ml to 1 l) per week
Bones	☑ Ideally from grass-fed cows, pastured chickens, or wild-caught white fish to make homemade bone broth	1 large or 2 small chicken carcasses or about 1-2 lbs of bones per week
Vegetables (always cooked at the beginning)	☑ Carrot ☑ Zucchini ☑ Spinach ☑ Green beans	Between ¼-¾ cup (60-175 ml) per meal (and possibly some at snack time) = 5-21 cups (1.2-5 l) per week
Seasonings (all optional with the exception of unrefined salt)	☑ Unrefined salt**** ☑ Chives ☑ Asafoetida powder ☑ Cinnamon ☑ Lemon juice ☑ Lime juice ☑ Apple cider vinegar ☑ Fresh herbs ☑ Green part of green onions ☑ Garlic-infused oil ☑ Herb-infused oil	Between ½-1 tsp. (2-5 ml) of unrefined salt a day = 3.5 to 7 tsp (18 to 35 ml) per week The other seasonings can be purchased as needed and as desired.
Beverages (optional)	☑ Sparkling water ☑ Lemon or lime juice to add to water ☑ Fresh herbs to add to water ☑ Rooibos tea	As needed and as desired

*The ideal is organic produce and animal protein, ghee, and butter from healthy, happy, pastured animals; **Avoid shrimp, smoked fish, and aged/cured meats (bacon, sausage, ham) at the beginning; ***Avoid animal protein that is marinated, in a sauce, or breaded; ****Unless you have been medically advised to avoid salt.

Appendix 5: Your List of Safe Foods*

Animal Protein	Traditional Fats	Vegetables
Chicken	Ghee	Zucchini
Duck	Coconut oil	Spinach
Beef	Extra-virgin olive oil	Carrots
Bison	Macadamia oil	Green beans
Venison	Avocado oil	
Pork	Palm oil	
Fish	Tallow	
Crab	Lard	
Liver	Duck fat	

Seasonings	Beverages	Non-Grain Carbs (fruits, tubers, sweeteners)
Unrefined salt	Water	
Chives	Homemade bone broth	
Green part of green onions	Rooibos tea	
Cinnamon	Green tea	
Apple cider vinegar	Sparkling water	
Lemon/lime juice	Water infused with fresh rosemary, mint, or other herbs	
Asafoetida powder		
Fresh herbs		
Garlic-infused oil		
Herb-infused oil		

Other (dairy, nuts, seeds, fermented foods, etc.)	Supplements

*Simply cross out foods you don't tolerate and add any safe foods you discover during the reintroduction phase.

Appendix 6: The Elimination, Reintroduction, and Your BYO Diet Phases

Your BYO Diet	Elimination Phase	Reintroduction Phase	Your BYO Diet
Description And Goal	The most restrictive phase in which you cut out all potentially problematic foods and ingredients to "reset" your digestive system (eliminate your symptoms).	This phase will help you start reintroducing foods and groups of foods you eliminated from your diet to determine the ones to which you are intolerant and increase your food variety. Go slowly be systematic.	Your BYO diet will help you manage your symptoms and allow your digestive system to heal to ultimately improve your health and food tolerance.
Rules	Follow this phase for a minimum of 3-4 weeks with at least 5 symptom-free days in a row.	Add a new food every 3-4 days. Add to your list of safe foods if tolerated or reset before trying another new food.	Focus on what you can eat and be creative with the food options that make you feel best.
How Long?	A minimum of 3-4 weeks; possibly 6-8 weeks in severe cases	You can reintroduce new foods every 3-4 days. If you experience symptoms, keep that food out of your diet for at least 2-3 symptom-free days to do a small "reset" before experimenting with another new food.	Forever! Your BYO diet can evolve over time, depending on your health, but you should always eat the foods that you tolerate and eliminate those you don't. Everyone should be on his or her own BYO diet!
Until What Point?	Until you're symptom free (or your symptoms are improved significantly) for at least 5 days in a row (don't wait for perfection).	Until you are happy with your food variety. You can switch to your BYO diet if you want to take a break from reintroducing new foods.	Until you feel better or feel like experimenting with a new food. You can switch between the reintroduction phase and your BYO diet.
What Might Happen?	Withdrawal, die-off, and detox symptoms or the low-carb flu.	You may react to some of the foods you reintroduce.	You will continue feeling good and your digestive system will continue healing.

Appendix 7: Reintroduction Protocol

Progression	Reintroduction Protocol	
First Day	• Eat a small serving of a new food	e.g. ¼ avocado
Second Day	• Double the serving size	e.g. ½ avocado
Third Day	• Double the serving size again	e.g. whole avocado
Fourth Day	• Eat the same serving size again (optional)	e.g. whole avocado
If Symptoms	• Stop eating the new food if you start experiencing symptoms • Go back to your safe foods • Reset your body until you have 2-3 days without symptoms	
If No Symptoms	• Keep the new food in your diet and try another new food	

Appendix 8: Your Food Trials

Food Trial	Trial Dates	Serving	Symptoms	Verdict
Avocado (example)	Mon, Sept 10, 2012	¼ avocado	Nothing the first 2 days, bloating on Wednesday after eating whole avocado	Unsure… seem to tolerate small amounts, but need to try again to determine if I tolerate ¼ to ½ avocado
	Tues, Sept 10, 2012	½ avocado		
	Wed, Sept 10, 2012	1 avocado		

Appendix 9: Food Categories to Challenge

Categories			Foods	
To Trial		Egg protein (in order of reintroduction)	Egg yolks Whole eggs	Yolks are usually better tolerated than whites If tolerated, try making homemade mayonnaise and hollandaise sauce
		Other animal protein options	Shrimp Jerky (without sugar and MSG) Smoked salmon and other smoked fish Bacon, ham, or sausages (ideally without sweeteners, MSG, or artificial ingredients; from pastured animals)	
		Fats	Avocado (and guacamole) Butter Olive (and tapenade) Homemade mayonnaise (if egg yolks tolerated) Coconut milk or coconut cream (without guar gum) Coconut butter (also called coconut cream concentrate or coconut manna)	
	Dairy	Casein (from least to most)	Butter Cream Yogurt Cheese Milk	A2 casein (goat, Jersey's cow, buffalo) is usually better tolerated than A1 casein (regular cows) Dairy products from raw milk are sometimes better tolerated than pasteurized dairy Dairy products made from the milk of grass-fed animals are sometimes better tolerated than regular milk from grain-fed animals
		Lactose (from least to most)	Homemade yogurt Cream Aged cheese Fresh cheese Milk	
	Vegetables	Cruciferous	Broccoli Cauliflower Kale Cabbage Bok choy More in Table 40 (p. 109)	
		Nightshades	Tomato Eggplant Bell pepper Chili powder Paprika Curry Hot pepper sauce (without added sugar or gum) More in Table 39 (p. 108)	
		High-FOD-MAPs	Onion Garlic Cruciferous vegetables Asparagus Avocado Mushroom More on p. 43-49	
		Raw	Lettuce Carrots Celery sticks Any kind of raw vegetables	
		Moderate carb content	Winter squashes (butternut squash, acorn squash, pumpkin) Beets Rutabaga More in Table 81 (p. 230)	

	Categories	Foods
Caution	Seasonings	Black pepper Onion and garlic powder Spices (curry, chili powder, hot pepper sauce, etc.) Balsamic vinegar (sugar free, naturally aged) Red wine vinegar (sugar free, naturally aged) Coconut aminos Tamari sauce (wheat and gluten free) Sea vegetables and seaweed (kelp, nori) Sun-dried tomatoes More in Table 50 (p. 137)
	Fermented foods	Fermented vegetables (sauerkraut, pickles, carrots, etc.) Homemade 24-hour yogurt or kefir Kombucha (fermented tea)
	Nuts	Coconut milk (or coconut cream; without guar gum) Nut butter (macadamia, cashew, hazelnut, coconut, etc.) Nut flour Nuts (ideally soaked and dehydrated) Unsweetened dried coconut (or coconut chips) Coconut flour
	Seeds	Sunflower seeds, pepitas, flaxseeds, chia seeds, sesame seeds Spices (nutmeg, celery seed, cumin seed, fennel seed, mustard seed, etc.) More in Table 37 (p. 104)
	Beverages	Other varieties of tea Coconut milk (without sweeteners or gums) Almond milk (without sweeteners or gums)
	Grain-free carb options — Fruits (from easier to hardest to digest/tolerate)	Bananas Cooked, puréed, and unsweetened apples and pears Raw fruits (berries, citrus fruits, melons, etc.) Dried fruits (without added ingredients)
Watch Out	Sweeteners	Honey Maple syrup Coconut sugar (or coconut nectar) Stevia Dextrose (glucose)
	Roots and tubers	Sweet potatoes White potatoes (peeled) Plantains Yucca/cassava More in Appendix 14 (p. 360)
	Caffeine and alcohol (only after at least 3-6 months without them)	Unsweetened cocoa powder Dark chocolate (at least 85% cocoa) Coffee Alcohol (gluten and sugar free: dry wine, hard liquor, gluten-free beer only)
Not Worth It	NOT food	Grains Gluten-containing foods Legumes (beans, lentils, soy, peanuts) Refined oils Processed ingredients (MSG, artificial sweeteners, etc.) Beer and other gluten-containing alcoholic beverages

Appendix 10: Potentially Problematic Foods (and Reasons to Avoid Them)

Food Groups	Problematic Compounds	Reasons To Avoid Them
Grains (wheat, barley, rye, oats, quinoa, amaranth, millet, teff, triticale, kamut, rice, corn, etc.)	Gluten and similar hard-to-digest proteins	• Can increase intestinal permeability • Can irritate your digestive system • Can trigger food-sensitivity reactions
	Carbohydrates (starches and sugars)	• Can feed a gut dysbiosis*
	Anti-nutrients	• Prevent the absorption of nutrients • Can irritate your digestive system
	Insoluble fiber	• Can irritate your digestive system
	Fructans (FODMAPs)	• Can feed a gut dysbiosis*
	Natural food chemicals	• Can irritate your digestive system
	Processed ingredients	• Can trigger food-sensitivity reactions • Can promote inflammation • Can irritate your digestive system
Dairy (except ghee)	Casein	• Can trigger food-sensitivity reactions
	Lactose (FODMAPs)	• Can feed a gut dysbiosis*
	Added sugars	• Can feed a gut dysbiosis*
Soy	Soy protein	• Can trigger food-sensitivity reactions
Peanuts	Peanut protein	• Can trigger food-sensitivity reactions
	Peanut lectins/aflatoxins	• Can irritate your digestive system
Legumes (beans and lentils)	Galactans (FODMAPs)	• Can feed a gut dysbiosis*
	Starches	• Can feed a gut dysbiosis*
	Natural food chemicals	• Can irritate your digestive system
	Processed ingredients	• Can trigger food-sensitivity reactions • Can promote inflammation • Can irritate your digestive system
Refined Oils (soybean oil, canola oil, corn oil, etc.)	High omega-6 fat content	• Can promote inflammation (especially if eaten in excess of omega-3) • Can contribute to intestinal permeability
Some Vegetables, Fruits and Tubers	Starches (in starchy vegetables)	• Can feed a gut dysbiosis*
	Sugars (in fruits)	• Can feed a gut dysbiosis*
	FODMAPs	• Can feed a gut dysbiosis*
	Cruciferous vegetables	• Can irritate your digestive system • Can feed a gut dysbiosis*
	Natural food chemicals	• Can irritate your digestive system
	Glycoalkaloids (in nightshades)	• Can promote inflammation • Can irritate your digestive system
	Insoluble fiber (especially in the skin, seeds, or membranes and/or in raw vegetables)	• Can irritate your digestive system
Processed Ingredients	Sugars, FODMAPs, food chemicals, problematic protein, etc.	• Can trigger food-sensitivity reactions • Can promote inflammation • Can irritate your digestive system
Sugars	Sugars	• Can feed a gut dysbiosis* • Can promote inflammation • Can slow down your immune system
	FODMAPs	• Can feed a gut dysbiosis*
Nuts and Seeds	Natural food chemicals	• Can irritate your digestive system
	High omega-6-to-omega-3 ratio	• Can promote inflammation
	FODMAPs	• Can feed a gut dysbiosis*
	Protein	• Can trigger food-sensitivity reactions
Spices	Natural food chemicals	• Can irritate your digestive system
Eggs	Egg proteins	• Can trigger food-sensitivity reactions

*Gut dysbiosis includes SIBO, candida overgrowth, and other gut-flora imbalances.

Appendix 11: List of Potentially Problematic Foods

	Food Groups		Foods
FODMAPs	FRUCTOSE	Fruits	Apple, boysenberries, cherries, figs, grapes, mango, pears, tamarillo, watermelon, dried fruits, canned fruits, fruit bars
		Vegetables	Artichoke, asparagus, sugar snap peas, tomato juice, tomato sauce, tomato paste
		Sweeteners	Agave syrup, honey, high-fructose corn syrup (HFCS), corn syrup solids
		Drinks	Fruit juices, fruit punches, soft drinks, energy drinks, sweeter wines, port wines, some ciders
	LACTOSE	High	Milk
		Moderate	Commercial yogurt and ice cream
		Low	Cheese and cream
	FRUCTANS	Grains	Wheat, rye, and barley (bread, pasta, couscous, gnocchi, muesli, wheat bran, and other foods derived from these grains), sweet corn
		Vegetables	Onion (all types, including brown onions, white onions, Spanish onions, red onions, shallots, leeks, and the white part of green onions), garlic, artichoke, asparagus, Jerusalem artichoke, beetroot, broccoli, Brussels sprouts, dandelion leaves, fennel, butternut squash, green peas, snow peas, cabbage, okra
		Fruits	Custard apples, nectarines, peaches, persimmon, pomegranate, rambutan, tamarillo, watermelon
		Nuts and seeds	Pistachios, cashews, almonds, hazelnuts, flaxseeds
		Seasonings	Onion powder, onion salt, garlic powder, garlic salt, bouillon cubes, broth, stock, chicken salt, vegetable salt, vegetable powder, dehydrated vegetables, gravies, soups, marinades, sauces, spices, and seasonings (often contain some form of onion or garlic)
		Sweeteners	Coconut sugar (also called coconut nectar or coconut crystals)
		Other	Inulin, chicory root, fructooligosaccharides (FOS), prebiotics
	SORBITOL	Fruits	Apple, apricot, avocado, blackberries, cherries, longan, lychee, nectarines, pears, plums, prunes, and juices from these fruits
		Sweeteners	Sugar alcohols such as sorbitol, mannitol, maltitol, xylitol, and isomalt
		Other	Gums, candies, and other sugar-free items containing sugar-alcohol sweeteners
	MANNITOL	Vegetables	Cauliflower, celery, mushrooms, snow peas, sweet potato, butternut squash, pumpkin
		Fruits	Peach, watermelon
		Sweeteners	Sugar alcohols such as sorbitol, mannitol, maltitol, xylitol, and isomalt
		Others	Some beers and wines
	GALACTANS	Legumes	Legumes, beans (chickpeas, red kidney beans, etc.), lentils, hummus, soy-based products (especially if made with whole soy beans or soy protein)
		Vegetarian foods	Soy-based products like tempeh, soy burgers, and soy yogurt (especially if made with whole soy beans or soy protein)
		Beverages	Soymilk (especially if made from whole soy beans)
		Vegetables	Broccoli, Brussels sprouts, cabbage, butternut squash, pumpkin, edamame

	Food Groups	Foods
NATURAL FOOD CHEMICALS / **SALICYLATES**	Vegetables	Avocado, bell pepper (capsicum), broccoli, cauliflower, cucumber (with peel), eggplant, mushrooms, nori, olives, onion, pickled vegetables, pumpkin, radicchio, radish, sauerkraut, spinach, spring onion, tomato, vegetable juices, soups, and stocks, zucchini with peel
	Fruits	Berries, cherries, citrus, dates, dried fruits, grapes, kiwi, mango, passion fruit, pineapple, plum, pomegranate, rhubarb, ripe banana, strawberry, watermelon, fruit juices
	Sweets	Chewing gums, honey, jams and jellies, licorice, mints, raw sugar
	Seasonings	Commercial gravies, sauces, stocks, herbs, spices, mustard, tomato sauce, ketchup, tomato paste, spices (cinnamon, anise, cloves, etc.), vinegar (balsamic, red wine, etc.)
	Animal protein	Beef (aged, corned, smoked, cured), commercial gravy, fish sauces, meat pies, sausages, stocks
	Legumes	Beans, falafel, hummus, textured vegetable protein (TVP)
	Nuts and seeds	Almonds, Brazil nuts, chestnuts, coconut, hazelnuts, macadamias, peanuts, pecans, pine nuts, pistachios, walnuts, and butters from these nuts, flaxseeds, pumpkin seeds, sesame seeds, sunflower seeds
	Fat	Almond oil, avocado oil, extra-virgin and regular olive oils, sesame oil, walnut oil, oils with added antioxidants, commercial marinades, salad dressings and mayonnaise, coconut milk, coconut cream, coconut oil, suet
	Grains and starchy foods	Breads (with corn, dried fruit, nuts, coconut, vinegar, and preservatives), breakfast cereals (with corn, cocoa, coconut, dried fruit, honey, nuts, artificial colors and flavors), potato chips, French fries, muesli, nachos, pasta, polenta, rice cakes, rice crackers
	Dairy	Flavored milk (chocolate, etc.), fruit-flavored yogurt
	Beverages	Coffee (regular and decaffeinated), herbal teas, teas, chai spiced tea, soft drinks
	Alcohol	Beer, champagne, cider, spirits, liqueurs, wines
	Other	Fermented foods, nutritional yeast, aspirin, natural flavorings, perfumes, botanical oils, liquid medications
AMINES	Vegetables	Avocado, broccoli, cauliflower, eggplant, olives, mushrooms, nori, pickled vegetables, radicchio, sauerkraut, spinach, tomato, vegetable soups and stocks
	Fruits	Berries, cherries, citrus, dates, dried fruits, grape, just-ripe banana, kiwi, mango, passion fruit, pineapple, plums, fruit juices
	Sweets	Chocolate, jams and jellies
	Seasonings	Commercial gravies, sauces, stocks, fish sauce, mustard, tomato sauce, ketchup, tomato paste, soy sauce, spices (cinnamon, anise, cloves), vinegar (balsamic, red wine, etc.)
	Animal protein	Anchovies, beef (aged, corned, smoked, cured), bacon, canned salmon, canned sardines, canned tuna, chicken skin, commercial gravies, fish fingers, fish sauce, game meat, ham, liver, meat pies, pork, turkey, sausages, shrimp, smoked fish, surimi (fake crab), stocks
	Legumes	Beans, falafel, hummus, textured vegetable protein (TVP)
	Nuts and seeds	Almonds, Brazil nuts, chestnuts, coconut, hazelnuts, macadamias, peanuts, pecans, pine nuts, pistachios, walnuts and butters from these nuts, flaxseeds, pumpkin seeds, sesame seeds, sunflower seeds
	Fat	Almond oil, avocado oil, extra-virgin and regular olive oil, sesame oil, walnut oil, oils with added antioxidants, commercial marinades, salad dressings and mayonnaise, coconut milk, coconut cream, coconut oil, suet
	Grains and starchy foods	Breads (with corn, dried fruit, nuts, coconut, vinegar and preservatives), breakfast cereals (with corn, cocoa, coconut, dried fruit, honey, nuts, artificial colors and flavors), potato chips, French fries, muesli, rice cakes, rice crackers
	Dairy	Flavored milk (chocolate, etc.), fruit-flavored yogurt, mild cheeses (cheddar, Swiss, feta, halloumi, etc.), strong-tasting cheeses (Brie, camembert, Parmesan, etc.)
	Beverages	Chai spiced tea, soft drinks
	Alcohol	Beer, champagne, cider, spirits, liqueurs, wines
	Other	Cocoa powder, fermented foods

Appendix 11: List of Potentially Problematic Foods (cont.)

Food Groups			Foods
OTHER VEGETABLES	**GOITROGENS**	Cruciferous vegetables	Bok choy, broccoli, Brussels sprouts, cabbage, cauliflower, collard greens, kale, kohlrabi, radishes, rapini, rutabaga, turnips (especially in their raw state or fermented)
		Produce	Spinach, sweet potato, some fruits (strawberries, pears, peaches)
		Other	Canola, soybeans, peanuts, millet
	NIGHTSHADES	Starches	Potato (but not sweet potato)
		Vegetables	Eggplant, tomato, tomatillo, bell pepper
		Fruits	Goji berries, ground cherries
		Spices and seasonings	Paprika, most kinds of pepper (chili pepper, chili powder, jalapeño, cayenne pepper, chipotle, hot pepper, Tabasco sauce), curry (often contains pepper); NOT black and white pepper
		Other	Ashwangandha (Ayurvedic supplement), nicotine
	CRUCIFEROUS	Vegetables	Kale, collard greens, broccoli (including Chinese broccoli, broccoflower, wild broccoli, broccoli romanesco, and rapini), cabbage (including Chinese cabbage, napa cabbage, red cabbage, and sauerkraut), Brussels sprouts, Kohlrabi, cauliflower, bok choy, pak choy, turnips, rutabaga, arugula (rocket lettuce), watercress, radish, daikon
		Other	Horseradish (including wasabi), maca, canola/rapeseed, mustard seed
NUTS AND SEEDS	**NUTS**	Tree nuts	Almonds, walnuts, cashews, chestnuts, macadamias, hazelnuts, pecans, Brazil nuts, pistachios, pine nuts, shea nuts
	SEEDS	Seeds	Flaxseeds (linseeds), chia seeds, hemp seeds, psyllium, sunflower seeds (including sunbutter), pumpkin seeds (pepitas), sesame seeds (including sesame oil and tahini), poppy seeds
		Seasonings	Nutmeg, anise seeds, black caraway seeds (regular caraway seed should be fine), celery seeds, cumin seeds, dill seeds, fennel seeds, fenugreek, mustard seeds (including mustard powder, prepared mustards, mustard oil, and mustard leaves)
		Other	Coffee and cacao
YEASTS, MOLDS, AND MYCOTOXINS		Plant foods	Some fruits (berries, melon, grapes, and dried fruits), overripe produce, refined vegetable oils, some nuts (cashews, pistachios), peanuts (including peanut butter)
		Seasonings	Vinegars (excluding apple cider vinegar), many condiments, MSG, citric acid, yeast extracts
		Fermented foods	Sauerkraut, kefir, miso, soy sauce, tamari sauce, cheeses
		Other	Aged and cured meats (sausage, bacon, ham), yeast spreads (Vegemite® or Marmite®), B vitamins and other supplements made from yeasts, grain products with baker's yeast, nutritional yeast, alcoholic beverages
CASEIN		A1 casein	Regular dairy products (from Holstein cows)
		A2 casein	From Jersey cows, goats, buffalo, camel, and a few other ancestral ruminant species

Appendix 12: Grain-Free Sources of Fiber

Food Group	REAL Food	Serving Size	Fiber (g)*
Veggies	Broccoli, cooked	1 cup	5.1
	Leafy greens, cooked	1 cup	4.3-5.1
	Brussels sprouts, cooked	1 cup	4.1
	Squash (spaghetti, butternut)	1 cup	2.2-6.6
	Onions, cooked	1 cup	2.9
	Cauliflower, cooked	1 cup	2.9
	Eggplant, cooked	1 cup	2.5
	Carrots, raw or cooked	1 cup	2.3
	Cabbage, raw or cooked	1 cup	1.8-2.8
	Leafy greens, raw	2 cups	1.3-2.1
	Sauerkraut, raw	¼ cup	0.9
Tubers	Sweet potato, cooked (without skin)	1 cup	8.2
	Plantain, cooked	1 cup	3.5-4.6
	Potato, cooked (without skin)	1 cup	3.1
Fruits	Berries	1 cup	3.6-8.0
	Pear	1 medium	5.5
	Mango	1 medium	5.4
	Apple	1 medium	4.4
	Dried figs	5	4.1
	Banana	1 medium	3.1
	Orange	1 medium	2.3
Nuts	Nuts	1 oz	1.9-3.5
	Nut butter	2 tbsp	3.2
	Almond flour	2 tbsp	1.5
	Coconut (unsweetened, dried)	2 tbsp	4.6
	Coconut flour	2 tbsp	6-10
Fats	Avocado	1 medium	13.5
	Olives	5 jumbo	1

Appendix 13: Dairy-Free Sources of Calcium

Food Groups	Food	Serving Size	Calcium Content*
Dairy	Milk	1 cup	352 mg
	Yogurt	½ cup	173-191 mg
	Cheese	1 oz	143-204 mg
Dairy Free	Homemade bone broth	1 cup	Unknown but highly bioavailable
	Sardines, canned with bones	3 oz	325 mg
	Collard greens, cooked	1 cup	266 mg
	Spinach, cooked	1 cup	245 mg
	Salmon, canned with bones	3 oz	203-249 mg
	Broccoli, cooked	2 cups	125 mg
	Almond butter	2 tbsp	111 mg
	Rhubarb	1 cup	105 mg
	Shrimp	4 oz	103 mg
	Chard, cooked	1 cup	102 mg
	Kale, cooked	1 cup	94 mg
	Almonds	1 oz (23 almonds)	75 mg
	Orange	1 large	74 mg
	Eggs	2	56 mg
	Dried figs	3	41 mg

Appendix 14: Grain-Free Sources of Carbohydrates

		Food	Serving Size	Total Carbs	Fiber
Roots and Tubers	Dense carbs	Sweet potatoes (skinless)	1 medium (5 oz or 150 g)	27 g	3.8 g
			1 cup (250 ml) mashed	58 g	8.2 g
		Yams (skinless)	1 cup (250 ml), cubed	38 g	5.3 g
		Potatoes (skinless)	1 cup (250 ml)	26 g	1.8 g
			1 medium	34 g	2.3 g
			1 cup (250 ml), mashed	36 g	3.2 g
		Plantains	1 cup (250 ml), mashed	62 g	4.6 g
			1 cup (250 ml), sliced	48 g	3.5 g
			1 cup (250 ml), green, fried	58 g	4.1 g
		Yucca (cassava root)	1 cup (250 ml)	78 g	3.7 g
	Moderate carbs	Taro root	1 cup (250 ml), sliced	46 g	6.7 g
		Parsnip	1 cup (250 ml), sliced	27 g	5.6 g
		Butternut squash	1 cup (250 ml)	22 g	6.6 g
		Turnip	1 cup (250 ml), sliced	8 g	3.1 g
		Rutabaga (swede)	1 cup (250 ml), sliced	15 g	3.1 g
		Jicama	1 cup (250 ml)	11-12 g	6-6.5 g
		Spaghetti squash	1 cup (250 ml)	10 g	2.2 g
		Pumpkin	1 cup (250 ml), mashed	12 g	2.7 g
		Beets	1 cup (250 ml), sliced	9 g	1.7 g
Fruits		Apple	1 medium (3"), with skin	25 g	4.4 g
		Apple sauce	1 cup (250 ml), unsweetened	28 g	2.7 g
		Banana	1 medium (7-8" long)	27 g	3.1 g
		Blueberries	1 cup (250 ml)	22 g	3.6 g
		Melon	1 cup (250 ml) cantaloupe	14 g	1.6 g
			1 cup (250 ml) watermelon	12 g	0.6 g
			1 cup (250 ml) honeydew	16 g	1.4 g
		Kiwi	1 fruit (2" diameter)	10 g	2.1 g
		Mango	1 cup (250 ml), diced (1/2 fruit)	25 g	2.6 g
		Orange	1 medium fruit (2.5-3")	15 g	3.1 g
		Peach	1 medium (2.5" diameter)	14 g	2.3 g
		Pears	1 medium or 1.3 cup slices	28 g	5.5 g
		Pineapple	1 cup (250 ml) chunks	22 g	2.3 g
		Strawberries	1 cup (250 ml) whole, ¾ cup (175 ml) whole or about 12 medium	11 g	2.9 g
Sugars		Honey	1 tablespoon (15 ml)	17 g	0 g
		Maple syrup	1 tablespoon (15 ml)	13 g	0 g
		Coconut crystals	1 tablespoon (15 ml)	7 g	0 g
		Coconut nectar	1 tablespoon (15 ml)	13 g	0 g
		Molasses	1 tablespoon (15 ml)	15 g	0 g
		Table sugar	1 tablespoon (15 ml)	13 g	0 g

*Peel your fruits if too much fiber bothers you; you can also cook them to make them easier to digest.

the 4 steps
{to better digestion and health}

1 control
digestive symptoms

- improve quality of life
- prevent further damage to the gut
- avoid further nutritional deficiencies
- support digestion
- soothe inflammation

2 repair
your gut

- control systemic symptoms
- improve digestion and absorption
- promote better food tolerance
- prevent/manage autoimmune conditions
- soothe inflammation

3 nourish
your body

- support gut repair
- improve digestion/absorption
- optimize overall health and well-being

4 prevent
recurrence

- correct gut dysbiosis
- maintain stomach-acid barrier
- promote regular cleansing waves
- strengthen your immune system

Appendix 16: Applying the Four Steps to Better Digestion and Health

	Steps	Goals	How?
1	Control Digestive Symptoms	• Improve quality of life • Prevent further damage to the gut • Avoid further nutritional deficiencies • Support digestion • Soothe inflammation	• Follow appropriate treatment per your doctor's recommendations • Follow the elimination diet protocol (eat REAL foods and avoid processed foods) • Manage your stress and sleep enough • Use digestive aids as needed (ox bile, betaine HCl, digestive enzymes)

2	Repair Your Gut	• Control systemic symptoms
		
		• Improve digestion/absorption
		
		• Promote better food tolerance
		
		• Prevent/manage autoimmune conditions
		
		• Soothe inflammation
			• Same as step 1
			
			• Eat nutrient-dense REAL foods
			
			• Manage your stress and sleep enough
			
			• Take homemade bone broth
			
			• Avoid food triggers
			
			• Supplement as needed:
			    ○ L-glutamine
			    ○ Zinc
			    ○ Vitamin A
			    ○ Omega-3 fats
			    ○ Probiotics

3	Nourish Your Body	• Support gut repair • Improve digestion/absorption • Optimize overall health and well-being	• Eat nutrient-dense REAL food • Avoid processed foods • Manage your stress and sleep enough
4	Prevent Recurrence	• Correct gut dysbiosis • Maintain stomach acid barrier • Promote regular cleansing waves • Strengthen your immune system	• Eat fermented foods or use probiotic supplements • Follow your BYO diet • Manage your stress and sleep enough • Use digestive aids as needed (betaine HCl, digestive bitters, ox bile) • Space your meals every 4-5 hours and fast 12 hours overnight if possible

Appendix 17: Digestive-Health Tests

Gastrointestinal Conditions			Digestive Health Tests	
SIBO (small intestinal bacterial overgrowth)			• Lactulose and/or glucose breath test • Organic urine acids (not validated) • Elimination diet with reintroduction challenges	
FODMAP Intolerance	Fructose malabsorption		• Fructose breath test	• Elimination diet with reintroduction challenges
	Lactose intolerance		• Lactose breath test	
	Mannitol/polyol intolerance		• Mannitol breath test	
	Fructan intolerance		• Elimination diet with reintroduction challenges	
	Galactan intolerance			
Low Stomach Acid (hypochlorhydria)			• Heidelberg test (stomach-acid test) • Baking soda test (not validated)	
IBDs	Crohn's disease		• Colonoscopy	
	Ulcerative colitis			
Colon Cancer				
Gastroparesis (slow gastric emptying)			• Gastric-emptying study	
GERD (gastroesophageal reflux disease)			• Upper endoscopy • Heidelberg test (stomach-acid test) • *H. pylori* test (antibodies in blood) • Ultrasound to look for hiatal hernia	
Gastrointestinal Infections (bacteria, virus, parasites and yeast, including candida overgrowth)			• DNA stool test • Culture tool tests • Urine organic acids (not validated)	
Celiac Disease			• Anti-gliadin antibodies (IgA and IgG) in the blood or stools • Anti-tissue transglutaminase antibodies • Intestinal biopsy • Wheat/gluten proteome reactivity and autoimmunity (not validated)	
Non-Celiac Gluten Sensitivity			• Wheat/gluten proteome reactivity and autoimmunity (not validated) • Elimination diet with reintroduction challenges	
Gallbladder Diseases and Gallstones			• Abdominal ultrasound	
Bowel Obstructions			• X-rays	
Hiatal Hernia (can be a cause of GERD)			• Other imaging techniques	
Increased intestinal permeability (leaky gut)			• Lactulose-mannitol intestinal permeability test	
Candida overgrowth			• Urine organic acids (not validated) • DNA stool test	
Food Sensitivities (to dairy, gluten, soy, grains, eggs, nuts, seeds, etc.)			• Skin prick (only detects food allergies) • IgG testing by ELISA (not always accurate) • Elimination diet with reintroduction challenges	
IBS (irritable bowel syndrome)			• Exclusion of all other conditions	

Appendix 18: Monitoring Your Health

Monitor Your Health		Target		Your Values	
		US values	Int'l values	Date: _____	Date: _____
Total Cholesterol		< 200 mg/dL	< 5.2 mmol/L		
LDL Cholesterol		< 100 mg/dL	< 2.6 mmol/L		
HDL Cholesterol		> 60 mg/dL	> 1.5 mmol/L		
Triglycerides (TG)		< 150 mg/dL	< 1.7 mmol/L		
Fasting Blood Sugar		< 100 mg/dL	< 6.1 mmol/L		
Post-Meal Blood Sugar (1-2 hours post-meal)		< 140 mg/dL	< 7.8 mmol/L		
Hemoglobin A1c		< 5.7%	< 5.7%		
C-Reactive Protein (CRP)		< 1.0 mg/dL	< 10 nmol/L		
Waist Girth	Women	< 35 in	< 88 cm		
	Men	< 40 in	< 102 cm		
Blood Pressure		< 130/90 mm Hg	< 130/90 mm Hg		
Glomerular Filtration Rate (GFR)		90 or above	90 or above		
Creatinine		0.5-1.2 mg/dL	0.044-0.107 mmol/L		

the poop chart

type		
1		separate hard lumps (hard to pass)
2		sausage shaped but lumpy (hard to pass)
3		like a sausage with cracks on the surface (easy to pass)
4		like a sausage, smooth and soft (easy to pass)
5		soft blobs with clear-cut edges (easy to pass)
6		fluffy pieces with ragged edges, mushy stools (easy to pass)
7		entirely liquid, no solid pieces, could be drunk with a straw! (easy to pass)

subtype		
a		fatty stool (steatorrhea): floats, has a chalky color and/or foul smell
b		undigested food particles seen in the stools

adapted from the Bristol Stool Chart © Aglaée Jacob

Appendix 20: The Mind-Body Connection

Taking Care Of Your Mind: Strategies
• Thinking positively!
• Belly breathing (p. 207)
• Going to your secret happy place (p. 207)
• Hanging out with Mother Nature (p. 208)
• Body scanning (p. 208)
• Writing a gratitude list (p. 208)
• Laughing! (p. 209)
• Smiling ☺ (p. 209)
• Practicing a hobby (p. 209)
• Doing what makes you feel good
• Allowing yourself to rest
• Living in the present
• Surrounding yourself with people you love
• Avoiding caffeine and foods to which you are sensitive
• Sleeping eight to nine hours per night (p. 210)
• Avoiding excessive and endurance exercise (p. 211)
• Addressing stressful situations (p. 210)

Add your own ways to help take care of your mind!

•

•

•

•

•

•

•

•

•

•

•

Appendix 21: Your Gratitude List

I Am Grateful For:

Appendix 22: Troubleshooting

Category	Possible Causes/Solutions	Page
Cravings	• Eat more, especially fat	222
	• Add unrefined salt	223
	• Avoid artificial sweeteners	223
	• Get enough sleep	223
	• Amino acids (L-glutamine and 5-HTP)	223
Fatigue	• Eat more fat	224
	• Get more sodium and water	224
	• Manage your stress	225
	• Sleep more	225
	• Increase your carb intake	225
Symptoms Returning	• Personal modifications	225
	• Cumulative effect	226
	• Slow down	226
	• Cross contamination	227
	• Personal hygiene products	227
	• Past exposure	227
	• Stress	228
	• Sleep	228
	• Biofilms	228
	• Too few carbs	228
	• Supplements	231
	• Medications	231
	• Plastics (BPA)	231
	• Chewing	231
	• Digestive aids	231
	• GI infections	231
	• Artificial sweeteners	232
	• Alcohol	232
	• Caffeine	232
	• Large servings of safe foods	232
	• Food quality	232
	• Remaining problematic foods	232
	• Hormonal changes in women	233
	• Normal part of condition progression	233
How to Alleviate Symptoms?	• Epsom salt baths	233
	• Activated charcoal	233
	• Hot water bottle or heating pad	233
	• Hydration	234
	• Rest	234
	• Turmeric	234
	• Peppermint oil, ginger, or chamomile	234
	• Avoid NSAIDs	234
Constipation	• Be patient	235
	• Eat more fat	235
	• Avoid trigger foods	235
	• SIBO	235
	• Probiotics	235
	• Fluids	236
	• Exercise	236
	• Stress management	236
	• Abdominal massage	236
	• Magnesium	237
	• Digestive aids	237
	• Castor oil packs	237
	• Ginger tea	237
	• Eat more carbs	237
	• See your doc (thyroid, diabetes, GI infection, etc.)	238
Diarrhea	• Avoid trigger foods	238
	• Supplements	238
	• Fat intake	239
	• Protein intake	239
	• Probiotics	236
	• Stress management	240
	• GI infections	240
	• Activated charcoal	240
	• Reset your digestive system	240

References

CHAPTER 1

★ Gropper SAS and Groff JL. Advanced Nutrition and Human Metabolism. Third Edition. 2000.

★ Mahan LK and Escott-Stump S. Krause's Food, Nutrition and Diet Therapy. 11th edition. 2003.

★ Maltby EJ. The Digestion of Beef Protein in the Human Stomach. J Clin Invest. 1934. 13(2): 193-207.

★ International Foundation for Functional Gastrointestinal Disorders. Facts About IBS. August 2012. Web August 2012. www.aboutibs.org/site/about-ibs/facts-about-ibs

★ Cunningham-Rundles S and Lin DH. Nutrition and the Immune System of the Gut. Nutr J. 1998. 14: 573–579.

★ Hanson LÅ. Immune Effects of the Normal Gut Flora. Monatsschr Kinderheilkd. 1998. 146 (Suppl 1): S2-S6.

★ Öhman L and Simrén M. Pathogenesis of IBS: Role of Inflammation, Immunity and Neuroimmune Interactions. Nat Rev Gastroenterol Hepatol. 2010; 7: 163-173.

★ Barbara G, et al. A Role for Inflammation in Irritable Bowel Syndrome? Gut. 2002; 51 (Suppl 1): i41-i44.

★ Akiho H, et al. Low-Grade Inflammation Plays a Pivotal Role in Gastrointestinal Dysfunction in Irritable Bowel Syndrome. World J Gastrointest Pathophysiol. 2010; 1(3): 97-105.

★ Philpott H, et al. Irritable Bowel Syndrome - An Inflammatory Disease Involving Mast Cells. Asia Pac Allergy. 2011; 1: 36-42.

★ Iliev ID, et al. Interactions between Commensal Fungi and the C-Type Lectin Receptor Dectin-1 Influence Colitis. Science. 2012; 336(6086): 1314-7.

★ Camilleri M, et al. The Confluence of Increased Permeability, Inflammation, and Pain in Irritable Bowel Syndrome. Am J Physiol Gastrointest Liver Physiol. 2012 Jul 26. (Epub ahead of print).

★ Madden JA and Hunter JO. A Review of the Role of the Gut Microflora in Irritable Bowel Syndrome and the Effects of Probiotics. Br J Nutr. 2002. 88 (Suppl. 1): S67-S72.

★ Dethlefsen L and Relman DA. Incomplete Recovery and Individualized Responses of the Human Distal Gut Microbiota to Repeated Antibiotic Perturbation. Proceedings of the National Academy of Sciences. 2011. 108 Suppl 1:4554-61.

★ Collins SM and Bercik P. The Relationship between Intestinal Microbiota and the Central Nervous System in Normal Gastrointestinal Function and Disease. Gastroenterology. 2009. 136(6): 2003-2014.

★ Othman M, et al. Alterations in Intestinal Microbial Flora and Human Disease. Curr Opin Gastroenterol. 2008. 24: 11-16.

★ Fasano A. Zonulin and its Regulation of Intestinal Barrier Function: The Biological Door to Inflammation, Autoimmunity, and Cancer. Physiol Rev. 2011. 91(1): 151-175.

★ Turner JR. Intestinal Mucosal Barrier Function in Health and Disease. Nat Rev Immunol. 2009. 9(11): 799-809.

★ Farhadi A, et al. Intestinal barrier: an interface between health and disease. J Gastroenterol Hepatol. 2003. 18(5): 479-497.

★ Groschwitz KR and Hogan SP. Intestinal Barrier Function: Molecular Regulation and Disease Pathogenesis. J Allergy Clin Immunol. 2009. 124(1): 3-20.

★ Wright J. Why Stomach Acid Is Good for You: Natural Relief from Heartburn, Indigestion, Reflux and GERD. 2001.

CHAPTER 2

Post-Infectious IBS

★ Ghoshal UC and Ranjan P. Post-Infectious Irritable Bowel Syndrome: The Past, the Present and the Future. J Gastroenterol Hepatol. 2011. 26 (Suppl. 3): 94-101.

★ Dupont AW. Postinfectious Irritable Bowel Syndrome. Clin Infect Dis. 2008. 46(4): 594-599.

Gluten Sensitivity

★ Cordain L. The Paleo Diet: Lose Weight and Get Healthy by Eating the Foods You Were Designed to Eat. 2002: 42.

★ Cordain L. Cereal Grains: Humanity's Double-Edged Sword. World Rev Nutr Diet. 1999. 84: 19–73.

★ Allam AH, et al. Atherosclerosis in Ancient Egyptian Mummies: the Horus Study. J Am Coll Cardiol Img. 2011; 4(4): 315-327.

★ Aris A and Leblanc S. Maternal and Fetal Exposure to Pesticides Associated to Genetically Modified Foods in Eastern Townships of Quebec, Canada. Reprod Toxicol. 2011. 31(4): 528-533.

★ Mesnage R, et al. Cytotoxicity on Human Cells of Cry1Ab and Cry1Ac Bt Insecticidal Toxins Alone or with a Glyphosate-Based Herbicide. J Appl Toxicol. February 2012.

★ Smith J. Genetically Modified Foods: What the People Want to Know. Underground Wellness Real Food Summit Presentation 2012. Web July 2012.

★ Davis W. Wheat Belly: Lose the Wheat, Lose the Weight, and Find your Path Back to Health. 2011.

★ Institute for Responsible Technology. Health Risks. Web August 2012. www.responsibletechnology.org/health-risks

★ Sapone A, et al. Divergence of Gut Permeability and Mucosal Immune Gene Expression in Two Gluten-Associated Conditions: Celiac Disease and Gluten Sensitivity. BMC Med. 2011. 9:23.

★ Sapone A, et al. Spectrum of Gluten-Related Disorders: Consensus on New Nomenclature and Classification. BMC Med. 2012. 10: 13.

★ Ventura A, et al. Duration of Exposure to Gluten and Risk for Autoimmune Disorders in Patients with Celiac Disease. Gastroenterology. 1999. 117(2): 297-303.

★ Biesiekierski JR, et al. Gluten causes gastrointestinal symptoms in subjects without celiac disease: a double-blind randomized placebo-controlled trial. Am J Gastroenterol. 2011. 106(3): 508-514.

★ Farrell RJ and Kelly CP. Celiac Sprue. New Engl J Med. 2002. 346(3): 180-188.

★ Carroccio A, et al. Non-celiac wheat sensitivity diagnosed by double-blind placebo-controlled challenge: exploring a new clinical entity. Am J Gastroenterol. 2012. 107(12):1898-1906.

★ Bernardo D, et al. Is Gliadin Really Safe for Non-Coeliac Individuals? Production of Interleukin 15 in Biopsy Culture from Non-Coeliac Individuals Challenged with Gliadin Peptides. Gut. 2007. 56(6): 889-890.

★ Catassi C, et al. Natural History of Celiac Disease Autoimmunity in a USA Cohort Followed since 1974. Ann Med. 2010. 42(7): 530-538.

★ Sapone A, et al. Differential Mucosal IL-17 Expression in Two Gliadin-Induced Disorders: Gluten Sensitivity and the Autoimmune Enteropathy Celiac Disease. Int Arch Allergy Immunol. 2010. 152(1): 75-80.

★ Hadjivassiliou M, et al. Gluten Ataxia in Perspective: Epidemiology, Genetic Susceptibility and Clinical Characteristics. Brain. 2003. 126(pt3): 685-691.

★ Hadjivassiliou M, et al. Neuropathy Associated With Gluten Sensitivity. J Neurol Neurosurg Psychiatry. 2006. 77(11):1262-1266.

★ Fine K. Early Diagnosis of Gluten Sensitivity: Before the Villi are Gone. 2003. Web September 2012. www.enterolab.com/StaticPages/EarlyDiagnosis.aspx

★ Drago S, et al. Gliadin, Zonulin and Gut Permeability: Effects on Celiac and Non-Celiac Intestinal Mucosa and Intestinal Cell Lines. Scand J Gastroenterol. 2006. 41(4): 408-419.

★ Zamakhchari M, et al. Identification of Rothia Bacteria as Gluten-Degrading Natural Colonizers of the Upper Gastro-Intestinal Tract. PLOS ONE. 2011. 6(9): e24455.

★ O'Bryan T. Gluten Sensitivity and Celiac Disease. DrLoRadio's podcast. Web July 2012. www.blogtalkradio.com/drloradio/2011/04/21/gluten-sensitivity-and-celiac-disease-with-dr-thomas-obryan

★ O'Bryan T. Autoimmune Disease. DrLoRadio's podcast. Web July 2012. www.blogtalkradio.com/undergroundwellness/2012/07/03/detecting-autoimmunity-early-w-dr-thomas-obryan

Fructose Malabsorption and FODMAPs

★ Shepherd SJ, et al. Dietary Triggers of Abdominal Symptoms in Patients with Irritable Bowel Syndrome: Randomized Placebo-Controlled Evidence. Clin Gastroenterol Hepatol. 2008. 6(7): 765-771.

★ Shepherd SJ and Gibson PR. Fructose Malabsorption and Symptoms of Irritable Bowel Syndrome: Guidelines for Effective Dietary Management. J Am Diet Assoc. 2006. 106(10): 1631-1639.

★ Ong DK et al. Manipulation of Dietary Short Chain Carbohydrates Alters the Pattern of Gas Production and Genesis of Symptoms in Irritable Bowel Syndrome. J Gastroenterol Hepatol. 2010. 25(8): 1366-1373.

★ Biesiekierski JR, et al. Gluten Causes Gastrointestinal Symptoms in Subjects without Celiac Disease: A Double-Blind Randomized Placebo-Controlled Trial. Am J Gastroenterol. 2011. 106(3): 508-514.

★ Barret JS and Gibson PR. Fermentable Oligosaccharides, Disaccharides, Monosaccharides and Polyols (FODMAPs) and Nonallergic Food Intolerance: FODMAPs or Food Chemicals? Therap Adv Gastroenterol. 2012. 5(4): 261-268.

★ Ventura EE, et al. Sugar Content of Popular Sweetened Beverages Based on Objective Laboratory Analysis: Focus on Fructose. Obesity. 2011. 19(4): 868-874.

★ Ledochowski M, et al. Fructose- and Sorbitol-Reduced Diet Improves Mood and Gastrointestinal Disturbances in Fructose Malabsorbers. Scand J Gastroenterol. 2000; 10: 1048-1052.

★ Ledochowski M, et al. Fructose Malabsorption is Associated with Early Signs of Mental Depression. Eur J Med Res. 1998; 3(6): 295-298.

★ Ledochowski M, et al. Fructose Malabsorption is Associated with Decreased Plasma Tryptophan. Scand J Gastroenterol. 2001; 36(4): 367-371.

★ Lustig RH. Sugar: The Bitter Truth. UCSF Mini Medical School for the Public. 2009. Web July 2012. www.youtube.com/watch?v=dBnniua6-oM

★ Shepherd SJ, et al. Dietary Triggers of Abdominal Symptoms in Patients with Irritable Bowel Syndrome: Randomized Placebo-Controlled Evidence. Clin Gastroenterol Hepatol. 2008. 6(7): 765-771.

★ Shepherd SJ and Gibson PR. Fructose Malabsorption and Symptoms of Irritable Bowel Syndrome: Guidelines for Effective Dietary Management. J Am Diet Assoc. 2006. 106(10): 1631-1639.

★ Gearry RB, et al. Reduction of Dietary Poorly Absorbed Short-Chain Carbohydrates (FODMAPs) Improves Abdominal Symptoms in Patients with Inflammatory Bowel Disease – A Pilot Study. J Crohns Colitis. 2009. 3(1): 8-14.

★ Eastern Health Clinical School (Monash University). The Low FODMAP Diet: Reducing Poorly Absorbed Sugars to Control Gastrointestinal Symptoms. 2010.

★ Biesiekierski JR, et al. Gluten Causes Gastrointestinal Symptoms in Subjects without Celiac Disease: A Double-Blind Randomized Placebo-Controlled Trial. Am J Gastroenterol. 2011. 106(3): 508-514.

★ Campbell AK, et al. Bacterial Metabolic "Toxins": A New Mechanism for Lactose and Food Intolerance, and Irritable Bowel Syndrome. Toxicology. 2010. 278(3): 268-276.

Small Intestinal Bacterial Overgrowth (SIBO)

★ Bures J, et al. Small Intestinal Bacterial Overgrowth Syndrome. World J Gastroenterol. 2010; 16(24): 2978-2990.

★ Siebecker A. Small Intestine Bacterial Overgrowth: Clinical Strategies. NCNM Continuing Education Online. October 2011. Recorded webinar ce.ncnm.edu/course/search.php?search=SIBO

★ Pimentel M. A New IBS Solution. 2005.

★ Gottschall E. Breaking the Vicious Cycle: Intestinal Health Through Diet. 2004.

★ Campbell-McBride N. Gut and Psychology Syndrome: Natural Treatment for Autism, Dyspraxia, A.D.D., Dyslexia, A.D.H.D., Depression, Schizophrenia. 2010.

★ Gasbarrini A, et al. Small Intestinal Bacterial Overgrowth: Diagnosis and Treatment. Dig Dis. 2007; 25(3): 237-240.

★ Giamarellos-Bourboulis EJ and Tzivras M. Small Intestinal Bacterial Overgrowth: Novel Insight in the Pathogenesis and Treatment of Irritable Bowel Syndrome. Annals of Gastroenterology. 2009; 22(2): 77-81.

★ Olendzki B, et al. Pilot Testing a Novel Treatment for Inflammatory Bowel Disease. University of Massachusetts Medical School and UMass Memorial Health Care. 2011. Web July 2012. www.umassmed.edu/uploadedFiles/MBD_Poster59_EDITED_5-15-2011.pdf

★ DiBaise JK. Nutritional Consequences of Small Intestinal Bacterial Overgrowth. Pract Gastroenterol. 2008. 69: 15-28.

★ Lin HC. Small Intestinal Bacterial Overgrowth: A Framework for Understanding Irritable Bowel Syndrome. JAMA. 2004. 292(7): 852-858.

★ Riordan SM, et al. Luminal Bacteria and Small-Intestinal Permeability. Scand J Gastroenterol. 1997. 32(6): 556-563.

★ Lauritano EC, et al. Small Intestinal Bacterial Overgrowth and Intestinal Permeability. Scand J Gastroenterol. 2010. 45(9): 1131-1132.

★ Sabaté JM, et al. High Prevalence of Small Intestinal Bacterial Overgrowth in Patients With Morbid Obesity: A Contributor to Severe Hepatic Steatosis. Obes Surg. 2008. 18(4): 371-377.

★ Riordan SM, et al. Luminal Antigliadin Antibodies in Small Intestinal Bacterial Overgrowth. Am J Gastroenterol. 1997. 92(8): 1335-1338.

★ Nucera G, et al. Abnormal Breath Tests to Lactose, Fructose and Sorbitol in Irritable Bowel Syndrome May Be Explained by Small Intestinal Bacterial Overgrowth. Aliment Pharmacol Ther. 2005. 21(11): 1391-1395.

★ Campbell AK, et al. Bacterial Metabolic "Toxins": A New Mechanism for Lactose and Food Intolerance, and Irritable Bowel Syndrome. Toxicology. 2010. 278(3): 268-276.

Bloating

★ Houghton LA et al. Relationship of Abdominal Bloating to Distention in Irritable Bowel Syndrome and Effect of Bowel Habit. Gastroenterology. 2006. 131(4): 1003-1010.

★ King TS, Elia M, and Hunter JO. Abnormal Colonic Fermentation in Irritable Bowel Syndrome. Lancet. 1998. 352(9135): 1187-1189.

Migrating Motor Complex (MMC)

★ Románski KW. Migrating Motor Complex in Biological Sciences: Characterization, Animal Models and Disturbances. Indian J Exp Biol. 2009. 47(4): 229-244.

★ Vasbinder GB, et al. Micturition is Associated with Phase III of the Interdigestive Migrating Motor Complex in Man. Am J Gastroenterol. 2003. 98(1): 66-71.

★ Husebye E, et al. Influence of Microbial Species on Small Intestinal Myoelectric Activity and Transit in Germ-Free Rats. Am J Physiol Gastrointest Liver Physiol. 2001. 280(3): G368-380.

★ Stotzer PO, Björnsson ES, and Abrahamsson H. Interdigestive and Postprandial Motility in Small-Intestinal Bacterial Overgrowth. Scand J Gastroenterol. 1996. 31(9): 875-880.

Food Chemicals

★ Allergy Unit, Royal Prince Alfred Hospital. RPAH Elimination Diet Handbook. 2011.

★ Breakey J. Dietitians Practice Manual – For Professionals. 2011.

★ Breakey J. Are You Food Sensitive? 2011.

★ Bold J. Considerations for the Diagnosis and Management of Sulphite Sensitivity. Gastroenterology and Hepatology From Bed to Bench. 2012. 5(1): 3-6.

★ Swain AR. The Role of Natural Salicylates in Food Intolerance. University of Sydney. 1988.

★ Breakey J. A Report on the Use of a Low Additive And Amine, Low Salicylate Diet in the Treatment of Behavior, Hyperactivity and Learning Problems in Children. Queensland University of Technology. 1995.

★ Dietitians Association of Australia. The Dietary Management of Food Allergy and Food Intolerance in Children and Adults. Australian Journal of Nutrition and Dietetics. 1996. 53(3): 89-98.

★ Maintz L and Novak N. Histamine and Histamine Intolerance. Am J Clin Nutr. 2007. 85(5): 1185-1196.

Celiac Disease

★ Fasano A. Physiological, Pathological, and Therapeutic Implications of Zonulin-Mediated Intestinal Barrier Modulation. The Am J Pathol. 2008. 173(5): 1243-1252.

★ Tursi A, Brandimarte G and Giorgetti G. High prevalence of small intestinal bacterial overgrowth in celiac patients with persistence of gastrointestinal symptoms after gluten withdrawal. Am J Gastroenterol. 2003. 98(4): 839-843.

★ Ghoshal UC, et al. Partially responsive celiac disease resulting from small intestinal bacterial overgrowth and lactose intolerance. BMC Gastroenterol.2004. 4: 10.

★ Fasano A, et al. Prevalence of Celiac Disease in At-Risk and Not-At-Risk Groups in the United States – a Large Multicenter Study. Arch Intern Med. 2003. 163(3):286-292.

★ National Foundation for Celiac Awareness. Celiac Disease Facts & Figures. Web July 2012. www.celiaccentral.org/celiac-disease/facts-and-figures/

★ Abdulkarim AS, et al. Etiology of Nonresponsive Celiac Disease: Results of a Systematic Approach. Am J Gastroenterol. 2002. 97(8): 2016-2021.

★ Gluten in gluten-free processed foods (not labeled GF): Thompson T, Lee AR and Grace T. Gluten Contamination of Grains, Seeds and Flours in the United States: A Pilot Study. J Am Diet Assoc. 2010. 110: 937-940.

★ Catassi C, et al. A Prospective, Double-Blind, Placebo-Controlled Trial to Establish a Safe Gluten Threshold for Patients With Celiac Disease. Am J Clin Nutr. 2007. 85: 160-166.

★ Rubio-Tapia A, et al. The Prevalence of Celiac Disease in the United States. Am J Gastroenterol. 2012 Jul 31. (Epub ahead of print). Doi: 10.1038/ajg.2012.219.

IBDs (Inflammatory Bowel Disorders)

★ Klaus J, et al. Small Intestinal Bacterial Overgrowth Mimicking Acute Flare as a Pitfall in Patients with Crohn's Disease. BMC Gastroenterol. 2009. 9: 61.

★ Shafran I and Burgunder P. Adjunctive Antibiotic Therapy with Rifaximin May Help Reduce Crohn's Disease Activity. Dig Dis Sci. 2010. 55: 1079-1084.

★ Shafran I and Johnson LK. An Open-Label Evaluation of Rifaximin in the Treatment of Active Crohn's Disease. Curr Med Res Opin. 2005. 21(8): 1165-1169.

★ Gerova VA, et al. Increased Intestinal Permeability in Inflammatory Bowel Diseases Assessed by Iohexol Test. World J Gastroenterol. 2011. 17(17): 2211-2215.

★ Olendski BC, et al. Pilot Testing a Novel Treatment for Inflammatory Bowel Disease. Clinical and Translational Science Research Retreat. May 2011. Web July 2012. www.umassmed.edu/uploadedFiles/MBD_Poster59_EDITED_5-15-2011.pdf

Gastroesophageal Reflux Disease (GERD)

★ Yarandi SS, et al. Overlapping Gastroesophageal Reflux Disease and Irritable Bowel Syndrome: Increased Dysfunctional Symptoms. World J Gastroenterol. 2010. 16(10): 1232-1238.

★ Reimer C, et al. Proton-Pump Inhibitor Therapy Induces Acid-Related Symptoms in Healthy Volunteers After Withdrawal of Therapy. Gastroenterology. 2009. 137(1): 80-87.

★ Urita Y, et al. High Incidence of Fermentation in the Digestive Tract in Patients with Reflux Oesophagitis. European Journal of Gastroenterol Hepatol. 2006. 18(5): 531-535.

★ Compare D, et al. Effects of Long-Term PPI Treatment on Producing Bowel Symptoms and SIBO. Eur J Clin Invest. 2010. 41(4): 380-386.

★ Wright J. Why Stomach Acid is Good for You: Natural Relief from Heartburn, Indigestion, Reflux and GERD. 2001.

★ Lombardo L, et al. Increased Incidence of Small Intestinal Bacterial Overgrowth during Proton Pump Inhibitor Therapy. Clin Gastroenterol Hepatol. 2010. 8(6): 504-508.

★ Mertz H. Helicobacter Pylori: Its Role in Gastritis, Achlorhydria, and Gastric Carcinoma. In: Holt P, Russell R. eds. Chronic Gastritis and Hypochlorhydria in the Elderly. 69-82. Boca Raton., FL. CRC Press. 1993.

★ NIH Consensus Conference. Helicobacter Pylori in Peptic Ulcer Disease. NIH Consensus Development Panel on Helicobacter Pylori in Peptic Ulcer Disease. JAMA. 1994. 272(1): 65-69.

★ Levie A, et al. Celiac-Associated Peptic Disease at Upper Endoscopy: How Common Is It? Scand J Gastroenterol. 2009. 44(12): 1424-1428.

★ Olson JW and Maier RJ. Molecular Hydrogen as an Energy Source for Helicobacter Pylori. Science. 2002. 298(5599): 1788-1790.

Gallbladder Issues

★ Maggiore G and Caprai S. Liver Involvement in Celiac Disease. Indian J Pediatr. 2006. 73(9): 809-811.

★ Fravel RC. The Occurrence of Hypochlorhydria in Gall-Bladder Disease. Am J Med Sci. 1920. 159: 512.-517.

★ Capper WM, et al. Gallstones, Gastric Secretion, and Flatulent Dyspepsia. Lancet. 1967. 1(7487): 413-415.

★ Breneman JC. Allergy Elimination Diet as the Most Effective Gallbladder Diet. Ann Allergy. 1968. 26(2): 83-87.

★ Liddle RA, Goldstein RB, and Saxton J. Gallstone Formation during Weight-Reduction Dieting. Arch Intern Med. 1989; 149(8): 1750-1753.

★ Tsai C-J, et al. Dietary Carbohydrates and Glycaemic Load and the Incidence of Symptomatic Gall Stone Disease in Men. Gut. 2005. 54(6): 823-828.

CHAPTER 3

History of Celiac Disease

★ Guandalini S. A Brief History of Celiac Disease. Impact. 2007. 7(3): 1-2.

★ Anderson CM, et al. Coeliac Disease; Gastrointestinal Studies and the Effect of Dietary Wheat Flour. Lancet. 1952. 1(6713): 836-842.

★ Gottschall E. Whatever Happened to the Cure for Celiac Disease? Nutritional Therapy Today. 1997. 7(1): 8-11.

SCD

★ Nieves R and Jackson RT. Specific Carbohydrate Diet in Treatment of Inflammatory Bowel Disease. Tenn Med. 2004. 97(9): 407.

★ Olendzki B, et al. Pilot Testing a Novel Treatment for Inflammatory Bowel Disease. University of Massachusetts Medical School and UMass Memorial Health Care. 2011. Web July 2012. www.umassmed.edu/uploadedFiles/MBD_Poster59_EDITED_5-15-2011.pdf

★ Gottschall EG. Breaking the Vicious Cycle: Intestinal Health Through Diet. 1994.

★ Gottschall EG. Digestion-Gut-Autism Connection: The Specific Carbohydrate Diet. Medical Veritas 1. 2004. 261-271.

★ Gordon D. The Specific Carbohydrate Diet: Does It Work? Crohn's & Colitis Foundation of America. Web July 2012. www.ccfa.org/resources/specific-carbohydrate-diet.html

GAPS Diet

★ Campbell-McBride, N. Gut and Psychology Syndrome: Natural Treatment Of Autism, ADD/ADHD, Dyslexia, Dyspraxia, Depression, Schizophrenia. 2004.

Paleo Diet

★ Wolf R. The Paleo Solution: The Original Human Diet. 2010.

★ Hartwig M and Hartwig D. It Starts with Food: Discover the Whole30 and Change Your Life in Unexpected Ways. 2012.

Weston A. Price Foundation (WAPF) Diet

★ Price WA. Nutrition and Physical Degeneration. 2003.

★ WAPF. Principles of Healthy Diets. The Weston A. Price Foundation for Wise Traditions in Food, Farming and Healing Arts. Web July 2012. www.westonaprice.org/basics/principles-of-healthy-diets

Ancestral Diets

★ Lindeberg S. Food and Western Disease: Health and Nutrition from an Evolutionary Perspective. 2009.

★ Cordain L, Eades MR, and Eades MD. Hyperinsulinemic Diseases of Civilization: More than just Syndrome X. Comp Biochem Physiology A Mol Integr Physiol. 2003. 136(1): 95-112.

★ Lindeberg S. Paleolithic Diets as a Model For Prevention and Treatment of Western Disease. Am J Hum Biol. 2012. 24(2): 110-115.

★ Cordain L, et al. Origins and Evolution of the Western Diet: Health Implications for the 21st Century. Am J Clin Nutr. 2005. 81(2): 341-354.

★ Spreadbury I. Comparison with Ancestral Diets Suggests Dense Acellular Carbohydrates Promote an Inflammatory Microbiota, and May Be the Primary Cause of Leptin Resistance and Obesity. Diabetes Metab Syndr Obes. 2012. 5: 175-189.

★ Lindeberg S, et al. A Palaeolithic Diet Improves Glucose Tolerance more than a Mediterranean-Like Diet in Individuals with Ischaemic Heart Disease. Diabetologia. 2007. 50(9): 1795-1807.

★ Cordain L. The Nutritional Characteristics of a Contemporary Diet Based upon Paleolithic Food Groups. J Am Neutraceut Assoc. 2002. 5(3): 15-24.

★ Frassetto LA, et al. Metabolic and Physiologic Improvements from Consuming a Paleolithic, Hunter-Gatherer Type Diet. Eur J Clin Nutr. 2009. 63(8): 1-9.

★ Milton K. The Critical Role Played by Animal Source Foods in Human (Homo) Evolution. J Nutr. 2003. 133(11 Suppl 2): 3886S-3892S.

★ Colagiuri S and Brand-Miller JC. The "Carnivore Connection"—Evolutionary Aspects of Insulin Resistance. Eur J Clin Nutr. 2002. 56 Suppl 1: S30-35.

★ Mummert A, et al. Stature and Robusticity during The Agricultural Transition: Evidence from the Bioarchaeological Record. Econ Hum Biol. 2011. 9(3): 284-301.

★ Carrera-Bastos P, et al. The Western Diet and Lifestyle and Diseases of Civilization. Research Reports in Clinical Cardiology. 2011. 2: 15-35.

★ Eaton SB, Cordain L, and Lindeberg S. Evolutionary Health Promotion: A Consideration of Common Counterarguments. Prev Med. 2002. 34(2): 119-123.

★ Gluckman PD and Bergstrom CT. Evolutionary Biology within Medicine: a Perspective of Growing Value. BMJ. 2011. 343: d7671.

★ Cordain L. Cereal Grains: Humanity's Double-Edged Sword. World Rev Nutr Diet. 1999. 84: 19-73.

Grains

★ Sapone A, et al. Divergence of Gut Permeability and Mucosal immune Gene Expression in Two Gluten-Associated Conditions: eliac Disease and Gluten Sensitivity. BMC Med. 2011; 9: 23.

★ Wangen S. Healthier Without Wheat – A New Understanding of Wheat Allergies, Celiac Disease, and Non-Celiac Gluten Intolerance. 2009.

★ Reddy NR and Sathe, SK. Food Phytates. 2001.

★ Gibson PR, et al. Review Article: Fructose Malabsorption and the Bigger Picture. Aliment Pharmacol Ther. 2006; 25: 349–363.

★ Zioudrou C, et al. Opioid Peptides Derived from Food Proteins. J Biol Chem. 1979; 254(7): 2446-2449.

★ Bijkerk CJ, et al. Soluble or Insoluble Fiber in Irritable Bowel Syndrome in Primary Care? Randomised Placebo Controlled Trial. BMJ. 2009. 339: b3154.

★ Stephen AM and Cummings JH. The Microbial Contribution to Human Faecal Mass. J Med Microbiol. 1980; 13(1): 45-56.

★ Schmidt RF and Thews G. Colonic Motility. Human Physiology. 1989; 29.7:733.

★ McClellan WS and Du Bois EF. Prolonged Meat Diets With a Study of Kidney Function and Ketosis. J Biol Chem. 1930. 87: 651-668.

★ Zevallos VG, et al. Variable Activation of Immune Response by Quinoa (Chenopodium Quinoa Willd.) Prolamins in Celiac Disease. Am J Clin Nutr. 2012. 96(2): 337-344.

★ Augustin LS, et al. Glycemic Index in Chronic Disease: A Review. Eur J Clin Nutr. 2002. 56(11): 1049-1071.

★ Foster-Powell K, Holt SHA, and Brand-Miller JC. International Table of Glycemic Index and Glycemic Load Values: 2002. Am J Clin Nutr. 2002. 76(1): 5-56.

★ The University of Sydney. Glycemic Index Database. Web July 2012. glycemicindex.com

Gluten-Free Grains

★ Cabrera-Chávez F, et al. Transglutaminase Treatment of Wheat and Maize Prolamins of Bread Increases the Serum IgA Reactivity of Celiac Disease Patients. J Agric Food Chem. 2008. 56(4): 1387-1391.

★ Davidson IW, et al. Antibodies to Maize in Patients with Crohn's Disease, Ulcerative Colitis and Coeliac Disease. Clin Exp Immunol. 1979. 35(1): 147-148.

★ Skerritt JH, et al. Cellular and Humoral Responses in Celiac Disease. 2. Protein Extracts from Different Cereals. Clin Chim Acta. 1991. 204(1-3):109-122.

★ Kristjánsson G, et al. Gut Mucosal Granulocyte Activation Precedes Nitric Oxide Production: Studies in Coeliac Patients Challenged with Gluten and Corn. Gut. 2005. 54(6): 769-774.

Dairy

★ Robinson J. Super Natural Milk. Web July 2012. eatwild.com/articles/superhealthy.html
WAPF. Fresh, Unprocessed (Raw) Whole Milk: Safety, Health and Economic Issues. 2009. Web July 2012. www.realmilk.com/safety/fresh-unprocessed-raw-whole-milk

★ FDA/Center for Food Safety and Applied Nutrition, USDA/Food Safety and Inspection Service. *Listeria* monocytogenes Risk Assessment: Interpretive Summary. September 2003. Web July 2012. www.fda.gov/Food/ScienceResearch/ResearchAreas/RiskAssessmentSafetyAssessment/ucm185291.htm

★ Reddy NR and Sathe, SK. Food Phytates. 2001

★ Bischoff-Ferrari HA, et al. Calcium Intake and Hip Fracture Risk in Men and Women: a Meta-Analysis of Prospective Cohort Studies and Randomized Controlled Trials. Am J Clin Nutr. 2007; 86(6): 1780–1790.

★ Bischoff-Ferrari HA, et al. Milk Intake and Risk of Hip Fracture in Men and Women: A Meta-Analysis of Prospective Cohort Studies. J Bone Miner Res. 2011; 26(4): 833-839.

★ Cordain L, Eades MR, and Eades MD. Hyperinsulinemic diseases of civilization: more than just Syndrome X. Comp Biochem Physiol A Mol Integr Physiol. 2003. 136(1): 95-112.

Soy

★ Daniel KT. The Whole Soy Story: The Dark Side of America's Favorite Health Food. 2005

★ Barrett JS and Gibson PR. Clinical Ramifications of Malabsorption of Fructose and Other Short-Chain Carbohydrates. Practical Gastroenterology. August 2007: 51-65.

Peanut

★ Cornell University Department of Animal Science. Aflatoxins: Occurrence and Health Risks. 2008. Web July 2012. www.ansci.cornell.edu/plants/toxicagents/aflatoxin/aflatoxin.html

★ Cordain L. Atherogenic Potential of Peanut Oil-Based Monounsaturated Fatty Acids Diets. Lipids. 1998; 33(2): 229-230.

Sugars

★ Dickinson S, et al. High-Glycemic Index Carbohydrate Increases Nuclear Factor-κB Activation in Mononuclear Cells of Young, Lean Healthy Subjects. Am J Clin Nutr. 2008. 87(5): 1188-1193.

★ Sørensen LB, et al. Effect of Sucrose on Inflammatory Markers in Overweight Humans. Am J Clin Nutr. 2005. 82(2): 421-427.

★ Sanchez A, et al. Roles of Sugars in Human Neutrophilic Phagocytosis. Am J Clin Nutr. 1973; 26(11): 1180-1184.

★ Lenoir M, et al. Intense Sweetness Surpasses Cocaine Reward. PLOS ONE. 2007. 2(8): e698.

Carbohydrates

★ Hite AH, et al. Low-Carbohydrate Diet Review: Shifting the Paradigm. Nutr Clin Pract. 2011; 26(3): 300-308.

★ Phinney SD and Volek JS. The Art and Science of Low Carbohydrate Living: An Expert Guide to Making the Life-Saving Benefits of Carbohydrate Restriction Sustainable and Enjoyable. 2011.

★ Institute of Medicine Food and Nutrition Board. Dietary Reference Intakes for Energy, Carbohydrate, Fiber, Fat, Fatty Acids, Cholesterol, Protein, and Amino Acids. 2005: 275.

★ Avena NM, et al. Evidence for Sugar Addiction: Behavioral and Neurochemical Effects of Intermittent, Excessive Sugar Intake. Neurosci Biobehav Rev. 2008; 32(1): 20-39.

★ Klement RJ and Kämmerer U. Is there a role for carbohydrate restriction in the treatment and prevention of cancer. Nutr Metab (Lond). 2011; 8: 75.

Fructose

★ Lustig RH. Sugar: The Bitter Truth. University of California Television. July 2009. Web July 2012. www.youtube.com/watch?v=dBnniua6-oM

★ Stanhope KL, et al. Consuming Fructose-Sweetened, Not Glucose-Sweetened, Beverages Increases Visceral Adiposity And Lipids And Decreases Insulin Sensitivity In Overweight/Obese Humans. J Clin Invest. 2009; 119(5): 1322-1344.

★ Gaby AR. Adverse Effects of Dietary Fructose. Altern Med Rev. 2005; 10(4): 294-306.

★ Teff KL, et al. Dietary Fructose Reduces Circulating Insulin and Leptin, Attenuates Postprandial Suppression of Ghrelin, and Increases Triglycerides in Women. J Clin Endocrinol Metab. 2004; 89(6): 2963–2972.

★ Suarez G, et al. Nonenzymatic Glycation of Bovine Serum Albumin by Fructose (Fructation). Comparison with the Maillard Reaction Initiated by Glucose. J Biol Chem. 1989; 264(7): 3674-3679.

★ Liu H, et al. Fructose Induces Transketolase Flux to Promote Pancreatic Cancer Growth. Cancer Res. 2010; 70: 6368-6376.

★ Shepherd SJ and Gibson PR. Fructose Malabsorption and Symptoms of Irritable Bowel Syndrome: Guidelines for Effective Dietary Management. J Am Diet Assoc. 2006; 106(10): 1631-1639.

* Barrett JS and Gibson PR. Clinical Ramifications of Malabsorption of Fructose and Other Short-Chain Carbohydrate. Practical Gastroenterology. August 2007: 51-65.

* Eastern Health Clinical School - Monash University. Low FODMAP Diet: Reducing Poorly Absorbed Sugars to Control Gastrointestinal Symptoms. 2010.

* Ledochowski M, et al. Fructose- and Sorbitol-reduced Diet Improves Mood and Gastrointestinal Disturbances in Fructose Malabsorbers. Scand J Gastroenterol. 2000; 35(10): 1048-1052.

* Ledochowski M, et al. Fructose Malabsorption Is Associated with Lower Plasma Folic Acid Concentrations in Middle-Aged Subjects. Clin Chem. 1999; 45(11): 2013-2014.

* Hitosugi T, et al. Tyrosine Phosphorylation Inhibits PKM2 to Promote the Warburg Effect and Tumor Growth. Sci Signal. 2009; 2(97): ra73.

Artificial Sweeteners

* Abou-Donia MB, et al. Splenda Alters Gut Microflora and Increases Intestinal P-Glycoprotein and Cytochrome P-450 In Male Rats. J Toxicol Environ Health A. 2008. 71(21): 1415-1429.

* Yang Q. Gain weight by "going diet?" Artificial Sweeteners and the Neurobiology of Sugar Cravings. Yale J Biol Med. 2010; 83(2): 101-108.

Refined Oils

* Cordain L, et al. Origins and Evolution of the Western Diet: Health Implications for the 21st Century. Am J Clin Nutr. 2005; 81: 341-354.

* Enig ME. Know Your Fats: The Complete Primer for Understanding the Nutrition of Fats, Oils and Cholesterol. 2000.

* Simopoulos AP. The Importance of the Ratio of Omega-6/Omega-3 Essential Fatty Acids. Biomed Pharmacother. 2002; 56(8): 365-379.

* Carrera-Bastos P, et al. The Western Diet and Lifestyle and Diseases of Civilization. Res Rep Clin Cardiol. 2011; 2: 15-35.

* Kirpich IA, et al. The Type of Dietary Fat Modulates Intestinal Tight Junction Integrity, Gut Permeability, and Hepatic Toll-Like Receptor Expression in a Mouse Model of Alcoholic Liver Disease. Alcoholism: Clin Exp Res. 2012. 36(5): 835-846.

* The IBD in EPIC Study Investigators, et al. Linoleic Acid, a Dietary N-6 Polyunsaturated Fatty Acid, and the Aetiology of Ulcerative Colitis: A Nested Case-Control Study with a European Prospective Cohort Study. Gut. 2009. 58(12): 1606-1611.

Nightshades

* Childers NF and Margoles MS. An Apparent Relation of Nightshades (Solanaceae) to Arthritis. Journal of Neurological and Orthopedic Medical Surgery. 1993. 12: 227-231.

* The Hayden Institute. Inflammatory Foods: Nightshades. Web July 2012. haydeninstitute.com/additional-resources/additional-resources-diet-and-nutrition/inflammatory-foods-nightshades

* Smith G. Nightshades. The Weston A. Price Foundation. 2010. Web July 2012. www.westonaprice.org/food-features/nightshades

* Siegmund B, Leitner E, and Pfannhauser W. Determination of the Nicotine Content of Various Edible Nightshades (Solanaceae) and Their Products and Estimation of the Associated Dietary Nicotine Intake. J Agric Food Chem. 1999. 47(8): 3113-3120.

★ Carreno-Gomes B, Woodley JF and Florence AT. Studies on the Uptake of Tomato Lectin Nanoparticles in Everted Gut Sacs. Int J Pharm. 1999. 183(1): 7-11.

★ Francis G, et al. The Biological Action of Saponins in Animal Systems: A Review. Br J Nutr. 2002. 88(6): 587-605.

★ Jensen-Jarolim E, et al. Hot Spices Influence Permeability of Human Intestinal Epithelial Monolayers. J Nutr. 1998. 128(3): 577-581.

Candida

★ Nieuwenhuizen WF, et al. Is Candida Albicans a Trigger in the Onset of Celiac Disease? Lancet. 2003. 361(9375): 2152-2154.

★ Muedin L. Candida. Website of Dr. Ronald Hoffman. Web July 2012. www.drhoffman.com/page.cfm/616

★ Crook WG. The Yeast Connection: A Medical Breakthrough. Yeast-Fighting Program: Healthy Diet. Web July 2012. yeastconnection.com/pdf/GroceryList.pdf

Alcohol

★ Purohit V, et al. Alcohol, Intestinal Bacterial Growth, Intestinal Permeability to Endotoxin, and Medical Consequences: Summary of a Symposium. Alcohol. 2008. 42(5): 349-361.

Caffeine

★ Mayo Clinic. Caffeine Content for Coffee, Tea, Soda and More. 2011. Web July 2012. www.mayoclinic.com/health/caffeine/AN01211

★ Simren M, et al. Food-Related Gastrointestinal Symptoms in the Irritable Bowel Syndrome. Digestion. 2001; 63(2):108-115.

★ Boekema PJ, et al. Coffee and Gastrointestinal Function: Facts and Fiction. A Review. Scand J Gastroenterol Suppl. 1999. 230: 35-9.

★ Rao, SS, et al. Is Coffee a Colonic Stimulant? Eur J Gastroenterol & Hepatol. 1998. 10(2):113-118.

★ Brown SR, Cann PA, and Read NW. Effect of Coffee on Distal Colon Function. Gut. 1990. 31(4): 450-453.

★ Lovallo WR, et al. Caffeine Stimulation of Cortisol Secretion Across the Waking Hours in Relation to Caffeine Intake Levels. Psychosom Med. 2005. 67(5): 734-739.

★ Zampelas A, et al. Associations between Coffee Consumption and Inflammatory Markers in Healthy Persons: The ATTICA Study. Am J Clinical Nutr. 2004. 80(4): 862-867.

CHAPTER 4

Bone Broth

★ Lubec G, Wolf C, and Bartosch B. Aminoacid Isomerisation and Microwave Exposure. The Lancet. 1989. 2(8676): 1392-1393.

★ Siebecker A. Traditional Bone Broth in Modern Health and Disease. Townsend Letter. February/March 2005. Web August 2012. www.townsendletter.com/FebMarch2005/broth0205.htm

★ Daniel KT. Why Bone Broth is Beautiful: Essential Roles for Proline, Glycine and Gelatin. The Weston A. Price Foundation. June 2003. Web August 2012. www.westonaprice.org/food-features/why-broth-is-beautiful

★ Gotthoffer NR. Gelatin in Nutrition and Medicine. 1945.

★ Shanahan C. Deep Nutrition: Why Your Genes Need Traditional Food. 2008.

★ Pottenger, FM. Hydrophilic Colloid Diet. Price-Pottenger Nutrition Foundation. 1997. Web August 2012. www.ppnf.org/about-ppnf/about-drs-price-and-pottenger/dr-pottenger/11-resources-section/50-hydrophilic-colloidal-diet

★ Samonina G, et al. Protection of Gastric Mucosal Integrity by Gelatin and Simple Proline-Containing Peptides. Pathophysiology. 2000. 7(1): 69-73.

★ Richardson, CT, et al. Studies on the Mechanism of Food-Stimulated Gastric Acid Secretion in Normal Human Subjects. J Clin Invest. 1976. 58(3): 623-631.

★ Wald A and Adibi SA. Stimulation of Gastric Acid Secretion by Glycine and Related Oligopeptides in Humans. Am J Physiol, 1982. 242(2), G85-88.

Fermented Foods

★ Plengvidhya V, et al. DNA Fingerprinting of Lactic Acid Bacteria in Sauerkraut Fermentations. Appl Environ Microbiol. 2007. 73(23): 7697-7702.

★ Gerstmar T. Everything You Always Wanted to Know about Probiotics. April 2002. Web July 2012. whole9life.com/2012/04/probiotics-101

★ Parkes GC, et al. Gastrointestinal Microbiota in Irritable Bowel Syndrome: Their Role in Its Pathogenesis and Treatment. Am J Gastroenterol. 2008. 103(6): 1557-1567.

★ Fanigliulo L, et al. Role of Gut Microflora and Probiotic Effects in the Irritable Bowel Syndrome. Acta Biomed. 2006. 77(2): 85-89.

Animal Protein

★ Groff JL and Gropper SS. Advanced Nutrition & Human Metabolism. 1999.

★ Keith L. The Vegetarian Myth: Food, Justice, and Sustainability. 2009.

★ Rule DC, et al. Comparison of Muscle Fatty Acid Profiles and Cholesterol Concentrations of Bison, Beef, Cattle, Elk and Chicken. J Anim Sci. 2002; 80(5): 1202-1211.

★ Karsten HD, et al. Vitamins A, E and Fatty Acid Composition of the Eggs of Caged Hens and Pastured Hens. Renewable Agriculture and Food Systems. 2010; 25(1): 45-54.

★ Cordain L, et al. Origins and Evolution of the Western Diet: Health Implications for the 21st Century. Am J Clin Nutr. 2005; 81(2): 341-354.

★ Harvard Health Publications. Understanding and Treating an Irritable Bowel. Web August 2012. www.health.harvard.edu/newsweek/Understanding_and_treating_an_irritable_bowel.htm

★ Pan A, et al. Red Meat Consumption and Mortality: Results from 2 Prospective Cohort Studies. Arch Intern Med. 2012. 172(7): 555-563.

★ Masterjohn C. The Incredible, Edible Egg Yolk. Cholesterol-and-health.com. July 2005. Web July 2012. www.cholesterol-and-health.com/Egg_Yolk.html

★ Robinson J. Health Benefits of Grass-Fed Products. EatWild. 2009. Web July 2012.
www.eatwild.com/healthbenefits.htm

Organic Produce

★ Environmental Working Group. Shoppers Guide to Pesticides in Produce. 2012. Web August 2012.
static.ewg.org/reports/2012/foodnews/pdf/2012-EWGPesticideGuide.pdf

Fats

★ Dean W and English J. Medium Chain Triglycerides (MCTs): Beneficial Effects on Energy, Atherosclerosis and Aging.
Nutrition Review. Web August 2012. www.nutritionreview.org/library/mcts.php

★ Phinney SD and Volek JS. The Art and Science of Low Carbohydrate Living: An Expert Guide to Making the Life-
Saving Benefits of Carbohydrate Restriction Sustainable and Enjoyable. 2011.

★ Siri-Tarino PW, et al. Meta-Analysis of Prospective Cohort Studies Evaluating the Association of Saturated Fat with
Cardiovascular Disease. Am J Clin Nutr. 2010; 91(3): 535-546.

★ Taubes G. Good Calories, Bad Calories: Fats, Carbs, and the Controversial Science of Diet and Health. 2008.

★ Volek JS and Forsythe CE. The Case for Not Restricting Saturated Fat on a Low Carbohydrate Diet. Nutr Metab. 2005.
2: 21.

★ Hite AH, Berkowitz VG, and Berkowitz K. Low-Carbohydrate Diet Review: Shifting the Paradigm. Nutr Clin Pract. 2011.
26(3): 300-308.

★ El-Salhy M, et al. The Role of Diet in the Pathogenesis and Management of Irritable Bowel Syndrome (Review). Int J
Mol Med. 2012. 29(5): 723-731.

★ Fife B. Coconut Oil and Medium-Chain Triglycerides. Coconut Research Center. 2003. Web August 2012.
www.coconutresearchcenter.org/article10612.htm

★ Fife B. Scientific Evidence regarding Coconut Oil. Healthy Ways Newsletter. 2011. Web August 2012.
www.naturepacific.com/contents/en-us/d252_Scientific_Evidence_regarding_Coconut_Oil_.html

★ Enig MG. A New Look at Coconut Oil. The Weston A. Price Foundation. 2000. Web August 2012.
www.westonaprice.org/know-your-fats/new-look-at-coconut-oil

★ Enig MG. Know Your Fats: The Complete Primer for Understanding the Nutrition of Fats, Oils, and Cholesterol. 2000.

★ Kabara JJ, et al. Fatty Acids and Derivatives as Antimicrobial Agents. Antimicrob Agents Chemother. 1972. 2(1): 23-28.

★ Brown MJ, et al. Carotenoid Bioavailability is Higher from Salads Ingested with Full-Fat than with Fat-Reduced Salad
Dressings as Measured with Electrochemical Detection. Am J Clin Nutr. 2004. 80(2): 396-403.

★ Clark RM, et al. A Comparison of Lycopene and Astaxanthin Absorption from Corn Oil and Olive Oil Emulsions. Lipids.
2000. 35(7): 803-806.

Butyrate

★ Thibault R, et al. Butyrate Utilization by the Colonic Mucosa in Inflammatory Bowel Diseases: A Transport Deficiency.
Inflamm Bowel Dis. 2010. 16(4): 684-695.

★ Smith JG, Yokoyama WH, and German JB. Butyric Acid from the Diet: Actions at the Level of Gene Expression. Crit
Rev Food Sci Nutr. 1998. 38(4): 259-297.

★ Wong JM, et al. Colonic Health: Fermentation and Short Chain Fatty Acids. J Clin Gastroenterol. 2006. 40(3): 235-243.

Salt and Sodium

★ Phinney SD and Volek JS. The Art and Science of Low Carbohydrate Living: An Expert Guide to Making the Live-Saving Benefits of Carbohydrate Restriction Sustainable and Enjoyable. 2011.

★ O'Donnell MJ, et al. Urinary Sodium and Potassium Excretion and Risk of Cardiovascular Events. JAMA. 2011. 306(20): 2229-2238.

★ Stolarz-Skrzypek K, et al. Fatal and Nonfatal Outcomes, Incidence of Hypertension, and Blood Pressure Changes in Relation to Urinary Sodium Excretion. JAMA. 2011. 305(17): 1777-1785.

★ Ekinci EI, et al. Dietary Salt Intake and Mortality in Patients with Type 2 Diabetes. Diabetes Care. 2011. 34(3): 703-709.

★ Garg R, et al. Low-Salt Diet Increases Insulin Resistance in Healthy Subjects. Metabolism. 2011. 60(7):965-968.

★ Satin M. Salt and our Health. The Weston A. Price Foundation. 2012. Web Augsut 2012. www.westonaprice.org/vitamins-and-minerals/salt-and-our-health

★ Taubes G. The (Political) Science of Salt. Science. 1998. 281(5379): 898-907.

★ Drake SL and Drake MA. Comparison of Salty Taste and Time Intensity of Sea and Land Salts from around the World. J Sens Stud. 2010. 26(1): 25-34.

Nutritional Adequacy

★ United States Department of Agriculture. USDA National Nutrient Database Food Search for Windows, Version 1.0, Database Version SR23.

Low-Carb Diets

★ Food and Nutrition Board of the Institute of Medicine. Dietary Reference Intakes for Energy, Carbohydrate, Fiber, Fat, Fatty Acids, Cholesterol, Protein and Amino Acids (Macronutrients). 2005. P.275. Web August 2012. www.nap.edu/openbook.php?record_id=10490&page=275

★ Nutrition & Metabolism Society. Top Ten Low Carb Myths. Web August 2012. www.nmsociety.org/low-carb-myths.html>Sokoloff L. Metabolism of Ketone Bodies by the Brain. Annu Rev Med. 1973; 24: 271-80.

★ Veech RL. The Therapeutic Implications of Ketone Bodies: The Effects of Ketone Bodies in Pathological Conditions: Ketosis, Ketogenic Diet, Redox States, Insulin Resistance, and Mitochondrial Metabolism. Prostaglandins Leukot Essent Fatty Acids. 2004; 70(3): 309–319.

★ Veech RL, et al. Ketone Bodies, Potential Therapeutic Uses. IUBMB Life. 2001; 51(4): 241–247.

Withdrawal Reaction

★ Loblay RH and Swain AR. Food Intolerance. Recent Advances in Clinical Nutrition. 1986. 2:169-177.

★ Hofmann-Smith E. Die-Off Reaction – What it is and How to Prevent it. Web August 2012. www.naturaldocs.net/handouts/die_off_reaction.pdf

★ Melos L. The Allergy/Addiction Syndrome: Are Your Favorite Foods Draining Your Vitality. Web August 2012. lindamelosnd.com/articles/the-allergyaddiction-syndrome-are-your-favorite-foods-draining-your-vitality

CHAPTER 5

★ Rowe, A. Elimination Diets and the Patient's Allergies. 2nd Edition. Lea & Febiger, Philadelphia, PA: 1944.

★ Clarke L, McQueen J, Samild A, Swain AR (1996). Dietitians Association of Australia Review Paper: The Dietary Management of Food Allergy and Food Intolerance in Children and Adults. Aust J Nutr Dietetics. 53 (3): 89–98.

★ Eastern Health Clinical School - Monash University. The Low FODMAP Diet: Reducing Poorly Absorbed Sugars to Control Gastrointestinal Symptoms. 2010.

★ Allergy Unit, Royal Prince Alfred Hospital. RPAH Elimination Diet Handbook. 2011.

★ MacDermott RP. Treatment of Irritable Bowel Syndrome in Outpatients with Inflammatory Bowel Disease Using a Food and Beverage Intolerance, Food And Beverage Avoidance Diet. Inflamm Bowel Dis. 2007; 13(1): 91-6.

★ United States Department of Agriculture. USDA National Nutrient Database Food Search for Windows, Version 1.0, Database Version SR23.

★ Mahan LK and Escott-Stump S. Krause's Food, Nutrition, & Diet Therapy. 2000.

★ Phinney SD and Volek JS. The Art and Science of Low Carbohydrate Living: An Expert Guide to Making the Life-Saving Benefits of Carbohydrate Restriction Sustainable and Enjoyable. 2011.

★ Campbell-McBride, N. Gut and Psychology Syndrome: Natural Treatment for Autism, Dyspraxia, A.D.D., Dyslexia, A.D.H.D., Depression, Schizophrenia. 2004.

★ Gottschall EG. Breaking the Vicious Cycle: Intestinal Health Through Diet. 1994

★ Rheaume-Bleue K. Vitamin K2 and the Calcium Paradox: How a Little-Known Vitamin Could Save Your Life. 2011.

CHAPTER 6

Digestive Support

★ Wright J. Why Stomach Acid is Good for You: Natural Relief from Heartburn, Indigestion, Reflux and GERD. 2001.

★ Wegener T. Anwendung eines Trockenextraktes aus Gentiana Lutea Radix bei Dyspeptischem Symptomenkomplex. Z Phytother. 1998. 19: 163-164.

★ Valussi M. Functional Foods with Digestion-Enhancing Properties. Int J Food Sci and Nutr. 2012. 63 Suppl 1: 82-89.

Cod Liver Oil

★ Fallon S and Enig MG. Cod Liver Oil Basics and Recommendations. 2009. Web August 2012. <http://www.westonaprice.org/cod-liver-oil/cod-liver-oil-basics>

★ Masterjohn C. The Benefits of Liver, Cod Liver Oil, and Desiccated Liver. 2008. Web August 2012. <http://www.cholesterol-and-health.com/Benefit-Of-Cod-Liver-Oil.html>

Glutamine

★ Van der Hulst RR, et al. Glutamine and the Preservation of Gut Integrity. Lancet. 1993(8857). 341: 1363-1365.

★ Den Hond E, et al. Effect of Long-Term Oral Glutamine Supplements on Small Intestinal Permeability in Patients with Crohn's disease. JPEN J Parenter Enteral Nutr. 1999. 23(1): 7-11.

★ Ross J. The Diet Cure: The 8-Step Program to Rebalance Your Body Chemistry and End Food Cravings, Weight Gain, and Mood Swings—Naturally. 2012.

Zinc

★ Sturniolo GC, et al. Zinc Supplementation Tightens "Leaky Gut" in Crohn's Disease. Inflamm Bowel Dis. 2001. 7(2): 94-98.

★ Office of Dietary Supplements, National Institutes of Health. Zinc. Web August 2012. <http://ods.od.nih.gov/factsheets/Zinc-HealthProfessional/>

★ MacKay D and Miller AL. Nutritional Support for Wound Healing. Altern Med Rev. 2003. 8(4): 359-377.

★ Marone G, et al. Physiological Concentrations of Zinc Inhibits the Release of Histamine from Human Basophils and Lung Mast Cells. Agents Actions. 1986. 18(1-2): 103-106.

Vitamin B_{12}

★ Pacholok SM and Stuart JJ. Could It Be B12?: An Epidemic of Misdiagnoses. 2011.

Vitamin A

★ Fallon S and Enig MG. Vitamin A Saga. The Weston A. Price Foundation. 2002. Web August 2012. www.westonaprice.org/fat-soluble-activators/vitamin-a-saga

★ Hedrén E, Diaz V, and Svanberg U. Estimation of Carotenoid Accessibility from Carrots Determine by an In Vitro Digestion Method. Eur J Clin Nutr. 2002. 56(5): 425-430.

★ Hickenbottom SJ, et al. Variability in Conversion of Beta-Carotene to Vitamin A in Men as Measured by Using a Double-Tracer Study Design. Am J Clin Nutr. 2002. 75(5): 900-907.

★ Myhre AM, et al. Water-Miscible, Emulsified, and Solid Forms of Retinol Supplements are More Toxic than Oil-Based Preparations. Am J Clin Nutr. 2003. 78(6): 1152-1159.

★ MacKay D and Miller AL. Nutritional Support for Wound Healing. Altern Med Rev. 2003. 8(4): 359-377.

Vitamin K_2

★ Rheaume-Bleue K. Vitamin K2 and the Calcium Paradox: How a Little-Known Vitamin Could Save Your Life. 2011.

Probiotics

★ World Gastroenterology Organisation. Probiotics and Prebiotics. 2008. Web August 2012. www.worldgastroenterology.org/assets/downloads/en/pdf/guidelines/19_probiotics_prebiotics.pdf

★ Husebye E, et al. Influence of Microbial Species on Small Intestinal Myoelectrical Activity and Transit in Germ-Free Rats. Am J Physiol Gastrointest Liver Physiol. 2001. 280(3): G368-380.

★ Ait-Belgnaoui A, et al. Prevention of Gut Leakiness by a Probiotic Treatment Leads to Attenuated HPA Response to an Acute Psychological Stress in Rats. Pshychoneuroendocrinology. 2012. 37(11):1885-1895.

★ Lee BJ and Bak Y-T. Irritable Bowel Syndrome, Gut Microbiota and Probiotics. J Neurogastroenterol Motil. 2011. 17(3): 252-266.

★ Madden JA and Hunter JO. A Review of the Role of the Gut Microflora in Irritable Bowel Syndrome and the Effects of Probiotics. Br J Nutr. 2002. 88 Suppl 1: S67-72.

★ Hanson LÅ. Immune Effects of the Normal Gut Flora. Monatsschr Kinderheilkd. 1998. 146 Suppl 1: S2-S6.

★ Swidsinski A, et al. Spatial Organization and Composition of the Mucosal Flora in Patients with Inflammatory Bowel Disease. J Clin Microbiol. 2005. 43(7): 3380-3389.

★ O'Hara AM and Shanahan F. The Gut Flora as a Forgotten Organ. EMBO Rep. 2006. 7(7): 688-693.

★ Kotowska M, et al. Saccharomyces Boulardii in the Prevention of Antibiotic-Associated Diarrhoea in Children: A Randomized Double-Blind Placebo-Controlled Trial. Aliment Pharmacol Ther. 2005. 21(5): 583-590.

★ McFarland LV, et al. Prevention of Beta-Lactam-Associated Diarrhea by Saccharomyces Boulardii Compared with Placebo. Am J Gastroenterol. 1995. 90(3): 439-448.

Magnesium

★ Agrios A. Magnesium is a Natural Way to Treat Constipation. Web August 2012. www.thenaturalguide.com/nd/ag-A-Magnesium-Supplement-Is-A-Natural-Way-To-Treat-Constipation-Insomnia-and-Muscle-Tension.html

Vitamin D

★ Kong J, et al. Novel role of the vitamin D receptor in maintaining the integrity of the intestinal mucosal barrier. Am J Physiol Gastrointest Liver Physiol. 2008. 294(1): G208-G216.

★ Vitamin D Council. Vitamin D Supplementation. Web August 2012. www.vitamindcouncil.org/about-vitamin-d/how-to-get-your-vitamin-d/vitamin-d-supplementation

★ UC Riverside. More than Half the World's Population Gets Insufficient Amounts of Vitamin D, Says UC Riverside Biochemist. 2010. Web August 2012.newsroom.ucr.edu/news_item.html?action=page&id=2376

★ Holick MF, et al. Vitamin D and Skin Physiology: a D-lightful Story. J Bone Miner Res. 2007. 22 Suppl 2: V28-V33.

★ Webb AR, Kline L, and Holick MF. Influence of Season and Latitude on the Cutaneous Synthesis of Vitamin D3: Exposure to Winter Sunlight in Boston and Edmonton will not Promote Vitamin D3 Synthesis in Human Skin. J Clin Endocrinol Metab. 1988. 67(2): 373-378.

Omega-3 Fats

★ Hussein N, et al. Long-Chain Conversion of [13C]Linoleic Acid and A-Linolenic Acid in Response to Marked Changes in their Dietary Intake in Men. J Lipid Res. 2005. 46(2): 269-280.

★ Pawlosky RJ, et al. Physiological Compartmental Analysis of Alpha-Linolenic Acid Metabolism in Adult Humans. J. Lipid Res. 2001. 42(8): 1257-1265.

Vitamin C

★ Patak P, Willenberg HS, and Bornstein SR. Vitamin C is an Important Cofactor for Both Adrenal Cortex and Adrenal Medulla. Endocr Res. 2004. 30(4): 871-875.

★ Wilson JL. Adrenal Fatigue: The 21st Century Stress Syndrome. 2001.

Multivitamin

★ Neuhouser ML, et al. Multivitamin Use and Risk of Cancer and Cardiovascular Disease in the Women's Health Initiative Cohorts. Arch Intern Med. 2009. 169(3): 294-304.

★ Bjelakovic G, et al. Mortality in Randomized Trials of Antioxidant Supplements for Primary and Secondary Prevention – Systematic Review and Meta-Analysis. JAMA. 2007. 297(8): 842-857.

CHAPTER 7

Stress

★ Konturek PC, Brzozowski T, and Konturek SJ. Stress and the Gut: Pathophysiology, Clinical Consequences, Diagnostic Approach and Treatment Options. J Physiol Pharmacol. 2011. 62(6): 591-599.

★ Alonso C, et al. Acute Experimental Stress Evokes a Differential Gender-Determined Increase in Human Intestinal Macromolecular Permeability. Neurogastroenterol Motil. 2012. 24(8): 740-746.

★ Söderholm JD and Perdue MH. II. Stress and Intestinal Barrier Function. Am J Physiol Gastrointest Liver Physiol. 2001. 280(1): G7-G13.

★ Øktedalen O, et al. Changes in the Gastrointestinal Mucosa after Long-Distance Running. Scand J Gastroenterol. 1992. 27(4): 270-274.

★ Pals KL, et al. Effect of Running Intensity on Intestinal Permeability. J Appl Physiol. 1997. 82(2): 571-576.

★ Kraft TL and Pressman SD. Grin and Bear It: The influence of manipulated positive facial expression on the stress response. Psychol Sci. 2012. 23(11): 1372-1378.

★ Bailey MT, et al. Exposure to a Social Stressor Alters the Structure of the Intestinal Microbiota: Implications for Stressor-Induced Immunomodulation. Brain Behav Immun. 2011. 25(3): 397-407.

★ Aronson D. Cortisol—Its Role in Stress, Inflammation, and Indications for Diet Therapy. Today's Dietitian. 2009. 11(11): 38.

★ Wooten P. Humor: An Antidote for Stress. Holist Nurs Pract. 1996. 10(2): 49-56.

★ Bennett MP and Lengacher C. Humor and Laughter May Influence Health IV. Humor and Immune Function. Evid Based Complement Alternat Med. 2009. 6(2): 159-164.

★ Bennett MP and Lengacher C. Humor and Laughter May Influence Health III. Humor and Immune Function. Evid Based Complement Alternat Med. 2008. 5(1): 37-40.

Earthing

★ Sokal K and Sokal P. Earthing the Human Body Influences Physiologic Processes. J Altern Complement Med. 2011. 17(4): 301-308.

★ Ghaly M and Teplitz D. The Biologic Effects of Grounding the Human Body During Sleep as Measured by Cortisol Levels and Subjective Reporting of Sleep, Pain, and Stress. J Altern Complement Med. 2004. 10(5): 767-776.

★ Ober C, Sinatra ST, and Zucker M. Earthing: The Most Important Health Discovery Ever? 2010.

Sleep

★ Wiley TS and Formby B. Lights Out: Sleep, Sugar, and Survival. 2001.

★ Cajochen C, Chellappa S, and Schmidt C. What Keeps Us Awake? The Role of Clocks and Hourglasses, Light, and Melatonin. Int Rev Neurobiol. 2010. 93: 57-90.

★ Hill EE, et al. Exercise and Circulating Cortisol Levels: The Intensity Threshold Effect. J Endocrinol Invest. 2008. 31(7): 587-591.

★ Blumenthal JA, et al. Effects of Exercise Training on Older Patients with Major Depression. Arch Intern Med. 1999. 159(19): 2349-2356.

★ Spiegel K, et al. Sleep Loss: A Novel Risk Factor for Insulin Resistance and Type 2 Diabetes. J Appl Physiol. 2005. 99(5): 2008-2019.

★ Donga E, et al. A Single Night of Partial Sleep Deprivation Induces Insulin Resistance in Multiple Metabolic Pathways in Healthy Subjects. J Clin Endocrinol Metab. 2010. 95(6): 2963-2968.

★ Morselli L, et al. Role of Sleep Duration in the Regulation of Glucose Metabolism and Appetite. Best Pract Res Clin Endocrinol Metab. 2010. 24(5): 687-702.

★ Ackermann K, et al. Diurnal Rhythms in Blood Cell Populations and the Effect of Acute Sleep Deprivation in Healthy Young Men. Sleep. 2012. 35(7): 933-940.

CHAPTER 8

Gluten-Free & Restaurants

★ National Foundation for Celiac Awareness (NFCA). National Foundation for Celiac Awareness Puts Restaurant Industry to the Test. May 2012. Web August 2012. www.celiaccentral.org/press-room/nfca-press-releases/national-foundation-for-celiac-awareness-puts-restaurant-industry-to-the-test-7944/

Traveler's diarrhea

★ Zanello G, et al. Saccharomyces Boulardii Effects on Gastrointestinal Diseases. Curr Issues Mol Biol. 2009. 11(1): 47-58.

★ McFarland LV. Meta-analysis of probiotics for the prevention of traveler's diarrhea. Travel Med Infect Dis. 2007. 5(2): 97-105.

CHAPTER 9

Biofilms

★ Gibson PR and Barrett JS. The Concept of Small Intestinal Bacterial Overgrowth in Relation to Functional Gastrointestinal Disorders. Nutrition. 2010. 26(11-12): 1038-1043.

★ Lewis K. Riddle of Biofilm Resistance. Antimicrob Agents Chemother. 2001. 45(4): 999-1007.

* Swidsinski A, et al. Spatial Organization and Composition of the Mucosal Flora in Patients with Inflammatory Bowel Disease. J Clin Microbiol. 2005. 43(7): 3380-3389.

* Batchelor SE, et al. Cell Density-Regulated Recovery of Starved Biofilm Populations of Ammonia-Oxidizing Bacteria. Appl Environ Microbiol. 1997. 63(6): 2281-2286.

* Bezkorovainy A. Biochemistry and Physiology of Bifidobacteria. 1989.

Ginger

* Wu KL, et al. Effects of Ginger on Gastric Emptying and Motility in Healthy Humans. Eur J Gastroenterol Hepatol. 2008. 20(5): 436-440.

* Hu ML, et al. Effects of Ginger on Gastric Motility and Symptoms of Functional Dyspepsia. World J Gastroenterol. 2011. 17(1): 105-110.

* Black CD, et al. Ginger (Zingiber Officinale) Reduces Muscle Pain Caused by Eccentric Exercise. J Pain. 2010. 11(9): 894-903.

* Shen YH and Nahas R. Complementary and alternative medicine for treatment of irritable bowel syndrome. Can Fam Physician. 2009. 55(2): 143-148.

* Yamahara J, et al. Cholagogic Effect of Ginger and its Active Constituents. J Ethnopharmacol. 1985. 13(2): 217-225.

Peppermint

* Cappello G, et al. Peppermint Oil (Mintoil) in the Treatment of Irritable Bowel Syndrome: A Prospective Double Blind Placebo-Controlled Randomized Trial. Dig Liver Dis. 2007. 39(6): 530-536.

* Wu JC. Complementary and Alternative Medicine Modalities for the Treatment of Irritable Bowel Syndrome: Facts or Myths? Gastroenterol Hepatol (N Y). 2010. 6(11): 705-711.

* Liu JH, et al. Enteric-Coated Peppermint-Oil Capsules in the Treatment of Irritable Bowel Syndrome: A Prospective, Randomized Trial. J Gastroenterol. 1997. 32(6): 765-768.

* Logan AC and Beaulne TM. The Treatment of Small Intestinal Bacterial Overgrowth with Enteric-Coated Peppermint Oil: A Case Report. Altern Med Rev. 2002. 7(5): 410-417.

Chamomile

* Gardiner P. Complementary, Holistic and Integrative Medicine: Chamomile. Pediatr Rev. 2007. 28(4): e16-18.

Turmeric

* Holt PR, Katz S, and Kirshoff R. Curcumin Therapy in Inflammatory Bowel Disease: A Pilot Study. Dig Dis Sci. 2005. 50(11): 2191-2193.

* Bundy R, et al. Turmeric Extract May Improve Irritable Bowel Syndrome Symptomology in Otherwise Healthy Adults: A Pilot Study. J Altern Complement Med. 2004. 10(6): 1015-1018.

* Gupta SC, et al. Multitargeting by Turmeric, the Golden Spice: From Kitchen to Clinic. Mol Nutr Food Res. 2012. (Epub ahead of print).

NSAIDs

★ Sigthorsson G, et al. Intestinal Permeability and Inflammation in Patients on NSAIDs. Gut. 1998. 43(4): 506-511.

★ Kerckhoffs AP, et al. Intestinal Permeability in Irritable Bowel Syndrome Patients: Effects of NSAIDs. Dig Dis Sci. 2010. 55(3): 716-723.

Birth Control Pill

★ Khalili H, et al. Oral Contraceptives, Reproductive Factors and Risk of Inflammatory Bowel Diseases. Gut. 2012. (Epub ahead of print).

★ Looijer-van Langen M, et al. Estrogen receptor-β signaling modulates epithelial barrier function. Am J Physiol Gastrointest Liver Physiol. 2011. 300(4): G621-G626.

BPAs

★ Braniste V, et al. Impact of Oral Bisphenol A at Reference Doses on Intestinal Barrier Function and Sex Differences after Perinatal Exposure in Rats. Proceedings of the National Academy of Sciences. 2010. 107(1): 448-453.

Bile and Constipation

★ Abrahamsson H, et al. Altered bile acid metabolism in patients with constipation-predominant irritable bowel syndrome and functional constipation. Scand J Gastroenterol. 2008. 43(12): 1483-1488.

Abdominal Massage

★ McClurg D and Lowe-Strong A. Does Abdominal Massage Relieve Constipation? Nurs Times. 2011. 107(12): 20-22.

Index

A

Abdominal self-massage 236, 368
Acid reflux (heartburn) 14, 15, 40, 43, 58, 74-76, 189
Acid-suppressing medications (PPIs) 74
Activated charcoal (charcoal) 157, 233, 240, 368
Adrenal glands 111, 138, 172, 182, 194, 200, 205, 210, 223
Agave nectar 45, 46, 62, 106, 355
Alcohol 22, 34, 36, 39, 55, 58, 89, 110, 139, 171, 172, 174, 214, 232, 248, 254, 286, 353, 356-357, 363, 368
Alcohol, beer 34, 35, 36, 39, 48, 55, 110, 174, 356
Alcohol, wine 34, 46, 48, 55, 110, 133, 172, 174, 193, 248, 254, 286, 355
Amines 54-56
Ancestral diet 86-87
Animal protein 86, 89, 92, 102, 114-119, 122, 126, 130, 149, 150, 151, 152, 160, 168, 176, 348, 349, 352, 356
Animal welfare 117-118
Antibiotics 18, 31, 33, 34, 61, 65-67, 72, 74, 75, 118, 156, 158, 172, 191, 228, 232, 235, 240
Artificial sweeteners 34, 55, 107, 171, 174, 223, 232, 353, 368
Atkins diet 140

B

B vitamins 194, 200
Belly breathing 206-207, 209, 211, 366
Betaine HCl 16, 25, 67, 115, 127, 164, 187-190, 224, 228, 231, 237, 362
Beverages 34, 89, 110, 111, 150, 171, 172, 174, 176, 232, 348, 349, 354, 355, 356, 357
Biofilms 228, 368
Body scanning 206, 208, 211, 366
Body-care products 227
Bone broth 22, 85, 89, 101, 118, 127-128, 130, 139, 150, 152, 154, 157, 161, 166, 176, 182, 188, 198-199, 201, 223, 224, 234, 236, 238, 240, 244, 248, 250, 252, 254, 286, 316, 341, 348, 349, 359, 362
BPA 22, 231, 368
Brassicaceae 89, 108-109, 129, 131, 136, 146, 167, 168, 173, 333, 352, 354, 357

BRAT diet 98
Breakfast 34-36, 55, 62, 69, 84, 85, 88, 91-94, 126, 152, 178, 243, 308, 339, 340
Breath testing 49, 60-61
Butyric acid 125-126
BYO diet 145, 147, 148, 163, 164, 174, 178, 179, 198, 202, 204

C

Caffeine 89, 110-111, 124, 155, 171, 172, 174, 204, 211, 232, 353, 366, 368
Calcium 15, 41, 70, 76, 94, 94, 100-102, 128, 138, 161-162, 182, 186, 199, 228, 244, 359
Candida overgrowth 15, 32, 46, 61, 78, 106, 109, 131, 136, 146, 163, 354, 363
Carbohydrates 10, 11, 13, 18, 22, 34, 43-49, 57, 58, 61, 63, 64, 66, 69, 70, 72, 73, 75, 82, 83, 84, 85, 86, 88, 91-94, 102, 129, 140-142, 156-158, 222, 225, 228, 237, 360
Carbohydrates, grain-free sources 360
Carbohydrate, low- 140, 142, 156
Carbohydrates, FODMAPs 43-53, 62, 73, 75, 78, 93-94, 106
Carbohydrates, short-chain fermentable 43-51, 62, 93-94, 106
Cardiovascular health 119-120, 137-139, 153, 195, 201, 211
Casein 39-41, 44, 99-100, 134, 146, 169, 173, 246, 352, 354, 357
Castor oil packs 237, 368
Celiac disease 18, 21, 22, 27, 30, 35, 36, 37, 38, 43, 58, 64, 69-73, 77, 78, 82-83, 93, 94, 105, 109, 185-186, 197, 214, 363
Celiac disease, non-responsive 70-73
Chamomile 139, 234, 368
Charcoal 157, 233, 240, 368
Cleansing waves 65, 67-68, 90, 135, 177, 183, 190, 199, 205, 224, 361, 362
Coconut oil 10, 16, 55, 68, 77, 86, 89, 93, 121, 122, 123, 124, 125, 127, 131, 150, 152, 154, 176, 215, 217, 222, 224, 227, 239, 246, 341, 346, 348, 349, 356
Coconut, foods 125
Cod liver oil 185-187
Coffee 34, 55, 73, 89, 103-104, 110-111, 128, 139, 171, 172, 174, 232, 353, 356, 357
Constipation 15, 16, 21, 23, 26, 27, 30-31, 34, 40, 43, 52, 58, 60, 65, 69, 72, 98, 139, 144, 156-157, 162, 189, 195, 206, 235-238, 368

Cravings 32, 58, 107, 121, 156, 157, 158, 193, 210, 222-224, 232, 338, 368
Crohn's disease 18, 21, 58, 67, 73-74
Cross contamination 70, 71-72, 112, 214, 215, 216, 217, 227, 368
Cruciferous vegetables (Brassicaceae) 89, 108-109, 129, 131, 136, 146, 167, 168, 173, 333, 352, 354, 357
Cumulative effect 44, 46, 52-53, 82, 130, 154, 226, 368

D

Dairy 15, 31, 34-35, 39-41, 43-44, 55, 73, 75, 76, 78, 79, 84, 85, 86, 88, 89, 99-102, 133, 144, 146-147, 169-170, 173, 183, 199, 306, 352, 354, 356, 357, 359
Dairy, pastured 99, 100
Dairy, unpasteurized 99, 133
Dehydration 27, 73, 157, 223-224, 238
Delayed response 52, 165
DHA see Omega fats
Diarrhea 15, 16, 18, 21, 26, 27, 30-31, 32-34, 36, 40, 43, 50-53, 56-60, 69, 73, 82-83, 110, 135, 138, 156, 163, 164, 190, 191, 193, 195, 206, 219, 236, 238-240, 368
Die-off reaction 155-158, 160, 178, 222, 225, 233, 350
Digestion 10-13, 27
Digestion, optimal 27
Digestive support (enzymes, betaine HCl, ox bile) 16, 25, 67, 115, 127, 164, 187-190, 224, 228, 231, 237, 362
Digestive system 10-13

E

Eating out 214-219
Eggs 15, 73, 78, 89, 95, 117, 118, 119, 122, 146, 164, 168, 173, 197, 200, 217, 225, 232, 235, 238, 242, 243, 312, 314, 316, 320, 346, 352, 354, 359, 363
Elemental diets 65-66
Elimination diet 40, 50, 78, 79, 86-90, 91, 140-142, 144-179, 338, 344, 352, 362, 363
Elimination diet, elimination phase 145-164
Elimination diet, reintroduction phase 164-174
Enzymes 16, 25, 67, 115, 127, 164, 187-190, 224, 228, 231, 237, 362

EPA See **Omega fats**

Epsom salt baths 85, 157, 195, 233, 368

Exercise (physical activity) 211

F

Family reunion 214
Fats 10-11, 89, 97, 104-105, 118, 119-127, 150, 151-153, 162, 163-164, 169, 173, 176, 185, 186, 187-190, 195-196, 198, 199, 201, 215, 216, 222-224, 235, 239, 346-349, 352, 356, 358, 362, 368
Fats, butyric acid 125-126
Fats, medium-chain triglycerides (MCTs) 77, 124-125, 127, 163, 164, 222, 224, 239
Fats, omegas 105-106, 185, 187, 195-196
Fats, refined oils 89, 104-105, 112, 122, 123, 126, 146, 172, 174, 268, 353-354
Fermented cod liver oil 185-187
Fermented foods 18, 22, 54-55, 68, 98, 110, 133-136, 170, 174, 183, 198, 199, 302-308, 353, 356, 357, 362
Fiber 10, 11, 13, 31, 48, 57, 62, 91-94, 97-98, 102, 107, 125, 129-130, 132, 146, 162, 167, 170, 188, 196, 230, 235, 354, 358, 360
Fluids (water, tea) 139
(see **Beverages**)
Flying, flights 217
FODMAPs 43-53, 62, 73, 75, 78, 93-94, 106
Food allergies 15, 18, 40
Food intolerances see **Food sensitivities**
Food journal 153, 154, 166, 175, 201, 225, 226, 345
Food sensitivities 15-18, 20-22, 25, 27, 31, 34, 40-42, 57-58, 72, 73, 75-79, 90, 91, 94, 102-103, 111, 144, 146, 172, 177, 194, 204, 205, 214, 235, 238, 354, 363
Foods, to avoid 91-112
Foods, to eat 114-139
FOS 18, 48, 62, 135, 193, 237, 238, 355
Fructans 43, 47-49, 51, 52, 61, 62, 78, 91, 93-94, 106, 128, 146, 167, 182, 226, 354, 355
Fructose 31, 34, 43, 44-47, 49-53, 62-63, 78, 106-107, 167, 355
Fructose malabsorption 44-47, 49-53, 78, 193, 363
Fruit 131-132

G

Galactans 43, 49, 51, 52, 61-62, 78, 102, 146, 354
Gallbladder 12, 13, 14, 16, 25, 64, 76-77, 78, 124, 126-127, 190, 231, 235, 237, 239, 363
Gallstones 76, 78, 363
GAPS 66, 85-86, 334
Garlic 33, 34, 47-48, 53, 65, 128, 129, 130, 131, 137, 150, 173, 176, 182, 226, 243, 284, 346, 348, 349, 352, 353, 355
Garlic-infused oil 284
Gastrointestinal infections (infections, SIBO, GI infections) 14-18, 22, 25, 27, 31, 32-34, 56-57, 58, 65, 67-68, 74-75, 77-78, 109, 124, 163, 188, 199, 204, 219, 228, 231-232, 238, 240, 363, 368
Gastrointestinal infections (parasite infections) 14, 15, 22, 25, 27, 31, 32-33, 78, 107, 124, 156, 163, 219, 228, 232, 238, 363
GERD 15, 16, 18, 43, 58, 74-76, 78, 363
Ginger 137, 139, 234, 237, 346, 368
Glutamine 54-56
Gluten 22, 31, 34-39, 69-73, 75, 79, 82-83, 86, 88-89, 91, 93-94, 98, 110, 137, 139, 140, 144-147, 148, 155, 157-158, 163, 168, 170, 172-174, 176, 177, 190, 201, 214-218, 227-228, 232, 234, 238, 244, 346, 353, 354, 363
Gluten contamination 70-71, 227
Gluten-containing grains 35
Gluten-free grains 53, 71, 72, 73, 94, 174
Glycemic index 91-93, 94, 98, 121, 140
Glycemic load 91-93
Goitrogenic foods 136
Grains 22, 31, 34-39, 48, 49, 53, 55, 57, 62, 69, 71-73, 75, 78, 82, 84, 86, 88-89, 91-98, 117-119, 146, 162, 172, 174, 353, 355, 363
Grass fed 86, 99, 116, 118, 122, 150, 160, 162, 169, 173, 185, 195-196, 200, 232, 246, 306, 348, 352
Gratitude 206, 208, 209, 211, 366, 367
Gut dysbiosis 16-18, 31, 34, 43, 47, 48, 51, 53, 61, 66, 69, 70, 72-74, 83-85, 88-90, 93, 94, 98, 106, 107, 111, 114-115, 121, 122, 131, 134-135, 136, 144, 146, 170, 172, 173, 183, 193, 194, 201, 222, 225, 228, 242, 354, 361, 362

Gut flora 16-18, 27, 31-34, 46, 47-49, 51, 53, 56-57, 59, 61-62, 65, 69, 84, 88, 90, 98, 106, 107, 125, 126, 130-131, 132, 134, 135, 144, 146, 156, 162, 165, 166, 169, 170, 183, 190-191, 205, 219, 228, 231-232, 236, 237, 302, 306
Gut-brain axis 19

H

Heartburn 14, 15, 40, 43, 58, 74-76, 189
Heart health 119-120, 137-139, 153, 195, 201, 211
High-fructose corn syrup 34, 45-46, 62, 88, 106, 355
Histamine 54-56
Honey 46-47, 55, 62-63, 84-85, 89, 106, 172, 174, 222, 225, 229, 230, 232, 234, 235, 237, 355, 356, 360
Hormones 102, 114-115, 118, 121-122, 196, 200, 205, 208-211, 231
Hydration see **Fluids**
Hypochlorhydria 13, 14-16, 18, 25, 27, 58, 67, 74-76, 78, 90, 111, 115, 127, 139, 182, 183, 188-189, 194, 199, 204-205, 231, 237, 361-363
Hypothyroidism 21, 34, 36, 58, 64, 102, 136, 166, 186, 224, 238, 368

I

IBDs (inflammatory bowel diseases) 73-74
IBS (irritable bowel syndrome) 30-32, 33-34, 56-67, 70-73
IBS, post-infectious 33-34
Intestinal permeability 17, 19-23, 27, 31, 64, 69, 74, 77, 78, 94, 103, 105, 108, 110, 125, 144, 146, 172, 193, 196, 200, 205, 211, 231, 232, 244, 354, 363
Intestinal villi 13, 37, 69, 71, 83
Inulin-FOS (fructooligosaccharides) 18, 48, 62, 135, 193, 237, 238, 355
Iodine 136, 139

J

Journaling (food journal) 153, 154, 166, 175, 201, 225, 226, 345

K

Ketoacidosis 141-142
Keto-adaptation 155, 222, 224

Notes:

Notes:

Appendices, References, Index